Evidence-based Clinical Chinese Medicine

Volume 9
Vascular Dementia

Evidence-based Clinical Chinese Medicine

Co Editors-in-Chief

Charlie Changli Xue
RMIT University, Australia

Chuanjian Lu
Guangdong Provincial Hospital of Chinese Medicine, China

Volume 9
Vascular Dementia

Lead Authors

Brian H May
RMIT University, Australia

Mei Feng
Guangdong Provincial Hospital of Chinese Medicine, China

World Scientific

NEW JERSEY • LONDON • SINGAPORE • BEIJING • SHANGHAI • HONG KONG • TAIPEI • CHENNAI • TOKYO

Published by

World Scientific Publishing Co. Pte. Ltd.

5 Toh Tuck Link, Singapore 596224

USA office: 27 Warren Street, Suite 401-402, Hackensack, NJ 07601

UK office: 57 Shelton Street, Covent Garden, London WC2H 9HE

Library of Congress Cataloging-in-Publication Data
Names: Xue, Charlie Changli, author. | Lu, Chuan-jian, 1964– author.
Title: Evidence-based clinical Chinese medicine / Charlie Changli Xue, Chuanjian Lu.
Description: New Jersey : World Scientific, 2016. | Includes bibliographical references and index.
Identifiers: LCCN 2015030389| ISBN 9789814723084 (v. 1 : hardcover : alk. paper) |
ISBN 9789814723091 (v. 1 : paperback : alk. paper) |
ISBN 9789814723121 (v. 2 : hardcover : alk. paper) |
ISBN 9789814723138 (v. 2 : paperback : alk. paper) |
ISBN 9789814759045 (v. 3 : hardcover : alk. paper) |
ISBN 9789814759052 (v. 3 : paperback : alk. paper)
Subjects: | MESH: Medicine, Chinese Traditional--methods. | Clinical Medicine--methods. |
Evidence-Based Medicine--methods. | Psoriasis. | Pulmonary Disease, Chronic Obstructive.
Classification: LCC RC81 | NLM WB 55.C4 | DDC 616--dc23
LC record available at http://lccn.loc.gov/2015030389

Volume 9: Vascular Dementia
ISBN 978-981-120-494-4 (hardcover)
ISBN 978-981-123-534-4 (paperback)
ISBN 978-981-120-495-1 (ebook for institutions)
ISBN 978-981-120-496-8 (ebook for individuals)

First published 2020
Reprinted 2021

British Library Cataloguing-in-Publication Data
A catalogue record for this book is available from the British Library.

For any available supplementary material, please visit
https://www.worldscientific.com/worldscibooks/10.1142/11403#t=suppl

Disclaimer

The information in this monograph is based on systematic analyses of the best available evidence for Chinese medicine interventions both historical and contemporary. Every effort has been made to ensure accuracy and completeness of the data of this publication. This book is intended for clinicians, researchers and educators. The practice of evidence-based medicine consists of consideration of the best available evidence, practitioners' clinical experience and judgment, and patients' preference. Not all interventions are acceptable in all countries. It is important to note that some of the substances mentioned in this book may no longer be in use, may be toxic, or be prohibited or restricted under the provisions of the Convention on International Trade in Endangered Species of Wild Fauna and Flora (CITES). Practitioners, researchers and educators are advised to comply with the relevant regulations in their country and with the restrictions on the trade in species included in CITES appendices I, II and III. This book is not intended as a guide for self-medication. Patients should seek professional advice from qualified Chinese medicine practitioners.

Foreword

Since the late 20th century, Chinese medicine, including acupuncture and herbal medicine, has been increasingly used throughout the world. The parallel development and spread of evidence-based medicine has provided challenges and opportunities for Chinese medicine.

The opportunities have been evidence-based medicine's emphasis on the effective use of the best available clinical evidence, incorporating the clinicians' clinical experience, subject to patients' preference. Such practices have a patient focus which reflects the historical nature of Chinese medicine practice. However, the challenges are also significant due to the fact that, despite the long term development and very rich literature accumulated over 2,000 years, there is an overall lack of high level clinical evidence for many of the interventions used in Chinese medicine.

To address this knowledge gap, we need to generate clinical evidence through high quality clinical studies and to evaluate evidence to enable effective use of such available evidence to promote evidence-based Chinese medicine practice.

Modern Chinese medicine is rooted in its classical literature and the legacies of ancient doctors, grounded in the practice of expert clinicians and increasingly informed by clinical and experimental research efforts. In recognition of the unique features of Chinese medicine, for each of the conditions in this series a 'whole-evidence' approach is used to provide a synthesis of different types and levels of evidence to enable practitioners to make clinical decisions informed by the current best evidence.

There are four main components of this 'whole-evidence' approach. Firstly, we present the current approaches to the diagnosis, differentiation and treatment of each condition based on expert consensus in published textbooks and clinical guidelines. This provides an overview of how the condition is currently managed. The second section provides an analysis of the condition in a historical context based on systematic searches of the *Zhong Hua Yi Dian* 中华医典, which includes the full texts of more than 1,000 classical medical books. These analyses provide objective views on how the condition has been treated over two millennia, reveal continuities and discontinuities between traditional and modern practice, and suggest avenues for future research.

The third component is the assessment of evidence derived from modern clinical studies of Chinese medicine interventions. The methods established by the *Cochrane Collaboration* are used as the basis for conducting systematic reviews and undertaking meta-analyses of outcome data for randomised controlled trials (RCTs). In addition, the clinical relevance of meta-analysis data is enhanced by examining the herbal formulae, individual herbs and acupuncture treatments that were assessed in the RCTs and the evidence base is broadened by the inclusion of data from controlled clinical trials and non-controlled studies. The fourth component is to determine how the herbal medicine interventions may achieve the effects indicated by the clinical trials. Thus for each of the most frequently used herbs we provide reviews of their effects in pre-clinical models and their likely mechanisms of action.

For each condition, this 'whole-evidence' approach links clinical expertise, historical precedent, clinical research data and experimental research to provide the reader with assessments of the current state of the evidence of efficacy and safety for Chinese medicine interventions using herbal medicines, acupuncture and moxibustion and other health care practices such as *tai chi* 太极.

Since these books are available in Chinese and English, they can benefit patients, practitioners and educators internationally and enable practitioners to make clinical decisions informed by the current best evidence.

These publications represent a major milestone in the development of Chinese medicine and make a significant contribution to the development of evidence-based Chinese medicine globally.

Co-Editors-in-Chief
Distinguished Professor Charlie Changli Xue,
RMIT University, Australia

Professor Chuanjian Lu,
Guangdong Provincial Hospital of Chinese Medicine, China

Purpose of the Monograph

This book is intended for clinicians, researchers and educators. It can be used to inform tertiary education and clinical practice by providing systematic, multi-dimensional assessments of the best available evidence for using Chinese medicine to manage each common clinical condition.

How to Use this Monograph

Some Definitions

A glossary is included, containing terms and definitions which frequently appear in the book. It also describes the definitions of statistical tests, methodological terms, evaluation tools and interventions. For example, in this book, Integrative Medicine refers to the combined use of a Chinese medicine treatment with conventional medical management, and Combination Therapies refers to two or more Chinese medicines from different therapy groups (Chinese herbal medicine, acupuncture or other Chinese medicine therapies) administered together. Terminology used throughout the monograph is based on the World Health Organisation's *Standard Terminologies on Traditional Medicine in the Western Pacific Region* (2007) where possible or is from the cited reference.

Data Analysis and Interpretation of Results

In order to synthesise the clinical evidence, a range of statistical analysis approaches are used. In general, the effect size for dichotomous data is reported as a risk ratio (RR) with 95% confidence intervals (CI), and for continuous data, they are reported as mean difference (MD) with 95% CI. Statistically significant effects are indicated with an asterisk*. Readers should note that statistical significance does not necessarily correspond with a clinically important effect. Interpretation of results should take into consideration of the clinical significance, quality of studies (expressed as high, low or unclear risk of bias in this book) and heterogeneity amongst the studies. Tests for heterogeneity are conducted using the I^2 statistic. An I^2 score greater than 50% may indicate substantial heterogeneity.

Use of Evidence in Practice

The Grading of Recommendations Assessment, Development and Evaluation (GRADE) approach was used to summarise the results and the certainty of the evidence for critical and important comparisons and outcomes. Due to the diverse nature of Chinese medicine practice, treatment recommendations are not included with the summary of findings tables. Therefore readers will need to interpret the evidence with reference to the local practice environment.

Limitations

Readers should note some of the methodological limitations on classical literature and clinical evidence.

- Search terms used to search the *Zhong Hua Yi Dian* 中华医典 database may not include all terms that have been used for the condition, which may alter the findings.
- Chinese language has changed over time. Citations have been interpreted for analysis, and such interpretations may be subject to disagreement.
- Chinese medicine theory has evolved over time. As such, concepts described in classical Chinese medical literature may no longer be found in contemporary works.
- Symptoms described in citations may be common to many conditions, and a judgment was required to determine the likelihood of the

citation being related to the condition. This may have introduced some bias due to the subjective nature of the judgment.

- The vast majority of the clinical evidence for Chinese medicine treatments has come from China. The applicability of the findings to other populations and other countries requires further assessment.
- Many studies included participants with varying disease severity. Where possible, subgroup analyses were undertaken to examine the effects in different sub-populations. As this was not always possible, the findings may be limited to the population included, and not to sub-populations.
- The potential risk of bias found in many included studies suggested methodological limitations. The findings for GRADE assessments based on studies of very low to moderate quality evidence should be interpreted accordingly.
- Nine major English and Chinese language databases were searched to identify clinical studies, in addition to clinical trial registers. Other studies may exist which were not identified through searches, and which may alter the findings.
- The calculation of frequency of herbal formula use was based on formula names. It is possible that studies evaluated herbal treatments with the same or similar herb ingredients, but which were given different formula names. Due to the complexity of herbal formulas, it was considered not appropriate to make a judgment as to the similarity of formulas for analysis. As such, the frequency of formulas reported in Chapter 5 may be underestimated.
- The most frequently utilised herbs which may have contributed to the treatment effect have been described in Chapter 5. These herbs may provide leads for further exploration. Calculation of the herbs with potential effect is based on frequency of formulae reported in the studies, and doesn't take into consideration the clinical implications and functions of every herb in a formula.

Authors and Contributors

Co-Editors-in-Chief

Dist. Prof. Charlie Changli Xue (*RMIT University, Australia*)
Prof. Chuanjian Lu (*Guangdong Provincial Hospital of Chinese Medicine, China*)

Co-Deputy Editors-in-Chief

Assoc. Prof. Anthony Lin Zhang (*RMIT University, Australia*)
Dr. Brian H May (*RMIT University, Australia*)
Prof. Xinfeng Guo (*Guangdong Provincial Hospital of Chinese Medicine, China*)
Prof. Zehuai Wen (*Guangdong Provincial Hospital of Chinese Medicine, China*)

Lead Authors

Dr. Brian H May (*RMIT University, Australia*)
Dr. Mei Feng (*Guangdong Provincial Hospital of Chinese Medicine, China*)

Co-Authors:

RMIT University (Australia):
Dr. Shefton Parker
Assoc. Prof. Anthony Lin Zhang
Dist. Prof. Charlie Changli Xue

Guangdong Provincial Hospital of Chinese Medicine (China):
Dr. Yuanqi Zhao
Dr. Jingsong You
Dr. Shaonan Liu
Prof. Xinfeng Guo

Member of Advisory Committee and Panel

Co-Chairs of Project Planning Committee

Prof. Peter J Coloe (*RMIT University, Australia*)
Prof. Yubo Lyu (*Guangdong Provincial Hospital of Chinese Medicine, China*)
Prof. Dacan Chen (*Guangdong Provincial Hospital of Chinese Medicine, China*)

Centre Advisory Committee (in Alphabetical order)

Prof. Keji Chen (*The Chinese Academy of Sciences, China*)
Prof. Aiping Lu (*Hong Kong Baptist University, China*)
Prof. Caroline Smith (*University of Western Sydney, Australia*)
Prof. David F Story (*RMIT University, Australia*)

Methodology Expert Advisory Panel (in Alphabetical order)

Prof. Zhaoxiang Bian (*Hong Kong Baptist University, China*)
Prof. Lixing Lao (*The University of Hong Kong, China*)
The Late Prof. George Lewith (*University of Southampton, United Kingdom*)
Prof. Jianping Liu (*Beijing University of Chinese Medicine, China*)
Prof. Frank Thien (*Monash University, Australia*)
Prof. Jialiang Wang (*Sichuan University, China*)

Content Expert Advisory Panel (in Alphabetical order)

Prof. Yefeng Cai (*Guangdong Provincial Hospital of Chinese Medicine, China*)
Prof. Yan Huang (*Guangdong Provincial Hospital of Chinese Medicine, China*)

Prof. Weixiong Liang (*Guangzhou University of Chinese Medicine, China*)
Prof. Jingbo Sun (*Guangdong Provincial Hospital of Chinese Medicine, China*)
Prof. Guoqing Zheng (*The Second Affiliated Hospital & Yuying Children's Hospital of Wenzhou Medical University, China*)

Distinguished Professor Charlie Changli Xue, PhD

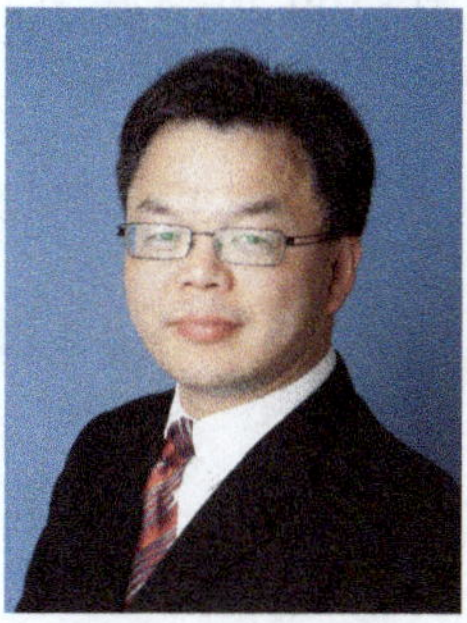

Distinguished Professor Charlie Changli Xue holds a Bachelor of Medicine (majoring in Chinese Medicine) from Guangzhou University of Chinese Medicine, China (1987) and a PhD from RMIT University, Australia (2000). He has been an academic, researcher, regulator and practitioner for almost three decades. Professor Xue has made significant contributions to evidence-based educational development, clinical research, regulatory framework and policy development and provision of high quality clinical care to the community. Professor Xue is recognised internationally as an expert in evidence-based traditional medicine and integrative healthcare.

Professor Xue is the Inaugural National Chair of the Chinese Medicine Board of Australia appointed by the Australian Health Workforce Ministerial Council (in 2011), and he was reappointed for the second term in 2014. Since 2007, he has been a Member of the World Health Organization (WHO) Expert Advisory Panel for Traditional and Complementary Medicine, Geneva. Professor Xue is also Honorary Senior Principal Research Fellow at the Guangdong Provincial Academy of Chinese Medical Sciences, China.

At RMIT, Professor Xue is Executive Dean, School of Health and Biomedical Sciences. He is also Director, World Health Organization (WHO) Collaborating Centre for Traditional Medicine.

Between 1995 and 2010, Professor Xue was Discipline Head of Chinese Medicine at RMIT University. He leads the development of five successful undergraduate and postgraduate degree programs in Chinese Medicine at RMIT University which is now a global leader in Chinese medicine education and research.

Professor Xue's research has been supported by over AU$15 million research grants including six project grants from the Australian Government's National Health & Medical Research Council (NHMRC) and two Australian Research Council (ARC) grants. He has contributed over 200 publications and has been frequently invited as keynote speaker for numerous national and international conferences. Professor Xue has contributed to over 300 media interviews on issues related to complementary medicine education, research, regulation and practice.

Professor Chuanjian Lu, MD

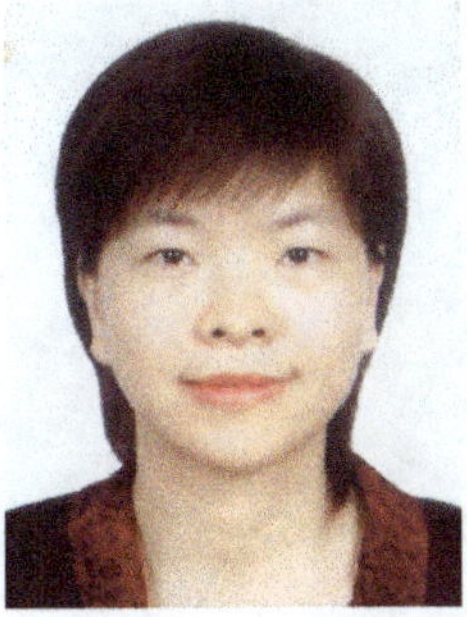

Professor Chuanjian Lu, Doctor of Medicine. She is the vice president of Guangdong Provincial Hospital of Chinese Medicine (Guangdong Provincial Academy of Chinese Medical Sciences, Second Clinical Medical College of Guangzhou University of Chinese Medicine). She also is the chair of the Guangdong Traditional Chinese Medicine (TCM) Standardization Technical Committee, and the vice-chair of the Immunity Specialty Committee of the World Federation of Chinese Medicine Societies (WFCMS).

Professor Lu has engaged in scientific research into TCM, clinical practice and teaching for some 25 years. Her research has been devoted to integrated traditional and western medicine. She has edited and published 12 monographs and 120 academic research articles as first author and corresponding author with over 30 articles being included in SCI journals.

She has received widespread recognition for her achievements with awards for "Excellent Teacher of South China", "National Outstanding Women TCM Doctor", and "National Outstanding Young Doctor of TCM". She also received "The Science and Technology Star of the Association of Chinese Medicine", the "National Excellent Science and Technology Workers of China Award" and the "Five-Continent Women's Scientific Awards of China Medical Women's Association".

Professor Lu has won the Award of Science and Technology Progress over 10 times from Guangdong Provincial Government, China Association of Chinese Medicine and Chinese Hospital Association.

Acknowledgements

The authors and contributors would like to acknowledge the valuable contributions of the following people who assisted with database searches, data extraction, data screening, data assessment, translation of documents, editing, and/or administrative tasks: Su-yueh Chang, Dr Meaghan Coyle, Jing Cui, Lin Dong, Dr Jhodie Duncan, Shengnan Gan, Dr Anna Hyde, Jingmin Lu, Wanxin Wen, Dr Claire Zhang, Shijie Zhang.

Contents

List of Figures

List of Tables

1

Introduction to Vascular Dementia

OVERVIEW

Vascular dementia is the second most common form of dementia after Alzheimer's Disease and bears a number of subtypes, most of which are more common in older people. Vascular dementia is associated with vascular disease and involves step-wise or progressive declines in cognitive functions. Although cognitive decline typically follows a stroke, not all people with vascular dementia have a clinical history of stroke. The brains of people with vascular dementia are characterised by: infarcts, vascular pathologies in large or small blood vessels, and shrinkage due to neuronal loss. Management with conventional medicine involves the control of cardiovascular and other risk factors, maintenance of cognitive function, and supportive care. This chapter describes the features of vascular dementia, pathological processes, diagnosis, and management with conventional medicine.

Definition of Vascular Dementia

Between 1991 to 1993, the National Institute of Neurological Disorders and Stroke (NINDS) and the Association Internationale pour la Recherche et l'Enseignement en Neurosciences (AIREN) developed a set of criteria for vascular dementia (VaD) specifying that:

- The patient must show dementia — a decline in memory and intellectual abilities leading to impaired functioning in daily living.
- There must be evidence of cerebrovascular disease (CVD) demonstrated by history, clinical examination, or brain imaging; and
- The two disorders must be reasonably related.[1]

In 1993, the International Classification of Diseases, Tenth Revision (ICD-10), and the Classification of Mental and Behavioural Disorders listed a code for VaD (f01), with additional codes for VaD of acute onset (f01.0), multi-infarct dementia (f01.1), subcortical VaD (f01.2), and mixed cortical and subcortical VaD (f01.3).[2] The Diagnostic and Statistical Manual of Mental Disorders (DSM) included a category for VaD in the 4th Edition (DSM IV-TR, 2000) but did not include the ICD-10 subtypes.[3]

It was proposed that VaD should be redefined to include a spectrum of disorders termed vascular cognitive impairment (VCI).[4] In this framework, a milder stage is recognised which can be called vascular mild cognitive impairment (VaMCI) or vascular cognitive impairment — no dementia (VCI-ND), while VaD is used to refer to more severe conditions.[5–7] In the American Heart Association/American Stroke Association Statement in 2011, the preferred terms were VCI for the condition in general and VaD for the most severe form.[8]

In 2013, the 5th edition of the DSM (DSM-5) reclassified the various forms of dementia as neurocognitive disorders (NCD) and also adopted a range from mild to severe disorders. In this framework, VaD became major vascular NCD while less severe conditions were classified as mild vascular neurocognitive disorder.[9] Other related terms include post-stroke dementia (PSD), ischemic vascular dementia (IVD), and vascular cognitive disorder (VCD).[6,10,11] The term "vascular dementia" will be used throughout this monograph unless specific sources are referenced or quoted, since this term has a long history of use and remains in currency.

Clinical Presentation

The main features of VaD are symptoms of dementia (major NCD), in which the dominant pathology is CVD. However, the presentation of VaD is heterogeneous due to the variety of vascular lesions that can develop and the parts of the brain that can be affected. VaD can progress in a step-wise fashion with a decline in cognition being temporally associated with cerebral infarctions (strokes), followed by periods of relative stability between infarctions. However, there may be gradual onset, slow progression, and complex presentations when small vessel disease or subcortical ischemic changes are present.[9]

Clinical symptoms include a significant decline in cognition with impairments in one or more cognitive domains (complex attention, executive function, learning and memory, language, perceptual-motor function, or social cognition). There may be personality and mood changes, abulia (diminished motivation), depression, and emotional lability. History of stroke is common and neurological assessment often reveals transient ischemic episodes and brain infarctions.[9]

Epidemiology of Dementia and Vascular Dementia

The prevalence of dementia (all types) in people aged 60 years and over has been estimated at 4.7%, although this varies by region.[12] The incidence of dementia is projected to increase as populations age, although the incidence rate may have stabilised in some high-income countries.[13] Alzheimer's disease (AD) is generally the most prevalent type of dementia, followed by VaD which can be present in up to 20% of cases of dementia, including cases with mixed types of dementia.[14,15]

In the United States (US), the prevalence of VaD has been estimated to be at 0.2% in individuals aged 65–70 years and 16% in people aged 80 years and older.[9] In Europe, VaD prevalence was reported as 1.6% in people aged 65 years and over.[15] In Africa, the prevalence in people aged 65 to 74 was estimated at 0.94%, increasing to 2.88% in people aged 85 years and over.[16] In China, a meta-analysis of 48 surveys found that the prevalence of VaD was 0.9% in people aged 60 years and over while AD prevalence was 1.9%. VaD was more prevalent in northern China (1.2%) than in southern China (0.6%), and was more prevalent in urban (0.9%) than in rural (0.4 %) areas. Prevalence increased gradually with age from 0.4% in those aged 60–64 years up to 2.0% at 85 years and over and was higher in males (2.2%) than in females (1.7%).[17] A subsequent population survey reported that in people aged 65 years and over, the overall prevalence of VaD was 1.5% with 1.59% in urban populations versus 1.36% in rural populations. The prevalence of VaD increased with age but the relationship was weak, unlike the prevalence of AD which increased markedly with age.[18]

Burden of Dementia and Vascular Dementia

Studies of community dwelling patients in the north-eastern US have compared the healthcare costs of VaD, CVD, AD and other dementias. These studies found that Medicare costs were highest for VaD, although the costs for physician visits and prescription drugs were lower for VaD than for CVD or AD. The main source of costs for VaD was hospital admissions, which were almost three times longer for VaD than for CVD and two times longer than for AD. Compared with AD patients, the prevalence rates in VaD patients were higher for the following comorbidities: CVD, congestive heart failure, hemiplegia and paraplegia, and myocardial infarction. In monetary terms, the per-annum cost for VaD was $14,387 US compared to $10,716 US for other dementias, $8,254 US for CVD, and $7,839 US for AD.[19,20]

Risk Factors

The main risk factors for VaD are the same as those for CVD and stroke: hypertension, diabetes, obesity, smoking, hyperlipidaemia (high cholesterol), high homocysteine, cardiac arrhythmia, atrial fibrillation, atherosclerosis, and arteriolosclerosis.[9,21] Lower education levels have also been associated with higher risks of dementia and VaD, but the cognitive tests used in assessing impairment have an educational component and lower educational level is difficult to disassociate from other socioeconomic factors, which may be confounders.[8]

High blood pressure is a cause of stroke and a risk factor for VaD. Mid-life hypertension is also an important modifiable risk factor for late-life cognitive decline including VaD. However, the evidence for late-life hypertension and cognitive decline is less clear.[8] The risk of VaD increases with age along with the risk of stroke and CVD, although VaD can also be present in young people. Following an ischaemic stroke, 20–30% of people will progress to vascular cognitive impairment or dementia within three months.[9,22] Following a stroke, both the severity and duration of ongoing hypertension increase the risk of VaD.[22] Coronary artery disease is also a risk factor for VaD, with or without coronary bypass surgery. Increased severity of peripheral arterial disease has been associated with lower cognitive function while reduced cardiac output has been associated with poorer executive function and white matter lesions. In addition, atrial fibrillation is a risk factor for stroke and VaD while chronic kidney disease is associated with cognitive impairment, hypertensive encephalopathy, increased stroke risk and higher VaD incidence.[8]

Hyperglycaemia, insulin resistance, metabolic syndrome, and diabetes are all associated with VCI and VaD; the longer the diabetes, the worse the effect on cognition. Also, recurrent hypoglycaemia has been associated with cognitive decline in the elderly.[8] The combination of hypertension and type two diabetes further increases the risk of VaD.[22] The presence of inflammation, as indicated by elevated levels of C-reactive protein and interleukin-6, has also been linked to substantially increased risk of VaD.[8] Furthermore, obesity and high waist-to-hip ratio in mid-life is associated with the development of hypertension and dementia. High cholesterol levels in mid-life increase the risk of developing VaD over a 30-year period, but these associations were less clear in older people.[8]

Smoking is associated with CVD and smokers show increased risk of cognitive decline. For alcohol intake, there is clear evidence that cognitive impairment is associated with heavy intake, but the results for other levels of intake have been inconclusive.[8] Long-term physical activity, including vigorous activity, has been associated with less cognitive decline and less VaD, but there is little data on the relationships between the type and amount of activity and brain health.[8] Work-related stress has also been associated with increased risk of VaD and AD.[23]

Dietary factors have been linked with CVD and Mediterranean dietary patterns have been associated with reductions in cognitive decline and cortical thinning.[8,24] A systematic review of the relationship between nutrition and reduced VaD found that the most convincing evidence was for micronutrients, including vitamins E and C.[25] Higher consumption of n-3 polyunsaturated fatty acids, which are found in fish and have been shown to have antioxidant and anti-inflammatory properties, has been associated with less cognitive decline in elderly men, and higher fish consumption is associated with lower dementia risk.[8,26]

Genetic factors that increase the risk of stroke and VaD include Notch-3 mutations on chromosome 19 which can lead to the rare disorder of cerebral autosomal-dominant arteriopathy with subcortical infarcts and leukoencephalopathy (CADASIL). This is associated with early onset of CVD and progression to a form of VaD.[8,27] Cerebral autosomal recessive arteriopathy with subcortical infarcts and leukoencephalopathy (CARASIL) is another rare disorder due to a mutation in the high-temperature requirement A serine peptidase 1 (HTRA1) gene leading to similar clinical presentation as CADASIL. Both conditions show small vessel disease and white matter injury.[27,28]

In China, epidemiological studies reported that the main risk factors for VaD in urban areas were hypertension, diabetes mellitus, or stroke, whereas in rural areas, the highest risk factors were illiteracy, alcohol consumption, and history of stroke.[18]

Pathological Processes

CVD is associated with cognitive impairment, VaD and AD, but CVD does not necessarily lead to dementia. In VaD, the presence of cerebral infarcts is a typical feature, but infarcts are also found in AD and in older people without dementia. Nevertheless, larger numbers and volumes of infarcts are associated with greater likelihood of dementia, although studies have not found consistent relationships between these factors and the severity of cognitive impairment. One reason is infarcts in certain locations, such as the angular gyrus, thalamus, and basal ganglia, have greater effects on cognition. Another reason is that multiple microscopic infarcts, which may not appear on imaging, can also lead to cognitive impairment.[8]

The typical process for the development of VaD progresses from vascular disease and hypertension to a stroke event with cerebral ischemia, followed by impairment of memory and other cognitive domains, which worsen with subsequent strokes. However, the current understanding of VaD allows for multiple pathological processes and multiple clinical presentations. In the case of microbleeds and diffuse white matter degeneration, there may have been no clinical stroke event, cognitive impairment may have been gradual, and memory impairment may not be a primary clinical feature.[8]

Another pathological process is accumulation of the peptide beta-amyloid within the arterioles and capillaries of the leptomeninges and cortex, leading to cerebral amyloid angiopathy (CAA). This involves damage to vessel walls, development of microaneurysms, splitting and necrosis of vessel walls, and leakage of red blood cells. Cerebral amyloid angiopathy can cause intra-cerebral haemorrhage and trigger vascular or perivascular inflammation. This pathology is common in the elderly and worse CAA has been associated with worse cognitive performance. This pathology is distinct from insoluble beta-amyloid plaques, which are deposited outside neurons in AD. However, CAA is often present in AD.[8]

Underlying the above processes are a range of changes in the vasculature associated with ageing, including thickening of the carotid artery wall (atherosclerosis), stiffening of the aorta (arteriosclerosis), and small-artery remodelling. These changes affect the regulation of blood pressure and can lead to cerebrovascular injuries, which in turn lead to inflammation, production of reactive oxygen species, endothelial dysfunction, and vascular leakage leading to further tissue damage.[8,27]

Diagnosis

The NINDS-AIREN criteria for the clinical diagnosis of VaD require all of the following:

1. The patient has dementia; that is, cognitive decline from a previous higher level of functioning with impairment in memory and at least two more abilities, including orientation, attention, language, visuospatial functions, executive functions, motor

control, and/or praxis. Preferably, these changes should be established through clinical examination and neuropsychological testing. Also, the cognitive deficits should be severe enough to impair activities of daily living.

Exclusion criteria include the physical effects of stroke alone, other types of dementia, delirium, disturbance of consciousness, psychosis, severe aphasia, and major sensorimotor impairment precluding neuropsychological testing.

2. There is evidence of CVD based on neurologic examination; that is, hemiparesis, lower facial weakness, Babinski sign, sensory deficit, hemianopia, and dysarthria consistent with stroke, although a history of stroke is not required. In addition, there is evidence of CVD based on brain imaging (CT or MRI) including multiple large-vessel infarcts or a single strategically placed infarct, as well as multiple basal ganglia and white matter lacunas or extensive periventricular white matter lesions, or some combination of these.
3. A relationship between these two disorders is manifest or can be inferred based on one or more of the following: onset of dementia within three months of a recognised stroke, abrupt deterioration in cognitive functions, or fluctuating, step-wise deterioration in cognition.[1]

The guideline produced by the National Collaborating Centre for Mental Health in 2007 (NICE-SCIE Guideline) listed the NINDS-AIREN criteria as preferred, but also mentioned the Modified Hachinski Ischaemic Score, which is an 8-point version of the earlier 13-point Hachinski Ischaemic Score[29,30] and the State of California Alzheimer's Disease Diagnostic and Treatment Centres (ADDTC) criteria for IVD.[10,14]

In 2011, the statement by the American Heart Association and American Stroke Association discussed the issues in defining VCI and its subtypes.[8] The diagnosis of VaD involved the following components:

- A diagnosis of dementia based on a decline in cognitive function from a prior baseline and deficits in two or more cognitive domains that are of sufficient severity to affect the subject's activities of daily living;

- The dementia diagnosis is based on cognitive testing which assessed a minimum of four cognitive domains: executive/attention, memory, language, and visuospatial functions;
- The deficits in activities of daily living are independent of the motor/sensory sequelae of the vascular event; and
- The person does not have delirium or an active diagnosis of drug or alcohol abuse/dependence.

In addition, for a diagnosis of 'probable VaD,' there is:

- Cognitive impairment and imaging evidence of CVD (e.g. cortical or subcortical infarcts or other stroke lesions);
  - A clear temporal relationship between a vascular event (e.g. clinical stroke) and onset of cognitive deficits; or
  - A clear relationship in the severity and pattern of cognitive impairment and the presence of diffuse, subcortical CVD pathology (e.g. as in CADASIL); and
- No history of gradually progressive cognitive deficits before or after the stroke that suggests the presence of a nonvascular neurodegenerative disorder.

Criteria for 'possible VaD' were also listed.[8]

DSM-5 Criteria

In the DSM-5[9] (2013), a diagnosis of major NCD due to vascular disease is required to satisfy: (1) the general diagnostic criteria for NCD and (2) the additional criteria for vascular NCD and additional criteria, as follows:

1. Neurocognitive disorder criteria: Significant cognitive decline from a previous level of performance in one or more cognitive domains (complex attention, executive function, learning and memory, language, perceptual-motor function, or social cognition) based on:
   - Concern of the individual, a knowledgeable informant, or the clinician that there has been a significant decline in cognitive function; and

- A substantial impairment in cognitive performance, preferably documented by standardized neuropsychological testing or, in its absence, another quantified clinical assessment.

2. Vascular NCD criteria: The cognitive deficits interfere with independence in everyday activities (i.e., at a minimum, requiring assistance with complex instrumental activities of daily living such as paying bills or managing medications).
3. The clinical features are consistent with a vascular aetiology as suggested by either of the following:
   - Onset of the cognitive deficits is temporally related to one or more cerebrovascular events; or
   - Evidence for decline is prominent in complex attention (including processing speed) and frontal-executive function.
4. There is evidence of the presence of CVD from history, physical examination, and/or neuroimaging that is considered sufficient to account for the neurocognitive deficits.
5. The symptoms do not occur exclusively in the context of a delirium and are not better explained by another brain disease or systemic disorder.

Additional criteria are required for a diagnosis of 'probable vascular neurocognitive disorder' as follows:

- Clinical criteria are supported by neuroimaging evidence of significant parenchymal injury attributed to CVD (neuroimaging-supported); and/or
- The neurocognitive syndrome is temporally related to one or more documented cerebrovascular events; and/or
- Both clinical and genetic, e.g. CADASIL, evidence of CVD are present.

If the clinical criteria are met but neuroimaging is not available and the temporal relationship of the neurocognitive syndrome with one or more cerebrovascular events is not established, the diagnosis should be 'possible vascular neurocognitive disorder'.[9]

Subtypes

The NINDS-AIREN criteria identified the following three subtypes based on the features of the lesions:

- Multi-infarct dementia: Which is characterised by multiple large infarcts usually as large-vessel occlusions in cortical and subcortical areas.
- Strategic single-infarct dementia: Characterised by small ischemic damage in cortical and subcortical areas whose functions are known and these result in specific impairments.
- Small-vessel disease with dementia: In which there are cortical and subcortical lesions, lacunas and white matter lesions (leukoencephalopathy).[1,31] This type also includes subcortical vascular encephalopathy (also known as Binswanger's disease) which is characterized by confluent central and peripheral white matter lesions associated with demyelination and axon loss.[1,27]

Assessment

The clinical assessment of VaD typically involves the presence of dementia based on performance on neurocognitive tests, a clinical history congruent with CVD and a temporal relationship between these two aspects, exclusion of other reasons for cognitive impairment, neuroimaging to detect cerebral lesions, and genetic testing.[1,8,9]

Commonly used clinical instruments for assessing the severity of cognitive impairment and its effects on daily living include:

- Mini-Mental State Examination (MMSE).
- Alzheimer's Disease Assessment Scale — cognitive subscale (ADAS-cog).
- Revised Hasegawa Dementia Scale (HDS-R).
- Montreal Cognitive Assessment (MoCA).
- Cognitive Capacity Screening Examination (CCSE).
- Clinical Dementia Rating (CDR).
- Blessed Dementia Scale (BDS).
- Global Deterioration Scale (GDS).
- Memory Quotient (MQ) of the Wechsler Memory Scale (WMS).

- Barthel Index (BI) and other measures of activities of daily living (ADL).
- Functional Activities Questionnaire (FAQ).

See Chapter 4 for details on these and other measures.

A history of stroke preceding the onset of dementia is suggestive of VaD but the cerebrovascular injuries may not have been clinically evident so magnetic resonance imaging (MRI) is recommended in order to detect the presence of brain atrophy, white matter hyperintensities, infarction, haemorrhage, masses, or other abnormalities. However, lesions are relatively common in older people and do not necessarily lead to cognitive impairment. Furthermore, multiple microscopic lesions not detected on MRI may be associated with dementia.[8,27]

Genetic testing is used to detect the gene mutations linked to CADASIL and CARASIL, which are associated with small-vessel disease and cognitive impairments that can progress to dementia.[8,27] Although biomarkers of VaD are not yet available, measures of beta-amyloid peptide in cerebrospinal fluid can be used to identify pathology. Cerebral amyloid angiopathy (CAA), which is associated with age-related small-vessel dysfunction, may be detected by amyloid ligand imaging. However, studies suggest that the most common type of dementia in the elderly may have mixed vascular and AD pathology and these may interact, so a positive test for AD may not rule out VaD.[21,32]

Differential Diagnosis

VaD needs to be differentiated from other age-related neurocognitive disorders, including:

- Alzheimer's disease (also known as major NCD due to AD).
- Frontotemporal dementia (also known as frontotemporal lobar degeneration, Pick's disease).
- Huntington's disease.
- Lewy body disease (also known as dementia with Lewy bodies).

- Creutzfeldt–Jakob disease (also known as NCD due to prion disease).
- Mild cognitive impairment (MCI, also known as mild NCD).

AD has insidious onset with gradual progression over a number of years without prolonged plateaus. Typical presentations include impairment in memory, learning and cognition, visuoconstructional/perceptual-motor ability, and language.[3,9,33]

Frontotemporal neurocognitive disorder is a rare disorder that can be difficult to distinguish from AD and has a number of variant forms:

- Behavioural-variant: Characterised by varying degrees of apathy, loss of interest in socialisation, self-care, and personal responsibilities, or disinhibition with display of socially inappropriate behaviours.
- Language-variant: Characterised by primary progressive aphasia with gradual onset, for which three subtypes have been identified: (1) semantic variant; (2) agrammatic/nonfluent variant; and (3) logopenic variant.[9]

In cases where the differential diagnosis of VaD, AD, and frontotemporal dementia is in doubt, perfusion hexamethylpropyleneamine oxime (HMPAO) single-photon emission computed tomography (SPECT) should be used to help differentiate these disorders.[14]

Lewy body disease develops following the onset of Parkinson's disease. Besides cognitive decline, there are recurrent complex visual hallucinations, concurrent symptoms of rapid eye movement (REM) sleep behaviour disorder, hallucinations in other sensory modalities, depression, and delusions.[9]

Huntington's disease is a genetic disorder for which there is family history and/or a positive genetic test. The motor symptoms of bradykinesia, such as slowing of voluntary movement and chorea (involuntary jerking movements), are distinctive.[9]

Creutzfeldt Jakob disease occurs mainly due to cross-species transmission of prion infections, although there are rare genetic types. It is characterised by rapid progressive dementia with ataxia and abnormal movements such as myoclonus, chorea, or dystonia.[9]

MCI is a transitional state between the cognitive changes of normal ageing and very early dementia. Some people with MCI will remain stable while others will progress to dementia. In particular, those with the amnestic subtype of MCI may progress to AD,[34–36] while those with vascular MCI (VaMCI), which is also called vascular cognitive impairment — no dementia (VCI-ND), may progress to VaD.[7,37]

Depression can be associated with impairments in cognition and ADL. In addition, depression may be associated with CVD and/or stroke. In some cases, post-stroke cognitive impairments and depression may improve during the stroke recovery process. Hence, the presence of depression does not rule out CVD as a likely cause of the cognitive impairment.[8]

Management

The 2007 NICE-SCIE guideline recommended that for people with VaD, their concurrent physical illnesses such as hypertension, diabetes, heart disease and hypercholesterolaemia should be treated using currently recommended interventions for these disorders. These treatments aim to reduce further damage to the brain, but the guideline noted that there was no evidence that these treatments could reduce cognitive impairments.[14]

Other aspects of management are the same as for AD. The guideline recommended that care of people with dementia should:

- Promote and maintain independence through care plans that provide adequate and consistent staffing, a stable environment, support with ADL, environmental modification to maintain independence, physical exercise, and support to participate in activities the person enjoys.
- Provide opportunity and support for non-pharmacological interventions to maintain cognitive function, such as structured group cognitive stimulation programmes.

For non-cognitive behavioural and psychological symptoms of dementia (BPSD) that are distressing to the person and/or pose challenges to care-givers, the NICE-SCIE guideline recommended individual assessment and a care-planning approach to address these factors, which may include undetected pain and discomfort. Non-pharmacological management should be provided in the first instance, unless there is severe distress or risk of harm that requires pharmacological management with benzodiazepines or antipsychotics. However, the guideline cautioned that antipsychotic drugs should not be prescribed to people with mild-to-moderate BPSD because of the possible increased risk of cerebrovascular adverse events and death.[14]

Pharmacological Interventions for Vascular Dementia

The 2007 NICE-SCIE guideline recommended that people with VaD should not be prescribed acetylcholinesterase inhibitors (AChEI) or memantine for the treatment of cognitive decline, except as part of properly constructed clinical studies, due the absence of evidence at the time.[14] A subsequent eight year review found that new evidence in this area was mixed but broadly supportive of the use of AChEI and memantine in VaD, particularly in improving cognition.[38]

In 2011, the World Federation of Biological Psychiatry (WFSBP) guidelines provided evidence-based assessments of AChEI for VaD, which indicated that studies of donepezil have shown superiority to placebo, but there were no comparable studies for galantamine or rivastigmine. Studies showed memantine to be superior to placebo. WFSBP recommended the use of the same pharmaceuticals as for AD, namely donepezil, galantamine, memantine, *Ginkgo biloba* extract, and rivastigmine.[31] The WFSBP guidelines noted that no drugs could be recommended for curing or arresting VaD or other types of degenerative dementias.[39]

The 2011 statement from the American Heart Association/American Stroke Association recommended that donepezil can be useful for cognitive enhancement in patients with VaD. Galantamine can be beneficial for patients with mixed AD/VaD, but the benefits of rivastigmine and memantine were not well established in VaD.[8] No drugs have been approved by the US Food and Drug Administration for the treatment of VaD.[40]

The following is a brief summary of the clinical evidence for the use of specific pharmacological interventions in the management of VCI and VaD (also see Table 1.1).

For the AChEI donepezil, analysis of the combined results of two VaD trials found improvement in cognition, global function, and ability to perform instrumental ADL (IADL).[41] Subsequent reports found improvements in cognition lasting for up to one year.[42,43] For CADASIL, one study found no significant effect for donepezil.[44] A Cochrane review of galantamine found two randomised controlled trials (RCTs)

Table 1.1 Summary of the Diagnosis and Management of Vascular Dementia

Definition of vascular dementia	• Decline in memory and intellectual abilities due to CVD; • Subtypes include: Multi-infarct dementia, small-vessel disease with dementia, subcortical vascular encephalopathy, and the genetic disorders CADASIL and CARASIL.
Diagnosis	• Presence of dementia based on clinical history and performance on neurocognitive tests; • Clinical presentation congruent with CVD and/or stroke; • Temporal relationship between cognitive decline and the development of CVD and/or specific cerebrovascular events; • Neuroimaging to detect cerebral lesions; • Genetic testing for CADASIL and CARASIL; • Exclusion of other reasons for cognitive impairment.
Management	• Pharmacological and/or non-pharmacological management of vascular risk factors including: High blood pressure, cardiac disorders, elevated cholesterol and lipid levels, and diabetes mellitus; • Acetylcholinesterase inhibitors or memantine for the treatment of cognitive decline; • Supportive care to maintain independence for as long as possible.

Abbreviations: CVD, cerebrovascular disease; CADASIL, cerebral autosomal-dominant arteriopathy with subcortical infarcts and leukoencephalopathy; CARASIL, cerebral autosomal recessive arteriopathy with subcortical infarcts and leukoencephalopathy.

References 1, 2, 3, 9, 14, 31, 39.

which suggested improvement for cognition and global scores relative to placebo[45] and a subsequent study reported improved cognition, including executive function.[46] For rivastigmine, a Cochrane review of three studies of VCI found evidence of cognitive improvement in the largest study[47], but not in the other two studies.[48] A meta-analysis of ADAS-cog and Clinician's Global Impression of Change (CGIC) scores from six studies of AChEI versus placebo found small but significant improvements in ADAS-cog for donepezil, galantamine, and rivastigmine, but no significant improvements in CGIC.[49]

Huperzine A is a novel AChEI derived from the Chinese herb: *Huperzia serrata* (Thunb. ex Murray) Trevis. (*she zu shi shan* 蛇足石杉), which has been tested in a number of clinical trials of dementia[50] and has shown cognitive benefits in VaD.[51,52]

The N-methyl-D-aspartate receptor antagonist memantine, which is used for severe AD, provided modest benefits on cognition as measured by ADAS-cog in two placebo-controlled clinical trials.[49,53]

The dihydropyridine calcium channel blocker nimodipine, which is used for stroke sequelae and hypertension, may slow the rate of decline in VaD and subcortical VaD.[53–55] Nicardipine, which is from the same drug class and is also used for hypertension, may slow cognitive decline in people with VCI[53] and flunarizine has been used for CVDs including migraine and dementia.[56,57]

Nicergoline is an ergot derivative that has been used for vascular and cognitive disorders and has been tested in placebo-controlled trials for multi-infarct dementia.[58] Reviews of clinical trials have reported evidence of positive effects for nicergoline on cognition and behaviour,[59] mild-to-moderate dementia, and vascular diseases.[60]

Piracetam and other nootropic drugs, including oxiracetam and aniracetam, have been used for age-related cognitive disorders since the 1980s.[61] A Cochrane review found no significant benefit in terms of cognition,[62] but other reviews have reported benefits in people with cognitive deficits due to ischemia.[63] Oxiracetam was reported to improve cognition compared with placebo in people with mild-to-moderate AD or multi-infarct dementia[64] in mixed dementia[65] as well as in tests of memory.[63] Aniracetam has also received clinical attention in MCI, AD, and VaD.[63,66] In one open label study of people with

MCI and various dementias, aniracetam was found to be more effective than AChEI for cognitive outcomes.[67]

Co-dergocrine mesylate (HYDERGINE®) is a mixture of the methane sulfonate salts of three dihydrogenated ergot alkaloids (dihydro-ergocristine, dihydroergocornine, and alpha- and beta-dihydroergocryptine). A Cochrane review found some evidence of benefit in dementia, but this was uncertain since the trials predated consensus guidelines on dementia diagnosis.[68] The peptide cerebrolysin has been used in the treatment of stroke. In VaD, a Cochrane review found benefits for cognition and global function in elderly patients, but concluded there was insufficient evidence to recommend the drug as a routine treatment for VaD.[69]

A standardised extract of *Gingko biloba* leaf (EGb 761) has been tested in a number of clinical trials of cognitive disorders and has been used in Germany and France, although it is not licensed in UK or the US.[70] Reviews of studies of EGb 761 have found improvements in cognition in dementia, including VaD.[71–73] The recent clinical guideline from the World Federation of Societies of Biological Psychiatry has included *Gingko biloba* leaf extract as an evidence-based intervention for VaD.[31,39]

The xanthine derivatives propentofylline and pentoxifylline have shown some evidence of benefit in VaD based on individual studies,[74] but the NICE-SCIE guideline concluded that the quality of the evidence was low and the benefits marginal.[14]

DUXIL® is the trade name for a combination of almitrine and raubasine. It has been reported to benefit age-related cerebral disorders and improve functional rehabilitation after stroke.[75,76] However, a Cochrane review concluded that there was insufficient evidence to support its use for the treatment of VaD.[77] It has been withdrawn from use in many countries, including China.

Although the NICE-SCIE guideline recommended measures to reduce cardiovascular and other risk factors for the prevention of VaD, the guideline found that drugs for hypertension, cholesterol, and diabetes did not appear to improve cognition in dementia.[14] The American Heart Association/American Stroke Association statement broadly concurred and recommended that: (1) lowering blood pressure in the middle-aged and young-elderly can be useful for the prevention of late-life dementia, but the evidence in people aged 80 years and over was not well established; (2) the evidence for treating diabetes/hyperglycaemia to prevent dementia was not well established; (3) the usefulness of hyperlipidaemia treatment for preventing of dementia was uncertain; and (4) the effectiveness of antiaggregant therapies (such as aspirin) for VCI was not well established.[8]

Non-pharmacological Interventions for Vascular Dementia

A Cochrane review of cognitive training and cognitive rehabilitation for dementia, including mild-to-moderate AD and VaD, found no significant benefit for these interventions.[78] Hyperbaric oxygen therapy, combined with donepezil, was reported to improve cognition in one study but a Cochrane review found the study to be of poor quality and the results to be inconclusive.[79] Although antiplatelet agents such as low-dose aspirin have shown evidence for stroke prevention, studies have not found evidence for reduction in cognitive decline in people with prior ischemic stroke. Similarly, although elevated homocysteine is a risk factor for CVD, trials of treatment with vitamin B and folic acid to lower homocysteine levels have not led to improvements in cognition.[53]

Limitations of Conventional Therapy

There is evidence of cholinergic impairment in VaD as well as in AD, but the cognitive benefits for the use of donepezil and other AChEIs as well as memantine are modest and these drugs do not appear to halt the progression of the disease.[8,31,40] Adverse effects in clinical trials of AChEI in VaD include gastrointestinal disorders, insomnia, and anorexia, with adverse events leading to significantly more withdrawals from AChEI groups than from placebo groups. Donepezil was associated with nausea, diarrhoea, and anorexia, which tended to be worse with higher doses (10 mg) compared to lower doses (5 mg); galantamine showed higher rates of nausea, vomiting, diarrhoea, anorexia, and insomnia; and rivastigmine was associated with nausea, vomiting, diarrhoea, and anorexia. Rates of stroke were similar in the AChEI and placebo groups, but there was higher mortality in the donepezil groups. For memantine, there were no significant increases in adverse events or mortality.[49]

Prognosis

The course of VaD can be variable. There may be acute onset associated with a stroke, followed by partial improvement or stepwise decline, with plateaus of variable durations or progressive decline. Subcortical types can have progressive decline which simulates AD. Physical deficits can impair functioning and additional pathologies and other types of dementia can also impair cognition in older people.[9] The control of hypertension, hyperlipidaemia, and/or diabetes may reduce damage to the brain, improve outcomes, and prevent further decline.[40]

Prevention

There has been a slowing or reversal of the trend towards increasing dementia incidence in some high-income countries, which may reflect greater awareness and better control of risk factors in mid-life over the last four decades. This suggests that public health measures may be able to reduce dementia prevalence. However, there have been increases in cardiovascular and metabolic risk factors in some middle-income countries, including China.[13]

An eight-year study found that medical interventions that identified and treated vascular risk factors in older people in Germany reduced dependence and the need for long-term care.[80] The WFSBP guidelines recommended the management of risk factors for VaD, including high blood pressure, cardiac disorders, elevated cholesterol and lipid levels, and diabetes mellitus, and other measures for the primary or secondary prevention of CVD.[31,39] A systematic review of antihypertensive medications found that these reduced the risk of both VaD and AD, with the best evidence being for calcium channel blockers and renin angiotensin system blockers.[81]

References

1. Roman GC, Tatemichi TK, Erkinjuntti T, *et al.* (1993) Vascular dementia: Diagnostic criteria for research studies. Report of the NINDS-AIREN International Workshop. *Neurology* **43**(2):250–260.
2. World Health Organisation. (1993) The ICD-10 classification of mental and behavioural disorders. World Health Organisation, Geneva.
3. American Psychiatric Association. (2000) Diagnostic and Statistical Manual of Mental Disorders, 4th ed., text revision (DSM IV-TR). American Psychiatric Association, Washington, DC.
4. Hachinski V. (1994) Vascular dementia: A radical redefinition. *Dementia* **5**(3–4):130–132.
5. Hachinski V, Iadecola C, Petersen RC, *et al.* (2006) National Institute of Neurological Disorders and Stroke — Canadian Stroke Network Vascular Cognitive Impairment Harmonization Standards. *Stroke* **37**(9):2220–2241.
6. Rojas-Fernandez CH, Moorhouse P. (2009) Current concepts in vascular cognitive impairment and pharmacotherapeutic implications. *Ann Pharmacother* **43**(7):1310–1323.
7. Stephan BCM, Matthews FE, Khaw KT, Dufouil C, *et al.* (2009) Beyond mild cognitive impairment: Vascular cognitive impairment, no dementia (VCIND). *Alzheimers Res Ther* **1**(1):4.
8. Gorelick PB, Scuteri A, Black SE, *et al.* (2011) Vascular contributions to cognitive impairment and dementia: A statement for healthcare professionals from the American Heart Association/American Stroke Association. *Stroke* **42**(9):2672–2713.
9. American Psychiatric Association. (2013) Diagnostic and Statistical Manual of Mental Disorders, 5th ed. (DSM V). American Psychiatric Association, Arlington, VA.
10. Chui HC, Victoroff JI, Margolin D, Jagust W, *et al.* (1992) Criteria for the diagnosis of ischemic vascular dementia proposed by the state of California Alzheimer's disease diagnostic and treatment centers. *Neurology* **42**(3 Pt 1):473–480.
11. Roman GC, Sachdev P, Royall DR, *et al.* (2004) Vascular cognitive disorder: A new diagnostic category updating vascular cognitive impairment and vascular dementia. *J Neurol Sci* **226**(1–2):81–87.
12. Prince M, Bryce R, Albanese E, Wimo A, *et al.* (2013) The global prevalence of dementia: A systematic review and metaanalysis. *Alzheimers Dement* **9**(1):63–75.

13. Prince M, Ali GC, Guerchet M, Prina AM, *et al.* (2016) Recent global trends in the prevalence and incidence of dementia, and survival with dementia. *Alzheimers Res Ther* **8**(1):23.
14. National Collaborating Centre for Mental Health. (2017) Dementia a NICE–SCIE guideline on supporting people with dementia and their carer in health and social care — Commissioned by the Social Care Institute for Excellence National Institute for Health and Clinical Excellence. The British Psychological Society and Gaskell, London.
15. Rizzi L, Rosset I, Roriz-Cruz M. (2014) Global epidemiology of dementia: Alzheimer's and vascular types. *Biomed Res Int* **2014**: 908915.
16. George-Carey R, Adeloye D, Chan KY, *et al.* (2012) An estimate of the prevalence of dementia in Africa: A systematic analysis. *J Glob Health* **2**(2):020401.
17. Zhang Y, Xu Y, Nie H, *et al.* (2012) Prevalence of dementia and major dementia subtypes in the Chinese populations: A meta-analysis of dementia prevalence surveys, 1980–2010. *J Clin Neurosci* **19**(10): 1333–1337.
18. Jia J, Wang F, Wei C, *et al.* (2014) The prevalence of dementia in urban and rural areas of China. *Alzheimers Dement* **10**(1):1–9.
19. Fillit H, Hill J. (2002) The costs of vascular dementia: A comparison with Alzheimer's disease. *J Neurol Sci* **203–204**:35–39.
20. Hill J, Fillit H, Shah SN, del Valle MC, *et al.* (2005) Patterns of healthcare utilization and costs for vascular dementia in a community-dwelling population. *J Alzheimers Dis* **8**(1):43–50.
21. Wiesmann M, Kiliaan AJ, Claassen JA. (2013) Vascular aspects of cognitive impairment and dementia. *J Cereb Blood Flow Metab* **33**(11): 1696–1706.
22. Kalaria RN, Akinyemi R, Ihara M. (2016) Stroke injury, cognitive impairment and vascular dementia. *Biochim Biophys Acta* **1862**(5): 915–925.
23. Andel R, Crowe M, Hahn EA, *et al.* (2012) Work-related stress may increase the risk of vascular dementia. *J Am Geriatr Soc* **60**(1):60–67.
24. Mosconi L, Murray J, Tsui WH, *et al.* (2014) Mediterranean diet and magnetic resonance imaging-assessed brain atrophy in cognitively normal individuals at risk for Alzheimer's disease. *J Prev Alzheimers Dis* **1**(1):23–32.
25. Perez L, Heim L, Sherzai A, Jaceldo-Siegl K, *et al.* (2012) Nutrition and vascular dementia. *J Nutr Health Aging* **16**(4):319–324.

26. Wu S, Ding Y, Wu F, Li R, *et al.* (2015) Omega-3 fatty acids intake and risks of dementia and Alzheimer's disease: A meta-analysis. *Neurosci Biobehav Rev* **48**:1–9.
27. Gorelick PB, Counts SE, Nyenhuis D. (2016) Vascular cognitive impairment and dementia. *Biochim Biophys Acta* **1862**(5):860–868.
28. Flanagan M, Larson EB, Latimer CS, *et al.* (2016) Clinical-pathologic correlations in vascular cognitive impairment and dementia. *Biochim Biophys Acta* **1862**(5):945–951.
29. Hachinski VC, Iliff LD, Zilhka E, *et al.* (1975) Cerebral blood flow in dementia. *Arch Neurol* **32**(9):632–637.
30. Rosen WG, Terry RD, Fuld PA, Katzman R, *et al.* (1980) Pathological verification of ischemic score in differentiation of dementias. *Ann Neurol* **7**(5):486–488.
31. Ihl R, Frolich L, Winblad B, *et al.* (2011) World Federation of Societies of Biological Psychiatry (WFSBP) guidelines for the biological treatment of Alzheimer's disease and other dementias. *World J Biol Psychiatry* **12**(1):2–32.
32. Snyder HM, Corriveau RA, Craft S, *et al.* (2015) Vascular contributions to cognitive impairment and dementia including Alzheimer's disease. *Alzheimers Dement* **11**(6):710–717.
33. Giannopoulos PF, Praticò D. Alzheimer's disease. In: Martin C, Preedy V. (eds.) (2015) *Diet and Nutrition in Dementia and Cognitive Decline.* Elsevier, Asterdam, pp. 13–21.
34. Petersen RC, Smith GE, Waring SC, Ivnik RJ, Tangalos EG, Kokmen E. (1999) Mild cognitive impairment: Clinical characterization and outcome. *Arch Neurol* **56**(3):303–308.
35. Petersen RC, Negash S. (2008) Mild cognitive Impairment: An overview. *CNS Spectr* **13**(1):45–53.
36. Gauthier S, Reisberg B, Zaudig M, *et al.* (2006) Mild cognitive impairment. *Lancet* **367**(9518):1262–1270.
37. Black SE. (2011) Vascular cognitive impairment: Epidemiology, subtypes, diagnosis and management. *J R Coll Phys Edinb* **41**(1):49–56.
38. National Institute for Health and Care Excellence. (2015) 8-year surveillance review of CG42: Dementia — Supporting people with dementia and their cares in health and social care. Centre for Clinical Practice — Surveillance Programme, London.
39. Ihl R, Bunevicius R, Frolich L, *et al.* (2015) World Federation of Societies of Biological Psychiatry guidelines for the pharmacological treatment of dementias in primary care. *Int J Psychiatry Clin Pract* **19**(1):2–7.

40. Alzheimer's Association. (2016) Vascular dementia (topic sheet). Alzheimer's Association, alz.org, pp. 1–4.
41. Roman GC, Wilkinson DG, Doody RS, Black SE, *et al.* (2005) Donepezil in vascular dementia: Combined analysis of two large-scale clinical trials. *Dement Geriatr Cogn Disord* **20**(6):338–344.
42. Roman GC, Salloway S, Black SE, *et al.* (2010) Randomized, placebo-controlled, clinical trial of donepezil in vascular dementia: Differential effects by hippocampal size. *Stroke* **41**(6):1213–1221.
43. Wilkinson D, Roman G, Salloway S, *et al.* (2010) The long-term efficacy and tolerability of donepezil in patients with vascular dementia. *Int J Geriatr Psychiatry* **25**(3):305–313.
44. Dichgans M, Markus HS, Salloway S, *et al.* (2008) Donepezil in patients with subcortical vascular cognitive impairment: A randomised double-blind trial in CADASIL. *Lancet Neurol* **7**(4):310–318.
45. Craig D, Birks J. (2006) Galantamine for vascular cognitive impairment. *Cochrane Database Syst Rev* (1):CD004746.
46. Auchus AP, Brashear HR, Salloway S, *et al.* (2007) Galantamine treatment of vascular dementia: A randomized trial. *Neurology* **69**(5):448–458.
47. Ballard C, Sauter M, Scheltens P, *et al.* (2008) Efficacy, safety and tolerability of rivastigmine capsules in patients with probable vascular dementia: The VantagE study. *Curr Med Res Opin* **24**(9):2561–2574.
48. Birks J, McGuinness B, Craig D. (2013) Rivastigmine for vascular cognitive impairment. *Cochrane Database Syst Rev* (5):CD004744.
49. Kavirajan H, Schneider LS. (2007) Efficacy and adverse effects of cholinesterase inhibitors and memantine in vascular dementia: A meta-analysis of randomised controlled trials. *Lancet Neurol* **6**(9):782–792.
50. Wang R, Yan H, Tang XC. (2006) Progress in studies of huperzine A, a natural cholinesterase inhibitor from Chinese herbal medicine. *Acta Pharmacol Sin* **27**(1):1–26.
51. Xu ZQ, Liang XM, Juan W, Zhang YF, *et al.* (2012) Treatment with huperzine A improves cognition in vascular dementia patients. *Cell Biochem Biophys* **62**(1):55–58.
52. Xing SH, Zhu CX, Zhang R, An L. (2014) Huperzine A in the treatment of Alzheimer's disease and vascular dementia: A meta-analysis. *Evid Based Complement Alternat Med* **2014**:363985.
53. Ritter A, Pillai JA. (2015) Treatment of vascular cognitive impairment. *Curr Treat Options Neurol* **17**(8):367.
54. Pantoni L, del Ser T, Soglian AG, *et al.* (2005) Efficacy and safety of nimodipine in subcortical vascular dementia: A randomized placebo-controlled trial. *Stroke* **36**(3):619–624.

55. Lopez-Arrieta JM, Birks J. (2002) Nimodipine for primary degenerative, mixed and vascular dementia. *Cochrane Database Syst Rev* (3): CD000147.
56. Jansen I, Tfelt-Hansen P, Edvinsson L. (1991) Comparison of the calcium entry blockers nimodipine and flunarizine on human cerebral and temporal arteries: Role in cerebrovascular disorders. *Eur J Clin Pharmacol* **40**(1):7–15.
57. Albizzati MG, Bassi S, Calloni E, Sbacchi M, *et al.* (1987) Cyclandelate versus flunarizine. A double-blind study in a selected group of patients with dementia. *Drugs* **33** (Suppl 2) pp. 90–96.
58. Herrmann WM, Stephan K, Gaede K, Apececche M. (1997) A multicenter randomized double-blind study on the efficacy and safety of nicergoline in patients with multi-infarct dementia. *Dement Geriatr Cogn Disord* **8**(1):9–17.
59. Fioravanti M, Flicker L. (2001) Efficacy of nicergoline in dementia and other age associated forms of cognitive impairment. *Cochrane Database Syst Rev* (4):CD003159.
60. Winblad B, Fioravanti M, Dolezal T, *et al.* (2008) Therapeutic use of nicergoline. *Clin Drug Investig* **28**(9):533–552.
61. Winblad B. (2005) Piracetam: A review of pharmacological properties and clinical uses. *CNS Drug Rev* **11**(2):169–182.
62. Flicker L, Grimley EG. (2004) Piracetam for dementia or cognitive impairment. *Cochrane Database Syst Rev* (2):CD001011.
63. Malykh AG, Sadaie MR. (2010) Piracetam and piracetam-like drugs: From basic science to novel clinical applications to CNS disorders. *Drugs* **70**(3):287–312.
64. Villardita C, Grioli S, Lomeo C, Cattaneo C, *et al.* (1992) Clinical studies with oxiracetam in patients with dementia of Alzheimer type and multi-infarct dementia of mild to moderate degree. *Neuropsychobiology* **25**(1):24–28.
65. Bottini G, Vallar G, Cappa S, *et al.* (1992) Oxiracetam in dementia: A double-blind, placebo-controlled study. *Acta Neurol Scand* **86**(3): 237–241.
66. Nakamura K. (2002) Aniracetam: Its novel therapeutic potential in cerebral dysfunctional disorders based on recent pharmacological discoveries. *CNS Drug Rev* **8**(1):70–89.
67. Koliaki CC, Messini C, Tsolaki M. (2012) Clinical efficacy of aniracetam, either as monotherapy or combined with cholinesterase inhibitors, in patients with cognitive impairment: A comparative open study. *CNS Neurosci Ther* **18**(4):302–312.

68. Olin J, Schneider L, Novit A, Luczak S. (2001) Hydergine for dementia. *Cochrane Database Syst Rev* (2):CD000359.
69. Chen N, Yang M, Guo J, Zhou M, *et al.* (2013) Cerebrolysin for vascular dementia. *Cochrane Database Syst Rev* **1**:CD008900.
70. Evans JG, Wilcock G, Birks J. (2004) Evidence-based pharmacotherapy of Alzheimer's disease. *Int J Neuropsychopharmacol* **7**(3):351–369.
71. Gauthier S, Schlaefke S. (2014) Efficacy and tolerability of *ginkgo biloba* extract EGB 761(r) in dementia: A systematic review and meta-analysis of randomized placebo-controlled trials. *Clin Interv Aging* **9**:2065–2077.
72. Hashiguchi M, Ohta Y, Shimizu M, Maruyama J, *et al.* (2015) Meta-analysis of the efficacy and safety of *ginkgo biloba* extract for the treatment of dementia. *J Pharm Health Care Sci* **1**:14.
73. Tan MS, Yu JT, Tan CC, *et al.* (2015) Efficacy and adverse effects of *ginkgo biloba* for cognitive impairment and dementia: A systematic review and meta-analysis. *J Alzheimers Dis* **43**(2):589–603.
74. Pantoni L. (2004) Treatment of vascular dementia: Evidence from trials with non-cholinergic drugs. *J Neurol Sci* **226**(1–2):67–70.
75. Li SW, Long J, Ma ZZ, Xu ZB, *et al.* (2004) Assessment of the therapeutic activity of a combination of almitrine and raubasine on functional rehabilitation following ischaemic stroke. *Curr Med Res Opin* **20**(3):409–415.
76. Allain H, Bentue-Ferrer D. (1998) Clinical efficacy of almitrine-raubasine. An overview. *Eur Neurol* **39** (Suppl 1) pp. 39–44.
77. Yang W, Liu M, Teng J, *et al.* (2011) Almitrine-raubasine combination for dementia. *Cochrane Database Syst Rev* (3):CD008068.
78. Bahar-Fuchs A, Clare L, Woods B. (2013) Cognitive training and cognitive rehabilitation for persons with mild to moderate dementia of the Alzheimer's or vascular type: A review. *Alzheimers Res Ther* **5**(4):35.
79. Xiao Y, Wang J, Jiang S, Luo H. (2012) Hyperbaric oxygen therapy for vascular dementia. *Cochrane Database Syst Rev* (7):CD009425.
80. Bickel H, Ander KH, Bronner M, *et al.* (2012) Reduction of long-term care dependence after an 8-year primary care prevention program for stroke and dementia: The INVADE trial. *J Am Heart Assoc* **1**(4):e000786.
81. Rouch L, Cestac P, Hanon O, *et al.* (2015) Antihypertensive drugs, prevention of cognitive decline and dementia: A systematic review of observational studies, randomized controlled trials and meta-analyses, with discussion of potential mechanisms. *CNS Drugs* **29**(2):113–130.

2

Vascular Dementia in Chinese Medicine

OVERVIEW

Although there are differences between the aetiology and pathogenesis of vascular dementia and Alzheimer's disease in modern medicine, in traditional Chinese medicine these diseases share similarities in terms of aetiology, pathogenesis, syndrome differentiation, and treatment. Deficiency of Kidney Essence leading to phlegm turbidity and stagnation of Blood is the main pathologic process. Major treatment methods include nourishing the Kidney, resolving phlegm, and activating blood. This chapter introduces the main aetiology, pathogenesis, and syndromes of vascular dementia in traditional Chinese medicine. Treatments are described based on practice guidelines, clinical texts, and scholarly papers and include Chinese herbal medicine and acupuncture as well as prevention, nursing, and dietary therapy.

Introduction

Vascular dementia (VaD) is a type of dementia associated with cerebrovascular disease that typically follows a stroke or cerebrovascular accident in the elderly.[1,2] In the ancient literature of Chinese medicine (CM), there was no specific term for VaD. This condition was included within the categories of *chi dai* 痴呆, *shan wang* 善忘, *jian wang* 健忘, *dai bing* 呆病, *zhong feng hou chi dai* 中风后痴呆, *zhong feng hou shan wang* 中风后善忘, and other related terms.[2,3] In modern Chinese, VaD is called *xue guan xing chi dai* 血管性痴呆.[2]

Aetiology and Pathogenesis

According to Chinese medicine (CM), VaD is mainly caused by dysfunction of the Brain and is also related to the Heart, Liver, Spleen, and Kidney.[1,3,4] When there is deficiency of the *sui hai* 髓海 'Sea of Marrow', which is transformed from the Kidney Essence, the Brain tissue is depleted and there is dysfunction of the *shen ming* 神明 'mental activity'.[5] In addition, phlegm turbidity and stagnation of Blood, which occur after a stroke, can obstruct the Brain Collaterals and impair the functioning of cognition and memory.[2,3] Hence, deficiency of Kidney Essence leading to phlegm turbidity and stagnation of Blood are the main pathologic changes in VaD.[1]

From another viewpoint, VaD shares similarities in pathogenesis with stroke (*zhong feng* 中风) in CM.[2] There have been two developmental stages in CM thought about stroke and its aetiology. In the Tang and Song dynasties (618–1279 AD) and before, the dominant etiological theory was 'external wind' attacking the body, but after the Tang and Song dynasties, especially since the Jin and Yuan dynasties (1127–1386 AD), many CM doctors believed that 'internal wind', which originates from the Liver, was the key trigger factor for the onset of stroke.[3,4] This change in theory also had a profound influence on the explanation of the pathogenesis and treatment of VaD.

Some modern CM experts have proposed that VaD could be divided into three stages according to the progress of VaD, namely the plateau stage, unstable stage, and decline stage. In the plateau stage, the disease manifests as Kidney deficiency with phlegm-stasis obstructing the collaterals; in the unstable stage, there is accumulated phlegm turbidity transforming into heat which engenders wind; in the decline stage, there are endogenous toxins damaging the body.[2,6] In addition, some modern CM clinicians have put forward another theory of pathogenesis called 'toxins damage the Brain collaterals' for VaD. They suggest that stasis, heat, phlegm, and toxins may occur after stroke, which cause damage to the Brain Marrow and collaterals leading to the malnourishment of the Brain and spirit. As a result, cognition and memory are impaired leading to the development of dementia.[2,7,8] Consequently, detoxification and dredging collaterals (i.e., improvement of Blood circulation) are the basic treatments.[9] This provides a new approach to the treatment of VaD and is also an important aspect of the integration of Chinese and Western medicine in VaD treatment.[10,11]

Syndrome Differentiation

As uniform standards for CM syndrome differentiation have not yet been established in VaD, the Internal Medicine Branch of the China Association of Traditional Chinese Medicine 中华全国中医学会内科分会 put forward standards for the diagnosis, syndrome differentiation, and evaluation of clinical effects for VaD.[12] This syndrome differentiation was based on the commonly applied approach to syndrome differentiation for VaD. On the basis of existing standards as well as the outcomes of the Delphi method judgments and expert consensus meetings, CM syndrome differentiation guidelines for dementia were developed and published in 2012 as the 'Chinese Guidelines for the Diagnosis and Treatment of Alzheimer's Disease and Other Dementias' 中国痴呆诊疗指南.[13]

Herbal Medicine Treatment Based on Syndrome Differentiation

The following main syndromes and herbal medicine treatments are based on the 'Chinese Guidelines for the Diagnosis and Treatment of Alzheimer's Disease and Other Dementias' 中国痴呆诊疗指南.[13]

Deficiency of 'Sea of Marrow' (*sui hai bu zu* 髓海不足)

Symptoms: Amnesia, fatigue, loosening of teeth, loss of hair, weakness and soreness of the lower back, difficulty with walking, inarticulate speech, inability in expressing oneself, impoverished vocabulary or speech, poor orientation, inability to do simple arithmetic calculations, agnosia or apraxia (in severe cases), pale and thin tongue with scant tongue coating, and deep, thin, and weak pulse.

Treatment principle: Nourish the Liver and Kidney (*ci bu gan shen* 滋补肝肾), nourish the Essence, and replenish Marrow (*sheng jing yang sui* 生精养髓).

Formula: Modified *Qi fu yin* 七福饮.

Herbs: *Ren shen* 人参, *shu di* 熟地, *dang gui* 当归, *bai zhu* 白术, *da zao* 大枣, *yuan zhi* 远志, *lu jiao jiao* 鹿角胶, *gui ban jiao* 龟板胶, *e jiao* 阿胶, and *zhi gan cao* 炙甘草.

Main actions of herbs: *Shu di* 熟地 nourishes the Kidney and replenishes *yin*; *lu jiao jiao* 鹿角胶, *gui ban jiao* 龟板胶, and *e jiao* 阿胶 replenish Kidney Essence; *dang gui* 当归 nourishes and regulates Blood; *ren shen* 人参, *bai zhu* 白术, and *zhi gan cao* 炙甘草 replenish *qi* and invigorate the Spleen; and *da zao* 大枣 and *yuan zhi* 远志 tranquilize the mind and improve intelligence.

Spleen and Kidney Dual Deficiency (*pi shen liang xu* 脾肾两虚)

Symptoms: Amnesia, expressionless face, quietness, slow movements, agnosia or inability to do simple arithmetic calculations, soreness of the lower back and knees, muscle atrophy, poor appetite, anorexia, shortness of breath, unwillingness to speak, drooling (sialorrhoea), coldness of the four limbs, loose stools, pale and enlarged tongue with white tongue coating, and deep, thin, and weak pulse, especially at both distal (*chi* 尺) positions.

Treatment principle: Warm the Spleen and tonify the Kidney (*wen bu pi shen* 温补脾肾) and nourish the Heart and tranquilize the mind (*yang yuan an shen* 养元安神).

Formula: Modified *Huan shao dan* 还少丹.

Herbs: *Shu di* 熟地, *gou qi zi* 枸杞子, *rou cong rong* 肉苁蓉, *ba ji tian* 巴戟天, *xiao hui xiang* 小茴香, *niu xi* 牛膝, *du zhong* 杜仲, *shan yu rou* 山萸肉, *fu ling* 茯苓, *wu wei zi* 五味子, *shan yao* 山药, *shi chang pu* 石菖蒲, *yuan zhi* 远志, and *chu shi* 楮实.

Main actions of herbs: *Shu di* 熟地, *gou qi zi* 枸杞子, and *shan yu rou* 山萸肉 nourish *yin* and tonify the Kidney; *rou cong rong* 肉苁蓉, *ba ji tian* 巴戟天, and *xiao hui xiang* 小茴香 warm the Life-gate fire and tonify Kidney *qi*; *niu xi* 牛膝, *du zhong* 杜仲, and *chu shi* 楮实 nourish the Liver and Kidney; *fu ling* 茯苓 and *shan yao* 山药 invigorate the Spleen and replenish *qi*; and *yuan zhi* 远志 and *shi chang pu* 石菖蒲 resolve phlegm and open the Orifices.

Deficiency of Qi and Blood (*qi xue kui xu* 气血亏虚)

Symptoms: Amnesia, apathy and lack of facial expression, shortness of breath, reluctance to communicate, pale complexion and lips, poor appetite, coldness of the four limbs, loose stools, pale tongue with tooth marks on the sides, white tongue coating, and thin and weak pulse.

Treatment principle: Tonify *qi* and invigorate the Spleen (*bu qi jian pi* 补气健脾) and nourish Blood and tranquilize the mind (*yang xue an shen* 养血安神).

Formula: Modified *Gui pi tang* 归脾汤.

Herbs: *Ren shen* 人参, *huang qi* 黄芪, *bai zhu* 白术, *dang gui* 当归, *fu ling* 茯苓, *long yan rou* 龙眼肉, *yuan zhi* 远志, *suan zao ren* 酸枣仁, *mu xiang* 木香, *sheng jiang* 生姜, *da zao* 大枣, and *zhi gan cao* 炙甘草.

Main actions of herbs: *Huang qi* 黄芪 tonifies *qi* and invigorates the Spleen; *long yan rou* 龙眼肉 nourishes Blood and tranquilizes the mind (both herbs play the role of monarch ingredient); *ren shen* 人参 and *bai zhu* 白术 nourish *qi* and invigorate the Spleen; *dang gui* 当归 and *long yan rou* 龙眼肉 generate Blood; *suan zao ren* 酸枣仁, *fu ling* 茯苓, and *yuan zhi* 远志 tranquilize the mind; *mu xiang* 木香 regulates *qi*, invigorates the Spleen, and prevents tonifying herbs from obstructing the Stomach; *sheng jiang* 生姜 and *da zao* 大枣 regulate the Spleen and Stomach; and *zhi gan cao* 炙甘草 regulates the middle-energizer and mediates the properties of the other herbs.

***Turbid Phlegm Obstructing the Orifices (tan zhuo meng qiao* 痰浊蒙窍)**

Symptoms: Amnesia, lack of facial expression, dizziness, heaviness in the body, obesity, productive cough with sputum in the mornings, poor appetite, nausea and vomiting, abdominal bloating, inability to look after oneself (in severe cases), pale complexion, shortness of breath, lethargy, enlarged tongue with tooth marks on the sides, white and greasy tongue coating, and slippery pulse.

Treatment principle: Resolve phlegm and open the Orifices (*hua tan kai qiao* 化痰开窍) and warm the *yang* and reinforce the healthy *qi* (*tong yang fu zheng* 通阳扶正).

Formula: Modified *Xi xin tang* 洗心汤.

Herbs: *Ren shen* 人参, *fu shen* 茯神, *ban xia* 半夏, *chen pi* 陈皮, *shen qu* 神曲, *fu zi* 附子, *shi chang pu* 石菖蒲, *hong zao* 红枣, and *gan cao* 甘草.

Main actions of herbs: *Ren shen* 人参 tonifies *qi* and invigorates the Spleen; *ban xia* 半夏 and *chen pi* 陈皮 eliminate dampness and phlegm and promote the flow of *qi*; *shi chang pu* 石菖蒲 resolves phlegm to open the Orifices; *fu shen* 茯神 and *hong zao* 红枣 calm the mind; *fu zi* 附子 warms and invigorates *yang qi*; *shen qu* 神曲 resolves food stagnation and harmonizes the Stomach; and *gan cao* 甘草 mediates the effects of the other herbs.

***Blood Stasis Obstructing the Brain Collaterals (yu zu nao luo* 瘀阻脑络)**

Symptoms: Amnesia, irritability, apathy, slow or delayed responses, quiet and seldom speaks, bizarre behaviour, headache, dull purplish tongue with spots or patches, thin and white tongue coating, uneven pulse, or thin, wiry, slow, and deep pulse.

Treatment principle: Activate Blood and resolve stasis (*huo xue hua tan* 活血化瘀) and open the Orifices and activate the mind (*tong qiao xing shen* 通窍醒神).

Formula: Modified *Tong qiao huo xue tang* 通窍活血汤.

Herbs: *Chi shao* 赤芍, *chuan xiong* 川芎, *tao ren* 桃仁, *hong hua* 红花, *hong zao* 红枣, *lao cong* 老葱, *sheng jiang* 生姜, *she xiang* 麝香, and *huang jiu* 黄酒.

Main actions of herbs: *Chi shao* 赤芍 and *chuan xiong* 川芎 activate Blood and promote Blood flow; *tao ren* 桃仁 and *hong hua* 红花 promote Blood circulation and remove Blood stasis; *lao cong* 老葱 and *sheng jiang* 生姜 warm the *yang* and open the Orifices; *she xiang* 麝香 opens the Orifices; *huang jiu* 黄酒 activates the collaterals; and *hong zao* mediates the properties of the other herbs/ingredients. Note: *she xiang* 麝香 is CITES listed and must be deleted or replaced.

Furthermore, modified *Bu yang huan wu tang* 补阳还五汤 (main ingredients: *Huang qi* 黄芪, *dang gui wei* 当归尾, *chi shao* 赤芍, *di long* 地龙, *chuan xiong* 川芎, *hong hua* 红花, and *tao ren* 桃仁) can be used for patients with the syndrome of *qi* deficiency with Blood stasis.[14]

Heart and Liver Fire (xing gan huo wang 心肝火旺)

Symptoms: Amnesia, cognitive impairment, and (1) self-centredness, irritability, proneness to anger, bitter taste in mouth, dizziness, headache, dry eyes, muscular twitching; or (2) dry mouth and throat, bad breath, mouth sores, dark urine and dry stool; or (3) red complexion, foul breath, sticky and greasy sensation in the mouth, mania (in severe cases). Dull red tongue, yellow and greasy tongue coating. Taut and slippery pulse, or taut, thin, and rapid pulse.

Treatment principle: Clear the Heart and pacify the Liver (*qing xin ping gan* 清心平肝) and settle the Heart and calm the mind (*an shen ding zhi* 安神定志).

Formula: Modified *Tian ma gou teng yin* 天麻钩藤饮.

Herbs: *Tian ma* 天麻, *gou teng* 钩藤, *shi jue ming* 石决明, *zhi zi* 栀子, *huang qin* 黄芩, *chuan niu xi* 川牛膝, *du zhong* 杜仲, *yi mu cao* 益母草, *sang ji sheng* 桑寄生, *ye jiao teng* 夜交藤, and *fu shen* 茯神.

Main actions of herbs: *Tian ma* 天麻 and *gou teng* 钩藤 are used as monarch drugs to expel the Liver-wind; *shi jue ming* 石决明 expels endogenous wind and suppresses hyperactive yang; *chuan niu xi* 川牛膝 directs Blood downwards (these two herbs are also used together to enhance the monarch herbs' ability to suppress hyperactive *yang* and expel endogenous wind); *du zhong* 杜仲 and *sang ji sheng* 桑寄生 nourish the Liver and Kidney; *zhi zi* 栀子 and *huang qin* 黄芩 clear heat from the Liver meridian; *yi mu cao* 益母草 and *chuan niu xi* 川牛膝 promote Blood flow and induce diuresis to treat the hyperactive and adverse ascent of *yang*; and *ye jiao teng* 夜交藤 and *fu shen* 茯神 tranquilize the mind.

Endogenous Toxins Damaging the Brain Collaterals (*du sun nao luo* 毒损脑络)

Symptoms: Blank facial expression, dull eyes, agnosia, dark complexion or red to slightly red complexion, foul breath, sticky and greasy sensation in the mouth, dark urine and dry stool, urine and bowel incontinence, tremor, loss of speech or disordered speech, manic and bizarre behaviour, bright red tongue with a scanty coat, or dull purple tongue with spots, thick, greasy, curdy tongue coat or turbid tongue coat, and slippery, rapid pulse.

Treatment principle: Clear heat and remove toxins (*qing re jie du* 清热解毒) and dredge collaterals and expel pathogens (*tong luo da xie* 通络达邪).

Formula: Modified *Huang lian jie du tang* 黄连解毒汤.

Herbs: *Huang lian* 黄连, *huang qin* 黄芩, *huang bai* 黄柏, *zhi zi* 栀子, *shui niu jiao* powder 水牛角粉, *quan xie* 全蝎, and *wu gong* 蜈蚣.

Main actions of herbs: *Huang lian* 黄连 purges Heart fire and fire in the middle-energizer (acting as the monarch herb); *huang qin* 黄芩 is an assistant herb that reduces the Lung fire in the upper-energizer; *huang bai* 黄柏 and *zhi zi* 栀子 function to purge fire in the lower-energizer and triple-energizer respectively, causing heat to descend; *quan xie* 全蝎 and *wu gong* 蜈蚣 resolve stasis and deobstruct

Table 2.1 Summary of Oral Chinese Herbal Medicine Treatments of Vascular Dementia

Syndrome Differentiation	Treatment Principle	Formula
Deficiency of 'Sea of Marrow'	Nourish the Liver and Kidney; nourish the Essence and replenish Marrow.	Modified *Qi fu yin* 七福饮加减
Spleen and Kidney dual deficiency	Warm the Spleen and tonify the Kidney; nourish the Heart and tranquilize the mind.	Modified *Huan shao dan* 还少丹加减
Deficiency of *qi* and Blood	Tonify *qi* and invigorate the Spleen; nourish Blood and tranquilize the mind.	Modified *Gui pi tang* 归脾汤加减
Turbid phlegm obstructing the Orifices	Resolve phlegm and open the Orifices; warm the *yang* and reinforce the healthy *qi*.	Modified *Xi xin tang* 洗心汤加减
Blood stasis obstructing the Brain collaterals	Activate Blood and resolve stasis; open the Orifices and activate the mind.	Modified *Tong qiao huo xue tang* 通窍活血汤加减
Heart and Liver fire	Clear the Heart and pacify the Liver; settle the Heart and calm the mind.	Modified *Tian ma gou teng yin* 天麻钩藤饮加减
Endogenous toxins damaging the Brain collaterals	Clear heat and remove toxins; dredge collaterals and expel pathogens.	Modified *Huang lian jie du tang* 黄连解毒汤加减

Notes: The use of some herbs may be restricted in some countries. Readers are advised to comply with relevant regulations.

collaterals; and *shui niu jiao* powder 水牛角粉 clears heat and endogenous toxins while opening the Orifices and tranquilizing the mind.

The main syndromes and formulae are summarized in Table 2.1.

Empirical Formulae

Suan zao ren shen bu nao tang 酸枣人参补脑汤[15]

Treatment principle: Powerfully tonify primordial *qi*, tranquilize the mind, and benefit cognitive function.

Method: Use 2–3 grams of *suan zao ren* 酸枣仁 and 10 grams of ginseng (*ren shen* 人参). First, grind the *suan zao ren* 酸枣仁 and then combine the *suan zao ren* 酸枣仁 and *ren shen* 人参 and simmer for one hour before finally adding honey. Consume in the morning.

Nv zhen zi jian 女贞子煎[1]

Treatment principle: Tonify the Liver and Kidney and benefit cognitive function.

Method: Put 15 grams of *nv zhen zi* 女贞子, 10 grams of black sesame (*hei zhi ma* 黑芝麻), 10 grams of *jue ming zi* 决明子, and 10 grams of goji berry (*gou qi zi* 枸杞子) into a pot and bring to boil and simmer for 30–40 minutes. Consume once a day. Suitable for people with Liver-Kidney *yin* deficiency.

Acupuncture and Related Therapies

As a specific treatment in CM, acupuncture therapy has been documented since at least the era of the *Huang Di Nei Jing* 黄帝内经. Acupuncture and related therapies, including body acupuncture, scalp acupuncture, electro-acupuncture, auricular acupuncture, and moxibustion have been commonly used to treat VaD and may help to alleviate some associated symptoms, such as physical disabilities and cognitive impairment. These are summarized in Table 2.2.

Other Management Strategies

Besides the use of Chinese herbal medicine and acupuncture therapies, other forms of physical and mental exercise, such as *tai chi* (*tai ji* 太极), 'eight pieces of brocade' (*ba duan jin* 八段锦), 'five-animal exercises' (*wu qin xi* 五禽戏), *qi gong* (气功), exercises for maintaining health (*dao yin yang sheng gong* 导引养生功), and Chinese massage therapies (*tui na* 推拿, *an mo* 按摩) are all important aspects of the management of VaD.[3,19] Patients can choose suitable

Table 2.2. Summary Table of Acupuncture and Related Therapies for Vascular Dementia

Intervention	Acupuncture Points/Body Area	Treatment Frequency
Body acupuncture[16]	**Main acupoints:** GV20 *Baihui* 百会, GV24 *Shenting* 神庭, GB20 *Fengchi* 风池, GV17 *Naohu* 脑户, HT7 *Shenmen* 神门, LU7 *Lieque* 列缺, ST40 *Fenglong* 丰隆, BL23 *Shenshu* 肾俞, KI4 *Dazhong* 大钟, ST36 *Zusanli* 足三里, SP6 *Sanyinjiao* 三阴交, HT5 *Tongli* 通里, LR3 *Taichong* 太冲, and KI3 *Taixi* 太溪.	Treatment is applied once a day, with 15 days as one treatment course.
Electro-acupuncture[1,2,16]	**Main acupoints:** 1. GV20 *Baihui* 百会, BL23 *Shenshu* 肾俞, and BL17 *Geshu* 膈俞;[1,2] 2. EX-HN1 *Sishencong* 四神聪, GV20 *Baihui* 百会, GB13 *Benshen* 本神 (bilateral), and GB20 *Fengchi* 风池 (bilateral).[16]	Treatment is applied for 20 minutes once per day, with 10 days as one treatment course.
Scalp acupuncture[1,2,16]	**Main acupoints:** MS5 *Dingzhongxian* 顶中线, MS1 *Ezhongxian* 额中线, MS2 *Epangxian 1* 额旁1线, MS3 *Epangxian 2* 额旁2线, MS4 *Epangxian 3* 额旁3线, MS10 *Nieqianxian* 颞前线, and MS11 *Niehouxian* 颞后线.	Treatment is applied for 30 minutes once per day, five times per week, with eight weeks as one treatment course.
Auricular acupuncture[17]	**Main acupoints:** TF4 *Shenmen* 神门, AT4 *Pizhixia* 皮质下 (subcortex), AT3 *Zhen* 枕 (occiput), CO15 *Xin* 心 (Heart), CO12 *Gan* 肝 (Liver), CO13 *Pi* 脾 (Spleen), and CO10 *Shen* 肾 (Kidney).	Treatment is applied for 15–20 minutes using 2–4 acupoints at a time, once a day or every other day, with 10–15 days as one treatment course.
Jin's three-needle therapy[2,17]	**Main combinations:** 1. *Sishenzhen* 四神针 (four points, 1.5 cun anterior, posterior and bilateral to GV20 *Baihui* 百会);	Treatment is applied once a day. There is no specific treatment course.

(*Continued*)

Table 2.2 (*Continued*)

Intervention	Acupuncture Points/Body Area	Treatment Frequency
	2. *Zhisanzhen* 智三针 ([GV24 *Shenting* 神庭, and GB13 *Benshen* 本神 (bilateral)].	
Moxibustion[18]	**Main acupoints:** HT3 *Shaohai* 少海, GV20 *Baihui* 百会, and ST36 *Zusanli* 足三里.	Treatment applied for 10–15 minutes once per day. There is no specific treatment course.

exercises or therapies according to their specific circumstances and preferences. Cognitive training is also important for VaD. Patients with mild VaD can read, sing, play chess, or partake in other mentally stimulating activities to improve cognition.[16]

Prevention and Nursing in Chinese Medicine

Due to the close relationship between VaD and cerebrovascular disease, CM nursing for VaD focuses strongly on rehabilitation in patients with physical disability, improving cognition, and prevention of a secondary stroke.

Nursing and Rehabilitation

Patients with VaD are recommended to remain emotionally stabile, lead a regular life, and get neurological rehabilitation treatments as soon as possible. Neurological rehabilitation treatments include not only physical therapy and language and cognitive training but also acupuncture, massage, Chinese herbal baths, and other CM therapies.[2] People with severe VaD should remain under the constant supervision of a reliable caregiver, as there is high chance that they may wander off, become lost, and meet with serious mishaps if left unsupervised. Furthermore, people who are bedridden with severe VaD should be given comprehensive care to prevent bedsores, infectious diseases, and other complications.[2,17]

Diet Therapy

Patients with VaD are recommended to follow a diet that is high in protein, vitamins, and fibre, and low in cholesterol, fat, glucose, and salt.[16] The diet should also include considerable amounts of fresh vegetables and fruits.[16] Alcohol and tobacco should be avoided.[16] In addition, some foods are said to benefit cognition and intelligence, such as glutinous rice (*nuo mi* 糯米), walnuts (*he tao ren* 核桃仁), longan fruit (*gui yuan rou* 桂圆肉), jujube (*da zao* 大枣), lily-bulbs (*bai he* 百合), yams (*huai shan yao* 淮山药), sesame seeds (*zhi ma* 芝麻), black beans (*hei dou* 黑豆), and black fungus (*hei mu er* 黑木耳). These may be consumed separately or added to decoctions.[20]

Prognosis

Vascular dementia is a chronic disease with step-wise or progressive declines in cognitive function. Good control of vascular risk factors and cardiovascular disease may reduce damage to the Brain, improve outcomes and prevent further decline.[21] Most patients with VaD die of acute cerebrovascular accidents or serious complications from their condition.[21]

References

1. 中华中医药学会. (2008) 中医内科常见病诊疗指南 西医疾病部分. 中国中医药出版社， 北京.
2. 王永炎, 张伯礼. (2003) 血管性痴呆现代中医临床与研究. 人民卫生出版社， 北京.
3. 周文泉, 李祥国. (2000) 实用中医老年病学. 人民卫生出版社， 北京.
4. 吴勉华， 王新月. (2012) 中医内科学. 全国高等中医药院校规划教材 (第九版). 中国中医药出版社, 北京.
5. 郭海英. (2005) 血管性痴呆中医治疗原则探讨. 南京中医药大学学报. **21**(4): 221–222.
6. 谢颖桢, 邹忆怀, 张云岭, 王永炎 (指导), 张伯礼 (指导). (2000) 血管性痴呆病因病机探讨. 北京中医药大学学报. **23**(6):1–3.
7. 王永炎. (1997) 关于提高脑血管疾病疗效难点的思考. 中国中西医结合杂志. **17**(4):195–196.

8. 杨辰华, 王永炎, 王新志. (2006) 血管性痴呆的证候要素与玄府病机. 北京中医药大学学报. **29**(10):665–667.
9. 韦云, 周文泉, 郭明冬. (2010) 络病理论与血管性痴呆相关性探讨. 中医杂志. **51**(7):584–585.
10. 冀宏, 黄启福. (2000) 中医对血管性痴呆的研究进展 (综述). 北京中医药大学学报. **23**(S1):80–83.
11. 朱世瑞, 马云枝. (2015) 从“毒损脑络”探讨血管性痴呆的机理. 河南中医. **35**(4):738–740.
12. 田金洲, 韩明向, 涂晋文, 杨承芝, *et al.* (2000) 血管性痴呆的诊断、辨证及疗效评定标准. 北京中医药大学学报. **23**(5):16–24.
13. 田金洲. (2012) 中国痴呆诊疗指南. 人民卫生出版社, 北京.
14. 周庚生, 胡纪明. (1985) 中西医临床精神病学. 中国中医药出版社, 北京.
15. 杨青选. (1994) 抗衰老食疗方. 中国医药科技出版社, 北京.
16. 中国中医科学院. (2011) 中医循证临床实践指南 中医内科. 中国中医药出版社, 北京.
17. 李建生. (2008) 临床中医老年病学. 人民卫生出版社, 北京.
18. 中华中医药学会. (2008) 中医内科常见病诊疗指南 中医疾病部分. 中国中医药出版社.
19. 中国记忆门诊指南专家编写组. (2014) 中国记忆门诊指南: 阿尔茨海默病全面纵向治疗计划. http://www.elseviermed.cn/news/detail/China_Memory_Clinic_Guide [accessed June 2016].
20. 刘文军, 刘月芝. (1999) 血管病中医食疗验方. 辽宁科学技术出版社, 沈阳.
21. 田金洲、 李曰庆. (2002) 中医老年病学. 上海科学技术出版社, 上海.

3

Classical Chinese Medicine Literature

OVERVIEW

The classical Chinese medicine literature is a valuable source of information on the signs and symptoms associated with post-stroke dementia and memory impairment and provides descriptions of the management of these disorders using Chinese herbal medicine, acupuncture, moxibustion, and other therapies. This chapter reports the results of a search of *Zhong Hua Yi Dian* 中华医典, one of the largest collections of classical Chinese medicine texts. A total of 2,207 citations were identified from a search of more than 50 dementia and memory impairment-related terms, of which 126 were identified as also relevant to stroke, paralysis, and/or hemiplegia. Of these, 92 reported the use of herbal formulae and 34 reported the use of acupuncture points for the treatment of memory impairment as well as stroke, paralysis, and/or hemiplegia.

Introduction

Disorders characterised by memory impairment appear in the *Huang Di Nei Jing Su Wen* 黄帝内经素问 (ca. first century BCE), which uses the terms *shan wang* 善忘 and *xi wang* 喜忘 to refer to the symptom 'frequent forgetting'. However, it can be difficult to determine the aetiology of these disorders since memory impairment may be indicative of dementia due to Alzheimer's disease, cerebrovascular disease, other types of dementia, a result of head injury, or psychiatric disturbance.[1] Nevertheless, when a classical text mentions other symptoms, it may be possible to infer the likely disorder from a modern perspective.

The modern Chinese medicine (CM) term for vascular dementia (VaD), *xue guan xing chi dai* 血管性痴呆, does not appear in the classical literature, but *chi dai* 痴呆 and related terms do appear and various terms referring to memory impairment are relatively frequent.[2] In addition, the term *zhong feng* 中风 'wind stroke', which is used in modern CM to refer to a stroke or cerebrovascular accident (CVA), appears multiple times in the *Huang Di Nei Jing* 黄帝内经 and is common throughout the classical literature. *Zhong feng* 中风 could be used to refer to a broad category of disorders characterised by sudden onset and severe manifestations,[3,4] so we cannot assume that all disorders described as *zhong feng* 中风 in the classical literature were instances of a CVA. However, when *zhong feng* 中风 is associated with symptoms of a CVA, such as hemiplegia and paralysis in a medical context, we can infer that a CVA was a likely cause.

Huang Di Nei Jing Su Wen 黄帝内经素问 Chapter 3 (*Sheng qi tong tian lun* 生气通天论) contains a description of a disorder that is consistent with a sudden CVA but does not mention the term *zhong feng* 中风. A passage which discusses normal and abnormal aspects of *yang qi* 阳气 describes a disorder of *yang qi* in a person who gets very angry, which then causes the *xing* 形 and *qi* 气 (i.e., *yin* and *yang*) to lose connection (allowing the *yang qi* to rush upwards), resulting in the Blood going up and accumulating in the upper body and causing the person to lose consciousness. This damage causes flaccidity of the tendons, which then cannot be used, and sweating on one side. Later, the person has hemiplegia. This passage suggests that CVAs were known in ancient China, but the absence of any cognitive symptoms precludes this as an example of VaD.

Huang Di Nei Jing Su Wen 黄帝内经素问 Chapter 42 (*Feng lun* 风论) describes multiple disorders due to wind (*feng* 风). In one passage, hemiplegia is caused by wind entering the internal organs. The same chapter later states that Brain wind occurs when wind enters the *feng fu* 风府 point and goes upwards, but because no symptoms are described, we do not know how the Brain was affected. The same chapter uses the term *zhong feng* 中风 a number of times. In one instance, it relates to a disorder due to alcohol consumption. In other passages in the *Huang Di Nei Jing* 黄帝内经, *zhong feng* 中风 is associated with wind cold 风寒 that is apparently of an external nature (see *Ling Shu Jing* 灵枢经 Chapter 10 *Jing mai* 经脉). Although there are no direct associations between the term *zhong feng* 中风 and CVAs in the *Huang Di Nei Jing* 黄帝内经, each passage is brief and *zhong feng* 中风 appears to refer to disorders with sudden onset, so we cannot rule out CVA as a possibility.

Perhaps the earliest example of a linkage between the symptom of hemiplegia and *zhong feng* 中风 is in the Han dynasty classic *Jin Gui Yao Lue* 金匮要略 (c. 206). Chapter 5, which is on *zhong feng* damaging the tendons (*zhong feng shang jie bing mai zheng bing zhi* 中风历节病脉证并治), includes a description of weakness on one side coupled with tension on the other, deviation of the face and eyes, and difficulty in speaking. These symptoms are consistent with a CVA but there is no mention of cognitive symptoms.

In order to investigate how disorders consistent with VaD were described and treated in the classical and pre-modern medical literature, we searched the *Zhong Hua Yi Dian* (ZHYD) 中华医典 'Encyclopaedia of Traditional Chinese Medicine', which is an electronic collection of more than 1,000 medical books spanning two millennia.[5] This collection is not only the largest available collection of classical and pre-modern CM literature but is also inclusive of much of the content of other large collections.[6,7]

Search Terms

From a clinical viewpoint, the presence of cognitive and/or memory impairment distinguishes VaD from the more general category of stroke and its sequelae. In traditional books, the cognitive impairments resulting from CVAs were likely to have been described as *jian wang* 健忘 'memory loss', *chi dai* 痴呆 'feeble mindedness', or other related terms.[3,4,8] Potential search terms for memory and cognitive impairment were identified by searching dictionaries and nomenclatures of CM terms[3,4,8–10] as well as discussions on the historical usage of terms for dementia in guidelines and clinical manuals.[11–21] Additional terms were identified from trial searches. These terms were in two main groups, namely *jian wang* 健忘 and associated terms and *chi dai* 痴呆 (also written as 癡呆) and associated terms. Terms were divided into subgroups for statistical purposes (Table 3.1).

A second set of terms for symptoms suggestive of a CVA were used to identify conditions possibly related to VaD from within the search results. These include hemiplegia (*ban shen bu sui* 半身不遂,

Table 3.1 Frequency of Citations Identified by the Search Terms

Search Term Group	Terms Included	No. of Hits	No. of Citations*
1: *Jian wang*	健忘	1860	1185
2: *Hao wang*	好忘	55	40
3: *Duo wang*	多忘	388	183
4: *Shan wang*	善忘	727	252
5: *Xi wang*	喜忘	830	309
6: *Bu wang* group	不忘, 不忘记, 不再忘, 止忘, and 不悟忘	590	120
7: Other *wang*	狂忘, 悸忘, 谬忘, 忘前失后, 忘誤, 失忘, 易忘, 忘记事, 迷忘, 错忘, 遗忘, 遇事則忘, 语后便忘, 眩忘, 忆忘, 怒忘, and 思忘	290	67
8: Weak memory group	强忘, 不记憶, 不能记, 不能记憶, 不记事, 失记, 不善记, 近事不记, 随说随忘, 无所记忆, and 记忆减弱	65	44
9. Strengthen memory group	强记, 记忆强, and 记忆自强	97	63
10: *Chi* group	癡/痴,[1] 神痴, 痴狂, 白痴, and 痴证	30	11
11: *Chi dai* group	痴呆 and 呆痴	180	144
12: *Chi bing*	痴病	7	7
13: *Ru chi*	如痴	253	2
14: *Dai bing* group	呆病, 人呆, 形呆, 神呆, and 呆证	269	8
Totals		5,641	2,207**

*After duplicate removal. **Citations may include multiple search terms. 1. Both characters were used for terms in groups 10–13.

pian ku 偏枯, etc.), paralysis or difficulty in moving the limbs (*si zhi bu sui* 四肢不遂, *shou zu bu ren* 手足不仁, etc.), deviation of the face, eye, or mouth (*kou yan wai xie* 口眼歪斜, etc.), difficulty in speaking (*yan yu jian se* 言语謇涩, etc.), and mention of *zhong feng* 中风 or related terms (*du feng* 毒风, etc.).

Procedures for Search, Data Coding, and Data Analysis

Each of the terms for memory and cognitive impairment was entered into the ZHYD search fields. The number of times the term appeared (i.e., 'hits') was calculated by summing the number of hits for the 'headings' and 'text' searches. All search results were downloaded onto spread sheets. Duplicates were identified and removed as were citations in books written after 1949. Codes were allocated for types of citations, book names, and the dynasties in which they were written based on the procedures described previously.[22] A 'citation' was defined as a distinct passage of text referring to one or more of the search terms that included a treatment for the disorder, and/or a definition or description of the aetiology or pathogenesis. When an extended passage referred to multiple treatments, each treatment was considered a separate citation.

To identify references to disorders that could now be considered VaD, we first searched for references to memory impairments and/or dementia. We then filtered these results based on the additional mention of *zhong feng* 中风 and/or observable physical sequelae of CVAs, such as paralysis and hemiplegia, deviation of the face, and the absence of symptoms indicating that the disorder could not have been VaD. Citations of conditions considered unlikely to have been related to VaD include disorders associated with fever (including *shang han* 伤寒, *wen bing* 温病, *yang ming bing* 阳明病, etc.), head injury, disorders of children or young people, and obstetric disorders. Following exclusion of these citations, the remaining citations were coded for references to *zhong feng* 中风, hemiplegia (*pian ku* 偏枯, *ban shen bu sui* 半身不遂, etc.), deviation of the face and/or mouth (*kou yan wai xie* 口眼歪斜, etc.), inability to use the arms and/or legs (*si zhi bu sui* 四肢不遂, etc.), and other descriptions of 'internal wind' or descriptions of other symptoms consistent with VaD.[3,4,8–21] Only citations that provided an intervention using herbal medicine, food, acupuncture, moxibustion, exercise, or therapeutic massage were included in the data analyses. Single herb entries in books on *materia medica* (*ben cao* 本草) that mentioned the search terms are not included in the analyses.

The group of citations that remained after the above exclusions that combined reference to cognitive impairment plus symptoms consistent with a CVA were considered to be 'possible' references to VaD (Figure 3.1). Of the symptoms listed in the classical literature that may have been a consequence of stroke, hemiplegia is perhaps the clearest and least ambiguous term. The term *zhong feng* 中风 can have a range of meanings. Deviation of the face may be due to Bell's palsy, while difficulty in moving may be due to multiple aetiologies, including arthritis. Consequently, the mention of hemiplegia, in addition to memory or cognitive impairment, as a symptom treated by the intervention was selected to further limit the data set and identify a subgroup of citations that were classified as more 'likely' to have referred to VaD. Using this procedure, it was possible to identify examples of conditions that could have been post-stroke VaD, but it was not possible to identify instances of small-vessel disease, VaD in

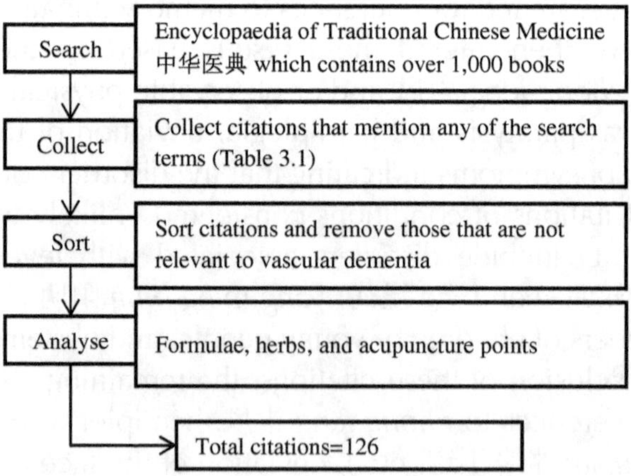

Figure 3.1 Search and Selection of Classical Literature Citations

which physical and/or mental symptoms were not remarkable, or VaD without memory impairment.

Search Results

The search terms identified 5,641 potential references. After removal of duplicates and citations not associated with an intervention for the search terms, 2,207 citations relating to the use of CM interventions for memory impairment or dementia remained. Some citations included multiple terms. The most productive search terms were *jian wang* 健忘 (1,185 citations) followed by *xi wang* 喜忘 (309 citations) and *shan wang* 善忘 (252 citations). Terms related to *chi dai* 痴呆 were less frequent with 144 potentially relevant citations of *chi dai* 痴呆 or *dai chi* 呆痴. The terms *bai chi* 白痴, *dai zheng* 呆证, and *chi zheng* 痴证 did not locate any relevant citations (Table 3.1).

After removing citations not relevant to dementia or VaD and only including citations in which there was a term or description associated with possible VaD, the remaining data set included 126 citations (Figure 3.1).

Definitions of the Condition and Aetiology

The modern conception of VaD has no direct counterpart in classical literature. The citations in this chapter mainly fall into the category of wind disorders (*feng men* 风门) or *zhong feng* 中风, with a few being listed under memory impairment (*jian wang* 健忘), dampness (*shi men* 湿门), and chronic debility (*xu lao* 虚劳). Essentially, this disorder is a subtype of *zhong feng* 中风 in which there are physicial signs and symptoms along with cognitive impairment. As VaD does not receive separate discussions of its aetiology and syndrome differentiation, we must rely upon the descriptions available in the citations.

In Chapter 5 of the *Jin Gui Yao Lue* 金匮要略 (c. 206), a section on *zhong feng* 中风 with hemiplegia describes the disorder as being due to cold, and emptiness. Blood emptiness and emptiness of the Collaterals (*luo mai* 络脉) allow pathogenic factors (wind, cold) to enter and not be expelled, thereby causing the various manifestations of *zhong feng* 中风, which can include hemiplegia and difficulty in speaking.

The earliest identified citations of Chinese herbal medicine (CHM) treatments for possible VaD are from *Bei Ji Qian Jin Yao Fang* 备急千金要方 (c. 652). The text for the formula *Da ba feng tang* 大八风汤 specifies that it is for treating toxic wind (*du feng* 毒风) and stubborn *bi* (*wan bi* 顽痹) with symptoms of paralysis and hemiplegia, and for wind entering the five *zang* 脏 organs with cognitive symptoms including memory impairment (*shan wang* 善忘). The citation for the formula *Pai feng tang* 排风汤 is more detailed. It states that the formula is for wind, emptiness, dampness, and cold (*feng xu shi leng* 风虚湿冷), and for pathogenic *qi* entering the *zang* 脏 organs. It then provides lists of signs and symptoms, including hemiplegia (*pian ku* 偏枯) which is a symptom of Liver wind, and frequent forgetting (*duo wang* 多忘). In the *Qian Jin Yi Fang* 千金翼方 (c. 682), the chapter on *zhong feng* 中风 includes the medicinal wine *Huang qi jiu* 黄芪酒. It is described as mainly for severe wind, emptiness, and cold with various symptoms, including hemiplegia (*pian ku* 偏枯), and can be used for memory loss (*duo wang* 多忘) when the herbs *chang pu* 菖蒲 and *zi shi ying* 紫石英 are added.

The *Wei Sheng Bao Jian* 卫生宝鉴 (c. 1343) citation for *Qiang huo yu feng tang* 羌活愈风汤 stated that this formula was for treating emptiness of Kidney and Liver (*shen gan xu* 肾肝虚), *zhong feng* 中风 with dampness and heat entering a weak person; and various symptoms including hemiplegia and forgetfulness (*jian wang* 健忘).

In most of the citations, the formulae are simply for pathogenic wind, *zhong feng* 中风, or specific symptoms. In the more detailed citations, the descriptions tend to reflect the *Jin Gui Yao Lue* 金匮要略 (c. 206) passage above and mention the concept of emptiness within the body that allows the penetration of pathogenic wind into the body. The pathogen may also affect one or more of the *zang* 脏 organs. In some cases, other pathogens including cold, dampness, phlegm, and heat are mentioned and some of the physical aspects of the disorder are described, such as hemiplegia and *bi* 痹.

Chinese Herbal Medicine

After the removal of duplicates, citations in books written after 1949, citations not associated with a Chinese herbal formula, and citations unlikely to refer to VaD, there were 92 citations of 'possible' references to VaD. Of these, 32 citations clearly specified hemiplegia as a symptom and were identified as 'likely' VaD.

Frequency of Treatment Citations by Dynasty

The 92 citations of formulae for 'possible' VaD are derived from 48 different books written from c. 652 to 1934 AD. More than half (53.3%) of the citations ($n = 49$) were from books written in the Ming dynasty and 14.1% were from books written during the Qing dynasty (Table 3.2). The most productive book, with 23 formulae citations, was the Ming dynasty work *Pu Ji Fang* 普济方 (c. 1406), which is the largest book in ZHYD and the largest of the classical CM encyclopaedia. The next most productive source book, with four citations, was *Zheng Zhi Zhun Sheng* 证治准绳 (c. 1604) which is a multi-volume work written by Wang Ken-Tang 王肯堂. Four other books provided three citations each, the earliest being from the Tang dynasty

Table 3.2 Citations of Chinese Herbal Formulae by Dynasty

Historical Period — Dynasty	'Possible' VaD — No. of Citations (%)	'Likely VaD' — No. of Citations (%)
Before Tang Dynasty (–617)	0 (0)	0 (0)
Tang and 5 Dynasties (618–959)	7 (7.6)	6 (18.8)
Song and Jin Dynasties (960–1271)	12 (13)	2 (6.3)
Yuan Dynasty (1272–1368)	8 (8.7)	6 (18.8)
Ming Dynasty (1369–1644)	49 (53.3)	16 (50)
Qing Dynasty (1645–1911)	13 (14.1)	0 (0)
Minguo period (1912–1949)	3 (3.3)	2 (6.3)
Total	**92 (100)**	**32 (100)**

Abbreviation: VaD, vascular dementia.

work, *Bei Ji Qian Jin Yao Fang* 备急千金要方 (c. 652), by Sun Si Miao 孙思邈.

The 32 citations that remained after hemiplegia was added as a criterion were from 19 different books written between c. 652 to 1934 AD, with 50% of the books having been written in the Ming dynasty (Table 3.2). Again, *Pu Ji Fang* 普济方 (c. 1406) provided the most citations ($n = 7$), followed by *Bei Ji Qian Jin Yao Fang* 备急千金要方 (c. 652) ($n = 3$).

Treatment with Chinese Herbal Medicine

Citations that included interventions using Chinese herbal formulae were identified and categorised into those that were considered 'possible' VaD, since they were used to treat memory impairment, *zhong feng* 中风, and symptoms of hemiplegia or paralysis, and there were no reasons to exclude the citation as unlikely to have been VaD. The subset of these citations that also specified the formula that was used to treat hemiplegia was considered to be likely to have referred to VaD, since this symptom is a common result of a CVA and was relatively frequently mentioned in the citations. This group was classified as 'likely' VaD.

Most Frequent Formulae in 'Possible' Vascular Dementia Citations

In the 92 citations for 'possible' VaD, there were eight un-named formulae and 50 named formulae. The most frequently cited formula was *Qiang huo yu feng tang* 羌活愈风汤 ($n = 7$). Its earliest citation was in the *Wei Sheng Bao Jian* 卫生宝鉴 (c. 1343) chapter on *zhong feng* 中风. Four formulae were cited four times each. Two of these were from the earliest book, *Bei Ji Qian Jin Yao Fang* 备急千金要方 (c. 652). One of these, *Da ba feng tang* 大八风汤, also appeared in *Wai Tai Mi Yao* 外台秘要 under the modified name *Shen shi da ba feng tang* 深師大八风汤. As this formula had the same ingredients, this citation was scored as *Da ba feng tang* 大八风汤. The formula ingredients that appear in Table 3.3 are based on the earliest book in each group of citations.

Table 3.3 Most Frequent Herbal Formulae for 'Possible' Vascular Dementia

Formula Name	Ingredients*	No. of Citations
Qiang huo yu feng tang 羌活愈风汤	*Qiang huo* 羌活, *gan cao* 甘草, *fang feng* 防风, *fang ji* 防己, *huang qi* 黄芪, *man jing zi* 蔓荆子, *chuan xiong* 川芎, *du huo* 独活, *xi xin* 细辛, *zhi ke* 枳壳, *ma huang* 麻黄, *di gu pi* 地骨皮, *ren shen* 人参, *zhi mu* 知母, *gan ju* 甘菊, *bo he* 薄荷, *bai zhi* 白芷, *gou qi zi* 枸杞子, *dang gui* 当归, *du zhong* 杜仲, *qin jiao* 秦艽, *chai hu* 柴胡, *ban xia* 半夏, *hou po* 厚朴, *qian hu* 前胡, *shu di huang* 熟地黄, *bai fu ling* 白茯苓, *huang qin* 黄芩, *sheng di huang* 生地黄, *cang zhu* 苍术, *shi gao* 石膏, *shao yao* 芍药, and *gui zhi* 桂枝. (*Wei Sheng Bao Jian* 卫生宝鉴 c. 1343)	7
Pai feng tang 排风汤	*Bai xian pi* 白藓皮, *bai zhu* 白术, *shao yao* 芍药, *gui xin* 桂心, *chuan xiong* 川芎, *dang gui* 当归, *xing ren* 杏仁, *fang feng* 防风, *gan cao* 甘草, *du huo* 独活, *ma huang* 麻黄, *fu ling* 茯苓, and *sheng jiang* 生姜. (*Bei Ji Qian Jin Yao Fang* 备急千金要方 c. 652)	4
Song jie san 松节散	*Xin mu* 心木, *ru xiang* 乳香, and *mu gua* 木瓜. (*Ben Cao Bei Yao* 本草备要 c. 1694) Note: *Xin mu* 心木 is also called *fu ling xin mu* 茯神心木 or *huang song jie* 黄松节.	4
Da ba feng tang 大八风汤	*Dang gui* 当归, *wu wei zi* 五味子, *sheng ma* 升麻, *wu tou* 乌头, *huang qin* 黄芩, *shao yao* 芍药, *yuan zhi* 远志, *du huo* 独活, *fang feng* 防风, *chuan xiong* 川芎, *ma huang* 麻黄, *qin jiao* 秦艽, *shi hu* 石斛, *ren shen* 人参, *fu ling* 茯苓, *xing ren* 杏仁, *huang qi* 黄芪, *zi wan* 紫菀, *shi gao* 石膏, *gan cao* 甘草, *gui xin* 桂心, *gan jiang* 干姜, and *da dou* 大豆. (*Bei Ji Qian Jin Yao Fang* 备急千金要方 *c. 652*, also called *Shen shi da ba feng tang* 深師大八风汤 in *Wai Tai Mi Yao* 外台秘要 c. 752)	4
Niu huang qing xin wan 牛黄清心丸	*Fang feng* 防风, *bai zhu* 白术, *bai shao* 白芍, *shan yang jiao* 山羊角, *she xiang* 麝香, *long nao* 龙脑, *mai men dong* 麦门冬, *huang qin* 黄芩, *ren shen* 人参, *shen qu* 神曲, *pu huang* 蒲黄, *gan cao* 甘草, *bai fu ling* 白茯苓, *chuan xiong* 川芎, *xing ren* 杏仁, *chai hu* 柴胡, *jie geng* 桔梗, *xiong huang* 雄黄, *niu huang* 牛黄, *shan yao* 山药, *bai lian* 白蔹, *gan jiang* 干姜, *dang gui* 当归,	4

(*Continued*)

Table 3.3 (*Continued*)

Formula Name	Ingredients*	No. of Citations
	da dou huang juan 大豆黄卷, *e jiao* 阿膠, *rou gui* 肉桂, *shui niu jiao* 水牛角, *da zao* 大棗, and *jin bo* 金箔. (*Wan Shang Ji Yao* 疠疡机要 c. 1529)	
Da ding xin tang 大定心汤	*Ren shen* 人参, *bai fu ling* 白茯苓, *fu shen* 茯神, *yuan zhi* 远志, *long gu* 龙骨, *gan jiang* 干姜, *dang gui* 当归, *gan cao* 甘草, *bai zhu* 白术, *shao yao* 芍药, *gui* 桂, *zi wan* 紫菀, *fang feng* 防风, and *chi shi zhi* 赤石脂. (*Sheng Ji Zong Lu* 圣济总录 c. 1117)	3
Ling bao dan 灵宝丹	*Liu huang* 硫黄, *zi ran tong* 自然銅, *xiong huang* 雄黄, *guang ming sha* 光明砂, *ci shi* 磁石, *zi shi ying* 紫石英, *yang qi shi* 阳起石, *chang li shi* 长理石, *wen nai qi* 膃肭脐, *long chi* 龙齿, *long nao* 龙脑, *she xiang* 麝香, *niu huang* 牛黄, *zhong ru* 钟乳, *tian ma* 天麻, *yuan zhi* 远志, *xian ling pi* 仙灵脾, *ba ji* 巴戟, *wu she* 乌蛇, *ku shen* 苦参, *rou gui* 肉桂, *lu rong* 鹿茸, *mu xiang* 木香, *rou dou kou* 肉豆蔻, *yan hu suo* 延胡索, *hu tong lu* 胡桐律, *ban xia* 半夏, *dang gui* 当归, *sheng di huang zhi* 生地黄汁, *tong zi xiao bian* 童子小便, *wu hui jiu* 无灰酒, and *zao jia ren* 皂荚仁. (*Tai Ping Hui Min He Ji Ju Fang* 太平惠民和剂局方 c. 1107)	3
Run ti wan 润体丸	*Fang feng* 防风, *bai long nao* 白龙脑, *ru xiang* 乳香, *shan yang jiao* 山羊角, *fu zi* 附子, *bai jiang can* 白僵蚕, *bing lang* 檳榔, *rou dou kou ren* 肉豆蔻仁, *chen xiang* 沉香, *ji li zi* 蒺藜子, *ding xiang* 丁香, *man jing zi* 蔓荊子, *niu huang* 牛黄, *huo xiang ye* 藿香叶, *ma huang* 麻黄, *shui niu jiao* 水牛角, *xiong huang* 雄黄, *she xiang* 麝香, *mu xiang* 木香, *chen sha* 辰砂, *fu ling* 茯苓, *bai fu zi* 白附子, *qiang huo* 羌活, *yuan can e* 原蚕蛾, *ren shen* 人参, *rou gui* 肉桂, *chuan xiong* 川芎, *zhen zhu* 真珠末, *du huo* 独活, *gan xie* 干蝎, *ban xia* 半夏, *chuan wu tou* 川乌头, *bai hua she* 白花蛇, *tian ma* 天麻, *hu po* 琥珀, *ni fen* 腻粉, *bai dou kou ren* 白豆蔻仁, and *jin bo* 金箔. (*Tai Ping Hui Min He Ji Ju Fang* 太平惠民和剂局方 c. 1107)	3

Table 3.3 (*Continued*)

Formula Name	Ingredients*	No. of Citations
Jia jian gu ben wan 加減固本丸	*Dan shen* 丹参, *tian men dong* 天门冬, *shu di* 熟地, *ren shen* 人参, *yuan zhi* 远志, *zhu sha* 朱砂, *shi chang pu* 石菖蒲, mai men dong 麦门冬, bai fu ling 白茯苓. (*Yi Xue Ru Men* 医学入门 c. 1575 and *Za Bing Yuan Liu Xi Zhu* 杂病源流犀烛 c. 1773)	3

Notes: *Formulae ingredients are based on the earliest book within the group of included citations; 1. Formulae with the same name can vary in their ingredients and the same combination of ingredients may have different names. In this data, formulae with the same name that have variations in a few ingredients are grouped together, while those with large variations in ingredients are separated. Also, formulae with the same ingredients but different names have been grouped together; 2. The use of some herbs/ingredients is restricted in some countries. Readers are advised to comply with relevant regulations.

Most Frequent Herbs in 'Possible' Vascular Dementia Citations

The 92 formulae for 'possible' VaD contained 1,593 ingredients which included around 200 different herbs. The herbs mostly commonly included in the formulae were tonic herbs, namely *fu ling* 茯苓 or *fu shen* 茯神 ($n = 60$), *gan cao* 甘草 ($n = 49$), *ren shen* 人參 ($n = 48$), *dang gui* 当归 ($n = 44$), *di huang* 地黄 ($n = 36$), *bai shao* 白芍 ($n = 33$), and *huang qi* 黄芪 ($n = 25$). Herbs for expelling wind included *fang feng* 防风 ($n = 44$), *du huo* 独活 ($n = 30$), *ma huang* 麻黄 ($n = 28$), *qin jiao* 秦艽 ($n = 18$), and *qiang huo* 羌活 ($n = 15$). Warming herbs that can be used for paralysis included *wu tou* 乌头 and *fu zi* 附子 ($n = 40$), *rou gui* 肉桂 ($n = 40$), and *gan jiang* 干姜 ($n = 17$) (Table 3.4). The herbs typically used for memory disorders that appeared in the list of most frequent herbs were *fu ling/fu shen* 茯苓/茯神 and *yuan zhi* 远志 ($n = 30$), while *chang pu* 菖蒲 was less frequent ($n = 15$). Some herbs that are used for hypertension appeared at medium frequencies including *tian ma* 天麻 ($n = 18$), *du zhong* 杜仲 ($n = 15$), *man jing zi* 蔓荆子 ($n = 14$), and *niu xi* 牛膝 ($n = 13$).

Table 3.4 Herbs Used in Formulae for 'Possible' Vascular Dementia

Herb Name	Scientific Name	Frequency of Use
Fu ling/shen 茯苓/神	*Poria cocos* (Schw.) Wolf	60 (*fu shen* 11)
Gan cao 甘草	*Glycyrrhiza uralensis* Fisch.	49
Ren shen 人参	*Panax ginseng* C.A. Mey.	48
Dang gui 当归	*Angelica sinensis* (Oliv.) Diels	44
Gui 桂 (rou gui 肉桂)	*Cinnamomum cassia* Presl	44 (*rou gui* 40)
Fang feng 防风	*Saposhnikovia divaricata* (Turcz.) Schischk.	44
Fu zi 附子/wu tou 乌头	*Aconitum* spp.	40 (*wu tou* 23)
Chuan xiong 川芎	*Ligusticum wallichii* Franch.	38
Di huang 地黄 (shu di 熟地, *sheng di* 生地)	*Rehmannia glutinosa* (Gaertn.) Libosch.	36 (*shu di* 19, *sheng di* 16)
Bai shao 白芍	*Paeonia lactiflora* Pall.	33
Yuan zhi 远志	*Polygala tenuifolia* Willd.	30
Du huo 独活	*Angelica pubescens* Maxim. *f. biserrata* Shan et Yuan	30
Ma huang 麻黄	*Ephedra sinica* Stapf	28
Huang qi 黄芪	*Astragalus membranaceus* (Fisch.) Bge. var. *mongholicus* (Bge.) Hsiao	25
Zhu sha 朱砂/*dan sha* 丹砂	Cinnabar	24
Ban xia (zhi) 半夏 (制)	*Pinellia ternata* (Thunb.) Breit.	22
Huang qin 黄芩	*Scutellaria baicalensis* Georgi	22
Chai hu 柴胡	*Bupleurum chinense* DC.	20
Bai zhu 白术	*Atractylodes macrocephala* Koidz.	20
Tian ma 天麻	*Gastrodia elata* Bl.	18
Qin jiao 秦艽	*Gentiana macrophylla* Pall., *G. crassicaulis* Duthie ex Burkill, *G. straminea* Maxim.	18

Notes: 1. The herbs *wu tou* 乌头, *fu zi* 附子, *zhu sha* 朱砂, and *dan sha* 丹砂 can be toxic. 2. The use of some herbs may be restricted in some countries. Readers are advised to comply with relevant regulations.

Most Frequent Formulae in 'Likely' Vascular Dementia Citations

When the 32 citations for 'likely' VaD that specifically mentioned hemiplegia in addition to memory impairment were considered as a subgroup, the most frequent formulae were similar to those in the more general 'possible' VaD group. *Qiang huo yu feng tang* 羌活愈风汤 (*n* = 6) remained the most frequent formula followed by *Da ba feng tang* 大八风汤 (*n* = 4) and *Pai feng tang* 排风汤 (*n* = 3). An additional 13 formulae were mentioned once or twice. Of these, *Ling bao dan* 灵宝丹 was listed in Table 3.3 and five additional formulae are listed in Table 3.5.

Most Frequent Herbs in 'Likely' Vascular Dementia Citations

The 32 citations of formulae for 'likely' VaD contained 690 ingredients derived from about 110 different herbs. The overall list was similar to Table 3.4 but herbs for expelling wind were more prominent, including *fang feng* 防风 (*n* = 25), *du huo* 独活 (*n* = 24), *ma huang* 麻黄 (*n* = 19), *qin jiao* 秦艽 (*n* = 18), *bai zhi* 白芷 (*n* = 13), and *qiang huo* 羌活 (*n* = 11) (Table 3.6). The tonic herbs and warming herbs were similar to Table 3.4 and the herbs for memory *fu ling/fu shen* 茯苓/茯神 (*n* = 18) and *yuan zhi* 远志 (*n* = 11) were lower on the list (Table 3.6).

Discussion of Chinese Herbal Medicine for Vascular Dementia

As the list of frequent formulae and herbs overlapped considerably between the group of 'possible' VaD and 'likely' VaD citations, restricting the data set to the formulae used for hemiplegia did not fundamentally change the nature of the Chinese herbal treatments included. When the herb frequencies were compared, the main difference was an increase in the relative importance of herbs for dispelling wind in the 'likely' VaD group (Tables 3.4 and 3.6).

Table 3.5 Most Frequent Formulae for 'Likely' Vascular Dementia

Formula Name	Ingredients*	No. of Citations
Qiang huo yu feng tang 羌活愈风汤	See Table 3.3	6
Da ba feng tang 大八风汤	See Table 3.3	4
Pai feng tang 排风汤	See Table 3.3	3
Ling bao dan 灵宝丹	See Table 3.3	2
Huang qi jiu (jia wei) 黄芪酒(加味)	*Huang qi* 黄芪, *du huo* 独活, *shan zhu yu* 山茱萸, *gui xin* 桂心, *shu jiao* 蜀椒, *bai zhu* 白术, *niu xi* 牛膝, *ge gen* 葛根, *fang feng* 防风, *chuan xiong* 川芎, *xi xin* 细辛, *fu zi* 附子, *gan cao* 甘草, *da huang* 大黄, *gan jiang* 干姜, *qin jiao* 秦艽, *dang gui* 当归, and *wu tou* 烏头, add *chang pu* 菖蒲 and *zi shi ying* 紫石英 for *duo wang* 多忘. (*Qian Jin Yi Fang* 千金翼方 c. 682)	2
Fu shen tang fang 茯神汤方	*Fu shen* 茯神, *fang feng* 防风, *niu xi* 牛膝, *zhi ke* 枳壳, *fang ji* 防己, *qin jiao* 秦艽, *xuan shen* 玄参, *shao yao* 芍药, *huang qi* 黄芪, *bai xian pi* 白藓皮, *ze xie* 泽泻, *du huo* 独活, *gui* 桂, *wu wei zi* 五味子, *ren shen* 人参, *yi yi ren* 薏苡仁, *mai men dong* 麦门冬, *shan yang jiao* 山羊角, *shi gao* 石膏, *gan cao* 甘草, and *ci shi* 磁石. (*Sheng Ji Zong Lu* 圣济总录 c. 1117)	2
Yu feng tang 愈风汤	*Qiang huo* 羌活, *gan cao* 甘草, *fang feng* 防风, *man jing zi* 蔓荆子, *chuan xiong* 川芎, *xi xin* 细辛, *zhi ke* 枳壳, *ren shen* 人参, *ma huang* 麻黄, *gan ju* 甘菊, *bo he* 薄荷, *gou qi zi* 枸杞子, *dang gui* 当归, *zhi mu* 知母, *di gu pi* 地骨皮, *huang qi* 黄芪, *du huo* 独活, *du zhong* 杜仲, *wu bai zhi* 吴白芷, *qin jiao* 秦艽, *chai hu* 柴胡, *ban xia* 半夏, *qian hu* 前胡,	2

Table 3.5 (*Continued*)

Formula Name	Ingredients*	No. of Citations
	hou po 厚朴, *shu di huang* 熟地黄, *fang ji* 防己, *fu ling* 茯苓, *huang qin* 黄芩, *shi gao* 石膏, *shao yao* 芍药, *sheng di huang* 生地黄, *cang zhu* 苍术, and *gui zhi* 桂枝 (another version of 愈风汤 uses gui 桂). (*Su Wen Bing Ji Qi Yi Bao Ming Ji* 素问病机气宜保命集 c. 1186)	
Bi feng dan 辟风丹	*Du huo* 独活, *fang feng* 防风, *wu bai zhi* 吴白芷, *gui* 桂, *gao ben* 蒿本, *ma huang* 麻黄, *bai shao yao* 白芍药, *tian ma* 天麻, *chuan wu tou* 川烏头, *huo xiang ye* 藿香叶, *chuan xiong* 川芎, *qiang huo* 羌活, *gan cao* 甘草, *bai hua she* 白花蛇, *jiang can* 白僵蚕, *quan xie* 全蝎, *zhu sha* 朱砂, *bai fu zi* 白附子, *tian nan xing* 天南星, and *yuan zhi* 远志. (*Yu Yao Yuan Fang* 御药院方 c. 1267)	2
Wu she wan 乌蛇丸	*Du huo* 独活, *fang feng* 防风, *wu bai zhi* 吴白芷, *ren shen* 人参, *gui xin* 桂心, *gao ben* 蒿本, *ma huang* 麻黄, *shao yao* 芍药, *tian ma* 天麻, *chuan wu tou* 川烏头, *huo xiang ye* 藿香叶, *wu she* 乌蛇, *quan xie* 全蝎, *gan cao* 甘草, *shui niu jiao* 水牛角, *chuan xiong* 川芎, *qiang huo* 羌活, *jiang can* 白僵蚕, *yuan zhi* 远志, *niu huang* 牛黄, *tian nan xing* 天南星, *bai fu zi* 白附子, *long nao* 龙脑, and *zhu sha* 朱砂. (*Yu Yao Yuan Fang* 御药院方 c. 1267)	2

Notes: *Formulae ingredients are based on the earliest book within the group of included citations; 1. Formulae with the same name can vary in their ingredients and the same combination of ingredients may have different names. In this data, formulae with the same name that have variations in a few ingredients are grouped together while those large variations in ingredients are separated. Also, formulae with the same ingredients but different names have been grouped together; 2. The use of some herbs/ingredients may be restricted in some countries. Readers are advised to comply with relevant regulations; 3. *Chuan wu tou* 川烏头 and *zhu sha* 朱砂 can be toxic.

Table 3.6 Herbs Used in Formulae for 'Likely' Vascular Dementia

Herb Name	Scientific Name	Frequency of Use
Fang feng 防风	*Saposhnikovia divaricata* (Turcz.) Schischk.	25
Gui 桂 (rou gui 肉桂)	*Cinnamomum cassia* Presl	25 (*rou gui* 23)
Gan cao 甘草	*Glycyrrhiza uralensis* Fisch.	24
Du huo 独活	*Angelica pubescens* Maxim. *f. biserrata* Shan et Yuan	24
Dang gui 当归	*Angelica sinensis* (Oliv.) Diels	23
Chuan xiong 川芎	*Ligusticum wallichii* Franch.	22
Bai shao 白芍	*Paeonia lactiflora* Pall.	21
Di huang 地黄 (*shu di* 熟地, *sheng di* 生地)	*Rehmannia glutinosa* (Gaertn.) Libosch.	21 (*shu di* 8, *sheng di* 12)
Ma huang 麻黄	*Ephedra sinica* Stapf	19
Ren shen 人参	*Panax ginseng* C.A. Mey.	18
Huang qi 黄芪	*Astragalus membranaceus* (Fisch.) Bge. var. mongholicus (Bge.) Hsiao	18
Fu ling/shen 茯苓/神	*Poria cocos* (Schw.) Wolf	18 (*fu shen* 2)
Qin jiao 秦艽	*Gentiana macrophylla* Pall., *G. crassicaulis* Duthie ex Burkill, *G. straminea* Maxim.	18
Fu zi 附子/*wu tou* 乌头	*Aconitum* spp.	15 (*wu tou* 11)
Huang qin 黄芩	*Scutellaria baicalensis* Georgi	13
Bai zhi 白芷	*Angelica dahurica* (Fisch. ex Hoffm.) Benth. et Hook. f.	13
Shi gao 石膏	*Gypsum fibrosum*	12
Xi xin 细辛	*Asarum sieboldii* Miq.	12
Yuan zhi 远志	*Polygala tenuifolia* Willd.	11
Qiang huo 羌活	*Notopterygium incisum* Ting ex H. T. Chang	11

Notes: 1. The use of some herbs may be restricted in some countries. Readers are advised to comply with relevant regulations; 2. *Wu tou* 乌头 and *Fu zi* 附子 can be toxic.

Formulae from the oldest book, *Bei Ji Qian Jin Yao Fang* 备急千金要方 (c. 652), appeared in Tables 3.3 and 3.5. *Da ba feng tang* 大八风汤 was used to treat toxic wind (*du feng* 毒风) causing paralysis and difficulty in moving the arms, wind entering the five *zang* 脏 organs causing dissociation, talking then forgetting, momentary fearfulness, dizziness, or stiff back and spine causing the person to be unable to bend forward or backward, hemiplegia, and a range of other symptoms. The formula *Pai feng tang* 排风汤 was also used for multiple disorders due to wind, including paralysis, muscle rigidity, inability to walk, dissociation and memory loss, and severe psychological symptoms such as delusions, crazed speech, and confusion. Another formula from Sun Si-Miao was *Huang qi jiu* 黄芪酒 from the *zhong feng* 中风 chapter in *Qian Jin Yi Fang* 千金翼方 (c. 682), which was for disorders due to severe wind, emptiness and/or cold including hemiplegia, weak legs, oedema, and multiple other disorders. It could be modified for memory impairment by adding *chang pu* 菖蒲and *zi shi ying* 紫石英. Each of these three formulae from the Tang dynasty included symptoms consistent with sequelae of CVAs as well as memory loss, so it is likely that these formulae could have been used for VaD as well as for other disorders.

The Song dynasty treatments included the two pills *Ling bao dan* 灵宝丹 and *Run ti wan* 润体丸. These include many ingredients, some of which are no longer used. *Ling bao dan* 灵宝丹 was for *zhong feng* 中风 with paralysis of the limbs and a variety of other symptoms, including difficulty in speaking and memory impairment (*jian wang* 健忘). *Run ti wan* 润体丸 was for wind paralysis and other post-stroke symptoms, such as drooling, difficulty in speaking, deviation of the mouth and eye, numbness, as well as memory impairment. The Ming dynasty pill *Niu huang qing xin wan* 牛黄清心丸 was for a similar list of symptoms.

The most commonly cited formula was *Qiang huo yu feng tang* 羌活愈风汤 (Tables 3.3 and 3.5). The earliest citation is in the *zhong feng* 中风 chapter of *Wei Sheng Bao Jian* 卫生宝鉴 (c. 1343) in which this formula is used for deficiency of Kidney and Liver 肾肝虚, various symptoms due to wind, and a range of symptoms consistent with post-stroke VaD including difficulty speaking, abnormal mental state, hemiplegia, and 'feeling frightened with memory loss'. The same formula appears in *Pu Ji Fang* 普济方 (c. 1406) with similar applications. However, some formulae mention a limited range of symptoms. *Da ding xin tang* 大定心汤 from *Sheng Ji Zong Lu* 圣济总录 (c. 1117) is for Heart empty wind stroke (心虚中风) with fright, dissociation, and memory impairment. *Fu shen tang fang* 茯神汤方 from the same book is for *zhong feng* 中风, inability to use the arms and legs on one side, and memory loss.

Jia jian gu ben wan 加减固本丸 was cited in three books for memory loss after *zhong feng* 中风 and for old people with senile debility. The first appearance with these indications was in the Ming dynasty book, *Yi Xue Ru Men* 医学入门 (c. 1575). The description in this book clearly indicates that the memory loss followed a stroke. These symptoms are consistent with VaD. This formula also has a more general application for *jian wang* 健忘 due to 'loss of connection between the Heart and Kidney' (*xin shen bu jiao bing* 心肾不交病). This formula is also cited during the Qing dynasty in the book *Za Bing Yuan Liu Xi Zhu* 杂病源流犀烛 (c. 1773) for memory loss following stroke (*zhong feng hou shan wang* 中风后善忘).

Song jie san 松节散 from *Ben Cao Bei Yao* 本草备要 (c. 1694) is a simple three-herb formula based around *xin mu* 心木 (also known as *huang song jie* 黄松节), which are the pine root inclusions in *fu shen* 茯神. It is used for symptoms of memory loss, anxiety and panic, frequent anger, and paralysis. This formula is more focused on clearing the mind than on wind symptoms. Although it may have been used for VaD, its applications are broader.

The most recent of the included citations is from the *Yi Xue Zhong Zhong Can Xi Lu* 医学衷中参西录 (1934) chapter on internal and external types of *zhong feng* 内外中風. *Jia wei bu xue tang* 加味补血汤 (*huang qi* 黄芪, *dang gui* 当归, *long yan rou* 龙眼肉, *lu jiao jiao* 鹿角膠, *dan shen* 丹参, *ru xiang* 乳香, *mo yao* 沒药, and *gan song* 甘松) was used for a range of disorders including unclear mind and *jian wang* 健忘, paralysis, hemiplegia, and muscle wasting over the whole body. The author explains that the formula is for internal *zhong feng* 内中风 that tends towards the 'empty cold type 虚寒'

(i.e., not for the type where the Liver effulgent generates wind) and recommends long-term consumption.

The formulae above may have been applicable in people who would now be classified as having VaD. In many cases, symptoms consistent with CVAs were mentioned, but some made more general mentions of impaired limb movement which could have been due to a diversity of causes. Those that clearly mentioned hemiplegia in addition to memory impairment were selected as more likely to have been intended for conditions consistent with post-stroke VaD, but none of the descriptions provided sufficient detail of the temporal relationships between symptoms to establish causal relationships. The closest were descriptions of post-stroke (*zhong feng hou* 中风后) memory impairment. Therefore, it is not possible to make a retrospective diagnosis of the conditions described in the citations with any certainty.

Acupuncture and Related Therapies

After the removal of duplicates, citations in books written after 1949, and citations unlikely to refer to dementia, there were 322 citations in the data set of which 34 were 'possible' references to VaD. When the data were limited to citations that mentioned hemiplegia, 22 citations considered 'likely' VaD remained.

Frequency of Treatment Citations by Dynasty

The 34 citations for 'possible' VaD were derived from 13 different books written from c. 1117 to 1883 AD. Most citations were in books written in the Ming dynasty (55.9 %), followed by the Song and Jin dynasties (23.5%) and the Qing dynasty (20.6 %); no citations were derived from the Tang dynasty or earlier or from the Minguo period (Table 3.7). The citations classified as 'likely' VaD were derived from 11 different books (c. 1117 to 1874 AD).

Almost half of the 34 citations judged as 'possible' references to VaD were derived from three books that provided five citations

Table 3.7 Citations of Acupuncture Points for VaD by Dynasty

Historical Period — Dynasty	'Possible' VaD — No. of Citations (%)	'Likely' VaD — No. of Citations (%)
Before Tang (–618)	0 (0)	0 (0)
Tang and 5 Dynasties (618–959)	0 (0)	0 (0)
Song and Jin (960–1271)	8 (23.5)	4 (18.2)
Yuan (1272–1368)	0 (0)	0 (0)
Ming (1369–1644)	19 (55.9)	15 (68.2)
Qing (1645–1911)	7 (20.6)	3 (13.6)
Minguo (1912–1949)	0 (0)	0 (0)
Total citations	34 (100)	22 (100)

Abbreviation: VaD, vascular dementia.

each, namely the *Zhen Jiu Zi Sheng Jing* 针灸资生经 (c. 1220), the acupuncture section of the Ming dynasty encyclopaedia *Pu Ji Fang* 普济方 (c. 1406), and the Ming dynasty acupuncture compendium *Zhen Jiu Da Cheng* 针灸大成 (c. 1601) by Yang Ji-Zhou 杨继洲. The earliest citations (*n* = 2) were from *Sheng Ji Zong Lu* 圣济总录 (c. 1117). In the 'likely' VaD subgroup, *Zhen Jiu Da Cheng* 针灸大成 and *Zhen Jiu Ju Ying* 针灸聚英 (c. 1529) provided four citations each, while *Pu Ji Fang* 普济方 (c. 1406) and *Lei Jing Tu Yi* 类经图翼 (c. 1624) provided three citations each.

Frequency of Acupuncture Points

In the 34 citations considered as 'possibly' referring to VaD, each mentioned at least one symptom relevant to VaD within a list of the various therapeutic applications for a single point. Seven different points were mentioned in total (Table 3.8). Most citations (*n* = 28) specified the use of acupuncture and 21 mentioned the use of moxibustion. There were no mentions of *tui na* 推拿 or other methods of point stimulation. The acupoint GV20 *Baihui* 百会 was the most frequently mentioned point (*n* = 17), followed by LU7 *Lieque* 列缺 (*n* = 9) and BL15 *Xinshu* 心俞 (*n* = 3). For acupuncture treatment, GV20 *Baihui* 百会 received more mentions (*n* = 14) than LU7 *Lieque* 列缺

Table 3.8 Most Frequently Used Acupuncture Points

'Possible' VaD		'Likely' VaD	
Point Name	**No. of Citations (%)**	**Point Name**	**No. of Citations (%)**
GV20 *Baihui* 百会	17 (50)	GV20 *Baihui* 百会	8 (36.4)
LU7 *Lieque* 列缺	9 (26.5)	LU7 *Lieque* 列缺	8 (36.4)
BL15 *Xinshu* 心俞	3 (8.8)	BL15 *Xinshu* 心俞	3 (13.6)
LI11 *Quchi* 曲池	2 (5.9)	LI11 *Quchi* 曲池	2 (9.1)
LU3 *Tianfu* 天府	1 (2.9)	GB39 *Xuanzhong* 悬钟	1 (4.5)
PC6 *Neiguan* 内关	1 (2.9)	—	—
GB39 *Xuanzhong* 悬钟	1 (2.9)	—	—

Abbreviation: VaD, vascular dementia.

($n = 7$), but for moxibustion, both GV20 *Baihui* 百会 and LU7 *Lieque* 列缺 had equal frequencies ($n = 8$). Moxibustion was not applied to LU3 *Tianfu* 天府 while GB39 *Xuanzhong* 悬钟 was only treated with moxibustion.

In the 22 citations that mentioned that a point was specifically for hemiplegia (classified as 'likely' VaD), the main points remained as GV20 *Baihui* 百会 ($n = 8$) and LU7 *Lieque* 列缺 ($n = 8$). Treatments were with acupuncture ($n = 19$) and moxibustion ($n = 16$). For both treatments, GV20 *Baihui* 百会 and LU7 *Lieque* 列缺 were the most frequently mentioned points.

Discussion of Acupuncture and Related Therapies

All of the citations that were included in the analysis were from lists of the various applications of individual points. None of the points were specific for VaD and each point had multiple uses.

In *Sheng Ji Zong Lu* 圣济总录 (c. 1117), there is a list of applications for GV20 *Baihui* 百会, including *zhong feng* 中风, talking in a disorderly manner, and memory impairment (*jian wang* 健忘). *Zhen Jiu Zi Sheng Jing* 针灸资生经 (c. 1220) mentioned its use for *zhong feng* 中风 with difficulty in speaking, hemiplegia, and the additional symptom of forgetting what happened earlier.

LU7 *Lieque* 列缺 is mentioned in *Sheng Ji Zong Lu* 圣济总录 for hemiplegia, memory impairment, and other disorders. Later books include similar lists.

Zhen Jiu Ju Ying 针灸聚英 (c. 1529) provided the first citation of BL15 *Xinshu* 心俞 for the symptoms of hemiplegia and *jian wang* 健忘. *Zhen Jiu Shen Shu* 针灸神书 (c. 1836) added the symptoms of severe chronic memory loss and numbness over half the body.

Similarly, *Zhen Jiu Ju Ying* 针灸聚英 (c. 1529) provided the first mention of the use of LI11 *Quchi* 曲池 for both hemiplegia and frequent forgetting (*shan wang* 善忘). The same applications are also recorded in *Zhen Jiu Da Cheng* 针灸大成 (c. 1601).

Lei Jing Tu Yi 类经图翼 (c. 1624) stated that PC6 *Neiguan* 内关 is a main point for treating stroke with loss of consciousness as well as for a range of mental disorders, including feeble mindedness or dementia, getting frightened and becoming crazy, inability in recognising familiar people, memory loss and confusion, and inability in remembering what was said. However, there was no mention of hemiplegia.

Zhen Jiu Zi Sheng Jing 针灸资生经 (c. 1220) provided a range of applications of GB39 *Xuanzhong* 悬钟 (also known as *Jue gu* 绝骨) including frequent unhappiness, memory loss and emotional lability, hemiplegia and contractures, paralysis and rigidity of the limbs, and multiple disorders characterised by weakness and debility. Moxibustion was particularly recommended for this point.

Regarding LU3 *Tianfu* 天府, amongst its indications *Zhen Jiu Da Cheng* 针灸大成 includes *zhong feng* 中风 and some mental disorders, including memory loss and talking to ghosts (i.e., people who are not there), but there is no mention of paralysis. Moxibustion was contraindicated for this point. For the other points, needles and moxibustion could both be used.

As with most common acupuncture points, all of the above points were used for a variety of disorders and not just for those consistent with VaD. Therefore, it is not possible to identify acupuncture points specific for VaD, only points used for treating the multiple symptoms and signs of VaD. It is important to note that these points were selected based on each point being applicable for symptoms associated with a CVA as well as for cognitive symptoms, since none of the citations provided multi-point prescriptions. Such an approach would not be used in clinical practice since separate points could be selected to address the paralysis and/or hemiplegia while other points could be selected to treat the cognitive symptoms and/or address the aetiology. If all of the points that have been used for a single symptom of VaD had been included in the analysis, a very large number of points would have been identified, although there would have been no means of prioritising them. Using the current approach, we can reasonably conclude that GV20 *Baihui* 百会, LU7 *Lieque* 列缺, BL15 *Xinshu* 心俞, LI11 *Quchi* 曲池, and GB39 *Xuanzhong* 悬钟 are all relevant to VaD, but we cannot say that these are the only or most relevant points.

The Classical Literature in Perspective

There is no direct one-to-one correspondence between modern disease categories and the classical terms used to describe similar conditions. For example, we cannot assume that a CVA was always described as *zhong feng* 中风 in the classical literature or that *zhong feng* 中风 always referred to CVAs. All we can establish is that there is a considerable degree of overlap. However, terms for certain symptoms can be interpreted with more confidence. The term *jian wang* 健忘 is clearly a disorder of memory impairment and *bàn shen bu sui* 半身不遂 refers to impaired movement of one half of the body. The co-occurance of these two symptoms is suggestive of a CVA but this is not sufficient to rule out other possibilities, nor do all CVAs result in hemiplegia.

In the classical literature, descriptions of the applications of herbal formulae and acupuncture points are often limited to lists of disorders, signs, and symptoms. These tend to accumulate over time as an intervention is reported to be effective for more and more conditions. Also, these classical descriptions seldom contain concrete examples of the temporal relationship between symptoms, so the reader can only infer that the intervention would have been used in people who had one or more of the listed symptoms. Since the readership of classical books on medicine would have been familiar with CM theory and with the arts of *materia medica* 本草 and formula construction, these lists of symptoms would have been read in this context, enabling the reader to form opinions about the relevance of a particular formula to a particular case, how the formula might function, and how the reader might modify it. In addition, formulae could be used for a diversity of disorders and symptoms provided they share similar aetiologies. For example, when the disorder was considered to be caused by wind, similar herbs could be used even when the disorders were as different as arthritis (*bi* syndrome 痹症) and stroke (*zhong feng* 中风) since wind is involved in both these disorders. The reader would have known this and interpreted the passage accordingly.

In the case of VaD, this modern disease category intersects with the traditional categories of *zhong feng* 中风, *chi dai* 痴呆, and *jian wang* 健忘 and can also include symptoms of *bi* syndrome 痹症, such as paralysis. In order to identify possible references to VaD, we used a multi-step process. First, we identified all references to *chi dai* 痴呆, *jian wang* 健忘, and related terms, eliminated those that were clearly not related to VaD, and selected those that included clinical symptoms associated with possible CVAs, including references to *zhong feng* 中风 'wind stroke' and symptoms suggestive of CVA sequelae, such as paralysis, hemiplegia, numbness, deviation of the face, drooling, and difficulty in speaking. This process reduced 2,207 citations to 126. In theory, we could have adopted a different order and started with *zhong feng* 中风 and other terms, but this would have identified a much larger initial data set. Finally, we used the symptom hemiplegia to limit the citations to those that combined this symptom with *jian wang* 健忘, *chi dai* 痴呆, or related terms to obtain the 'likely' VaD data set. This symptom was selected since it was relatively unambiguous and more indicative of CVAs than any of the other symptoms individually, but it cannot be considered definitive. That is, we cannot rule out hemiplegia as being due to other causes. Alternative approaches would have been to use *zhong feng* 中风 as the criterion or score citations based on multiple symptoms. Each of these alternatives proved to be equally or more problematic. Although the citations in the 'likely' VaD group are more focused on particular VaD symptoms than those in the larger 'possible' VaD group, they are not necessarily the most likely examples of VaD. This is due to the fact that VaD has a diversity of clinical presentations and there may not be any signs of hemiplegia. What they provide is a subset of citations for the purposes of comparison. As the results for herbal medicine and acupuncture show, the 'likely' VaD subgroups reflected the main features of the larger 'possible' VaD groups.

When compared to the formulae recommended for dementia in modern clinical guidelines,[11] many of the formulae used for possible VaD in the classical literature were quite different. None of the formulae listed in the guidelines appeared in the classical literature results (Chapter 2). One reason for this is that the guidelines provide formulae for dementia in general based on syndrome differentiation rather than for VaD with symptoms of paralysis and/or hemiplegia. Second, the modern conceptions of the aetiology of dementia differ from those in the classical literature. Whereas classical explanations focus on wind as a primary external pathogen, which can attack deeply due to deficiency within the body, modern explanations focus on internally generated wind, phlegm, Blood stasis, and toxins, in addition to deficiency. Nevertheless, a number of the classical formulae show similarities with those in the guidelines. For example, *Dang gui san* 当归散 (from *Pu Ji Fang* 普济方) contains many of the ingredients of *Gui pi tang* 归脾汤 (i.e., *ren shen* 人参, *huang qi* 黄芪, *bai zhu* 白术, *dang gui* 当归, *fu ling* 茯苓, *yuan zhi* 远志, and *gan cao* 甘草) plus herbs to expel wind (e.g. *fang feng* 防风, *du huo* 独活), mobilise Blood (e.g. *chi shao* 赤药, *chuan xiong* 川芎), and warm and unblock the channels 温经通络 (e.g. *chuan wu tou* 川乌头). Also, *Bu shen fu ling wan* 补肾茯苓丸 (from *Pu Ji Fang* 普济方) focuses on tonifying *qi* and Kidney like *Huan shao dan* 还少丹 and contains many similar ingredients, including *du zhong* 杜仲, *shan yu rou* 山萸肉, *fu ling* 茯苓, *rou cong rong* 肉苁蓉, and *shu yu* 薯蓣. So, although these formula names are different, they are based on similar combinations of ingredients.

Another issue is that some formulae for post-stroke hemiplegia that are now used for VaD were not indicated for dementia or memory impairment in the source text. For example, *Bu yang huan wu tang* 补阳还五汤 was used for hemiplegia with deviation of the eye and mouth in the Qing dynasty book, *Yi Lin Gai Cuo* 医林改错 (c. 1830), but there was no mention of cognitive symptoms and, thus, it was excluded from the data set.

Of the seven different acupuncture points identified in the 'possible' VaD group, GV20 *Baihui* 百会, LU7 *Lieque* 列缺, and PC6 *Neiguan* 内关 all mention multiple disorders or symptoms characteristic of VaD. Acupoint PC6 *Neiguan* 内关 was specified as being particularly useful for mental disorders resulting from stroke. Acupoints LI11 *Quchi* 曲池 and GB39 *Xuanzhong* 悬钟 appear to be more for paralysis, including that which is associated with stroke. Of these, GV20 *Baihui* 百会 and LU7 *Lieque* 列缺 are mentioned for VaD in modern books (See Chapter 2, Table 2.2).

From a clinical perspective, it is also important to consider the differences between historical use and contemporary guidelines for traditional CM treatment. A number of the medical substances used in pre-modern formulae cannot be used in modern traditional CM and some of the methods recorded in classical books have been superseded. Therefore, the findings provided in this chapter should not be used to guide clinical practice.

References

1. American Psychiatric Association. (2013) Diagnostic and Statistical Manual of Mental Disorders, 5th ed. (DSM V). American Psychiatric Association, Arlington, VA.
2. May BH, Mei FM, Zhou IW, Chang SY, *et al.* (2016) Memory impairment, dementia and Alzheimer's disease in classical and contemporary traditional Chinese medicine. *J Altern Complement Med.* **22**(9): 695–705.
3. 林昭庚, ed. (2002) 中西医病名对照. 人民卫生出版社, 北京.
4. 李经纬, 余瀛鳌, 蔡景峰, 张志斌, *et al.* (2005) 中医大辞典 (第二版). 人民卫生出版社, 北京.

5. Jia Hong Science and Technology Development Co. Ltd., 嘉鸿科技开发有限公司. (2014) Zhong Hua Yi Dian 中华医典 (ZHYD) Encyclopaedia of Traditional Chinese Medicine. 5 ed., Hunan Electronic and Audio-Visual Publishing House, Changsha.
6. May BH, Lu CJ, Xue CCL. (2012) Collections of traditional Chinese medical literature as resources for systematic searches. *J Altern Complement Med.* **18**(12):1101–1107.
7. May BH, Lu YB, Lu CJ, Zhang AL, *et al.* (2013) Systematic assessment of the representativeness of published collections of the traditional literature on Chinese Medicine. *J Altern Complement Med.* **19**(5):403–409.
8. 国家技术监督局. (1996) 中医病证分类与代码. 北京: 中国标准出版社.
9. World Health Organisation. (2007) WHO International Standard Terminologies on Traditional Medicine in the Western Pacific Region. World Health Organisation, Manila, Western Pacific Region.
10. Wiseman N. (1996) English-Chinese Chinese-English dictionary of Chinese medicine. Hunan Science and Technology Press, Changsha.
11. 田金洲. (2012) 中国痴呆诊疗指南, 第一版. 人民卫生出版社， 北京. pp. 108–114.
12. 陈辉, ed. (1993) 实用中医脑病学. 第一版. 学苑出版社， 北京.
13. 高福安, eds. (1995) 实用中医老年内科病学. 第一版. 安徽科学技术出版社， 合肥.
14. 周文泉, 高普, ed. (1995) 中医老年病临床研究. 第一版. 北京出版社, 北京.
15. 许沛虎, ed. (1998) 中医脑病学. 中国医药科技出版社， 北京.
16. 李求兵, 梅嵘, eds. (1999) 老年痴呆症的中西医诊断与治疗. 中国医药科技出版社， 北京.
17. 张登本, ed. (2000) 中医神经精神病学. 中国医药科技出版社， 北京.
18. 张瞀, eds. (2000) 实用中医老年病学. 人民军医出版社， 北京.
19. 李勇, 谢冬梅, ed. (2000) 古今中医脑病辨治精要. 人民军医出版社， 北京.
20. Flaws B, Lake J. (2003) Chinese Medical Psychiatry: A Textbook and Clinical Manual, 2nd ed. Blue Poppy Press, Boulder.
21. 盛树力, ed. (2006) 老年痴呆及相关疾病. 科学技术文献出版社， 北京.
22. May BH, Lu YB, Lu CJ, Zhang AL, *et al.* (2015) The systematic assessment of traditional evidence from the premodern Chinese medicinal literature: A text-mining approach. *J Altern Complement Med.* **20**(12):937–942.

4

Methods for Evaluating Clinical Evidence

OVERVIEW

This section describes the methods used to identify and evaluate clinical studies of Chinese medicine interventions for vascular dementia. Studies identified through a comprehensive search strategy were assessed against eligibility criteria, followed by a review of each study's methodological quality using standardised methods. Results from included studies were evaluated to provide an estimate of the effects of each type of Chinese medicine therapy.

Introduction

The use of Chinese medicine (CM) for vascular dementia (VaD) has been extensively researched in clinical studies. In the following chapters, the efficacy, effectiveness, and safety of CM interventions are evaluated using meta-analytic methods (where possible) for controlled clinical trials, while a descriptive approach is used for non-controlled clinical studies. The evidence is presented for the following main types of CM interventions:

- Chinese herbal medicine (CHM) (Chapter 5);
- Acupuncture and related therapies (Chapter 7);
- Other CM therapies (Chapter 8); and
- Combination CM therapies (e.g. CHM plus acupuncture) (Chapter 9).

Published data on clinical trials were obtained from databases and other sources and assessed by an expert review group comprised of researchers, clinical physicians, CM experts, and methodologists. All included studies are referenced at the end of each chapter.

Randomised controlled trials (RCTs), non-randomised controlled clinical trials (CCTs), and non-controlled studies were evaluated separately. Meta-analyses were conducted for RCTs and CCTs using the methods described below. This approach was not suitable for evidence from non-controlled studies. Therefore, the characteristics of the studies, details of the interventions, and any adverse events were described and summarised. References to included studies are indicated by a letter followed by a number. Specifically, studies of CHM are indicated by an 'H' (e.g. H1), studies of acupuncture and related therapies are indicated by an 'A' (e.g. A1), studies of other CM therapies are indicated by an 'O' (e.g. O1), and studies of combinations of CM therapies are indicated by a 'C' (e.g. C1).

Search Strategy

Comprehensive searches were conducted on multiple English - and Chinese-language databases using the methods outlined in the Cochrane Handbook of Systematic Reviews.[1] English-language databases included PubMed, Excepta Medica Database (Embase), Cumulative Index of Nursing and Allied Health Literature (CINAHL), Cochrane Central Register of Controlled Trials (CENTRAL) (including the Cochrane Library), and Allied and Complementary Medicine Database (AMED). Chinese-language databases included China Biomedical Literature (CBM), China National Knowledge Infrastructure (CNKI), Chongqing VIP (CQVIP), and Wanfang. Databases were searched from their respective inceptions to May 2014. No restrictions were applied. Search terms were mapped to controlled vocabulary (where applicable), in addition to being searched as keywords.

Search terms were grouped into blocks of terms for: (1) the disease (dementia and synonyms); (2) the CM intervention and (3) the type of study (e.g. clinical trial, RCT, etc.). The three search blocks were combined using "AND" (or a database-specific variant). Consequently, the following nine searches were conducted in each of the nine databases:

1. CHM — reviews
2. CHM — controlled trials (randomised and non-randomised)

3. CHM — non-controlled studies
4. Acupuncture and related therapies — reviews
5. Acupuncture and related therapies — controlled trials (randomised and non-randomised)
6. Acupuncture and related therapies — non-controlled studies
7. Other CM therapies — reviews
8. Other CM therapies — controlled trials (randomised and non-randomised), and
9. Other CM therapies — non-controlled studies.

Studies of combination CM therapies were identified from the above searches. In addition to electronic databases, reference lists of systematic reviews and included studies were searched for additional publications. Clinical trial registries were searched to identify clinical trials that were ongoing or completed and, where required, trial investigators were contacted to obtain further data. The searched trial registries included the Australian New Zealand Clinical Trial Registry (ANZCTR), Chinese Clinical Trial Registry (ChiCTR), EU Clinical Trials Register (EU-CTR), and ClinicalTrials.gov.

Inclusion Criteria

Study Type

Controlled prospective studies with or without randomisation (including parallel groups and cross-over studies) and uncontrolled studies (cohort and case series) that employed a CM therapy as a test intervention and reported an outcome of relevance to VaD.

Participants

People diagnosed with VaD based on one or more of the following guidelines including specific diagnostic criteria for VaD:

- International Classification of Diseases, Tenth Revision (ICD-10) or the Chinese version 国际疾病分类-10 for VaD.

- Diagnostic and Statistical Manual of Mental Disorders (DSM) or the Chinese version 美国精神病学会制定的《精神障碍诊断和统计手册》(any version) for VaD.
- National Institute of Neurological Disorders and Stroke and the Association Internationale pour la Recherche et l'Enseignement en Neurosciences (NINCDS-AIREN) citeria or the Chinese version 美国国立神经病与卒中研究所/瑞士神经科学研究国际会议 forVaD;
- Classification and Diagnostic Criteria of Mental Disorders in China (CCMD) 中国精神疾病分类 criteria for the diagnosis of VaD.

Interventions

Studies that employed a CM therapy as a test intervention including:

- CHM: Administered orally and/or topically.
- Acupuncture: With or without skin penetration, including ear acupuncture, ear acupressure, or laser therapy.
- Moxibustion: Applied directly or indirectly, using various heat sources.
- Manual therapies: Including *tui na* 推拿 and *an mo* 按摩 (massage);
- Other CM therapies: Including *tai chi* 太極, *qi gong* 气功, and dietary therapy (Table 4.1).

Table 4.1 Chinese Medicine Interventions Included in Clinical Evidence Evaluation

Category	Included Intervention
Chinese herbal medicine	Orally administered
Acupuncture and related therapies	Acupuncture, acupressure, ear acupuncture, ear acupressure, electroacupuncture, moxibustion, and scalp acupuncture therapy.
Other Chinese medicine therapies	Chinese massage (*tui na* 推拿, *an mo* 按摩), *tai chi* therapy 太極, diet therapy, and Chinese medicine psychological intervention.
Combination Chinese medicine	Two or more Chinese medicine interventions from different categories administered together: Oral Chinese herbal medicine plus acupuncture, oral Chinese herbal medicine plus *tai chi* therapy 太極, and diet therapy plus moxibustion therapy.

Co-interventions were allowed as long as the same intervention was used in at least two arms of the study.

Comparators in Controlled Trials (Randomised Controlled Trials and Controlled Clinical Trials)

Control interventions included:

- No treatment, supportive care, or placebo.
- Conventional therapy (using pharmacotherapies, manual methods, and psychological methods aimed at treating VaD).
- Combinations of CM interventions with conventional therapies in an integrative medicine (IM) approach. Note: The combination of CM with usual supportive care that was not specific for VaD (such as the use of anti-platelet aggregation drugs, anti-hypertension drugs, or hypoglycemic drugs) was not considered to be an IM approach.

Settings

In-patients or out-patients treated in hospitals, clinics, aged care facilities, or in their own homes.

Outcomes

Studies reported at least one of the following outcomes:

- Primary outcome assessments: At least one of the pre-specified outcome measures (Table 4.2); and/or
- Secondary outcome assessments: Incidence and type of adverse events during treatment.

The outcome measure instruments listed are not the only scales used for assessing people with VaD. Describing every scale and every variation is beyond the scope of this chapter. The included scales are ones that feature in the subsequent chapters. In addition to clinical scales, outcomes in dementia research include imaging and serological measures. These aspects are not assessed in the following meta-analyses.

Table 4.2 Clinical Outcome Measures

Outcome Categories	Outcome Measures	Units; Direction for Improvement
Cognition	Mini-Mental State Examination (MMSE)[2,3]	30 points, higher is better
	Hasegawa's Dementia Scale (HDS, HDS-R)[4,5]	30 points, higher is better
	Alzheimer's Disease Assessment Scale — cognitive subscale (ADAS-cog)[6]	11 items, 70 points, lower is better
	Vascular Dementia Assessment Scale — cognitive subscale (VaDAS-cog)[7]	14 items, 90 points, lower is better
	Montreal Cognitive Assessment (MoCA)[8]	30 points, higher is better
	Cognitive Capacity Screening Examination (CCSE)[9]	30 points, higher is better
	Memory Quotient (MQ)[10,11]	100 points, higher is better
	Wechsler Adult Intelligence Scale (WAIS), Wechsler Memory Scale (WMS), WAIS-Revised by China (WAIS-RC)[11,12]	100 points, higher is better
Global scales	Clinical Dementia Rating (CDR)[13–15]	3 points, lower is better
	Global Deterioration Scale (GDS)[14,16]	7 stages, lower is better
	Blessed Dementia Scale (BDS)[17,18]	22 items, lower is better
	Blessed Behaviour Scale (BBS)[17,18]	22 items, lower is better
Activities of daily living (ADL)	Barthel Index (BI)[19]	100 points, higher is better
	Alzheimer Disease Cooperative Study — ADL inventory (ADCS-ADL)[20]	19 items, 54 points, higher is better
	Other ADL scales (Robert)[21,22]	Various scoring systems
	Functional Activities Questionnaire (FAQ)[23]	30 points, lower scores indicate less dependence

(*Continued*)

Table 4.2 (*Continued*)

Outcome Categories	Outcome Measures	Units; Direction for Improvement
Behavioural and psychological symptoms of dementia (BPSD)	Neuropsychiatric Inventory (NPI)[24,25]	144 points (NPI-12), lower is better
	ADAS non-cognitive section (ADAS-noncog)[26]	50 points, lower is better
	Behavioural Pathology in Alzheimer's Disease Rating Scale (BEHAVE-AD)[27]	75 points, lower is better
	Cornell scale for depression in dementia (CSDD)[28]	19 items, lower is better
	Hamilton Depression Rating Scale (HAM-D, HDRS)[29]	17 items, 50 points, lower is better
	Cohen-Mansfield Agitation Inventory (CMAI)[30]	29 items, lower is better
Adverse events	Adverse events (as reported in studies)	Number and type of adverse events in each group

Note: 1. Although some studies mentioned HDS while others mentioned the revised version HDS-R, all studies used the same revised-version scale, so Hasegawa's Dementia Scale (HDS) was used throughout.

Exclusion Criteria

Study Type

Retrospective controlled studies, epidemiological studies, and studies that used the following designs:

- CM versus other CM therapy;
- CM plus other therapy versus CM; or
- CM plus pharmacotherapy versus CM.

Participants

- The participant group included people with: other forms of dementia, such as Alzheimer's disease, mild cognitive impairment (MCI), vascular cognitive impairment with no dementia (VCI-NO), other diseases such as Parkinson's disease (PD), or people with stroke sequelae who did not have concurrent probable VaD.

- History of hypertension, hyperlipidemia, diabetes, or depression were not considered as exclusion criteria.

Interventions

- Synthetic compounds or isolated chemical compounds, homeopathic preparations, nutritional supplements, and plant-based products that are not used in Chinese traditional medicine.
- Studies of modified *Gingko biloba* L. leaf extracts (such as EGb 761) and huperzine A used as test interventions were excluded. Studies were not excluded when *Gingko biloba* seed (*bai guo* 白果) was used as in traditional CHM, or when *Gingko biloba* was one component of a multi-component CHM intervention.

Comparators in Controlled Trials (Randomised Controlled Trials and Controlled Clinical Trial)

- Control groups that employed an intervention that was not used in the conventional care of VaD (in China or other countries) or was another CM intervention.
- Controls using another CM intervention, other herbal products, or *Gingko biloba* leaf extract.
- DUXIL® (almitrine/raubasine), which is not recommended for dementia treatment in the current guideline.[31]
- Comparisons with huperzine A were included since huperzine A is currently used as an acetylcholinesterase inhibitor in conventional medicine in China.

Outcomes

For missing data and data errors, if we failed to obtain sufficient data after contacting authors or retrieving related articles, the studies were excluded.

Risk of Bias

Risk of bias was assessed for RCTs using the Cochrane Collaboration's tool.[1] Risk of bias was assessed for the following domains: sequence generation, allocation concealment, blinding of participants and personnel, blinding of outcome assessors, incomplete outcome data, and selective reporting. Each domain was assessed to determine whether the risk of bias was 'low', 'high', or 'unclear'. Risk of bias assessment was verified by two independent researchers and disagreement was resolved by discussion and consultation with a third person.

Risk of bias is categorised using the following six domains:

- Sequence generation: The method used to generate the allocation sequence is given in sufficient detail to allow an assessment of whether it should produce comparable groups. 'Low' risk of bias refers to a random number table or computer random generator. 'High' risk of bias includes studies that describe a non-random sequence generation, such as odd or even date of birth or date of admission.
- Allocation concealment: The method used to conceal the allocation sequence is given in enough detail to determine whether intervention allocations could have been foreseen before or during enrolment. 'Low' risk of bias includes central randomisation or sealed envelopes while 'high' risk of bias includes allocation approaches such as open random sequence or date of birth.
- Blinding of participants and personnel: Measures used to describe if the study participants and personnel are blind to the intervention received. In addition, information relating to whether the blinding was effective is also assessed. Studies that ensure blinding of participants and personnel are at 'low' risk of bias. If the study is not blind or incompletely blind, it is at 'high' risk of bias.
- Blinding of outcome assessors: Measures used to describe if the outcome assessors are blind to knowledge of which intervention a participant received. In addition, information relating to whether the blinding was effective is also assessed. Studies that ensure

blinding of outcome assessors are at 'low' risk of bias. If the study is not blind or incompletely blind, it is at 'high' risk of bias.
- Incomplete outcome data: Completeness of outcome data for each main outcome, including drop outs, exclusions from the analysis with numbers missing in each group, and reasons for drop outs or exclusions. Studies with 'low' risk of bias would include all outcome data or, if there is missing data, such data is unlikely to relate to the true outcome or is balanced between groups. Studies at 'high' risk of bias would have unexplained missing data.
- Selective reporting: The study protocol is available and the pre-specified outcomes are included in the report. Studies with a published protocol that includes all pre-specified outcomes in their report would be at 'low' risk of bias. Studies are at 'high' risk of bias if they do not include all pre-specified outcomes or the outcome data is reported incompletely.

Statistical Analyses

Frequency of CM syndromes, CHM formulae, herbs, and acupuncture points reported in included studies were presented using descriptive statistics. CM syndromes reported in two or more studies were presented. In Chapter 5, the 20 most frequently reported CHM formulae and herbs presented were used in at least two studies. The top 10 acupuncture points used in two or more studies were presented when available. Where data were limited, reports of single CM syndromes or acupuncture points were provided as a guide for the reader.

Definitions of statistical tests and results are described in the glossary. Meta-analysis of outcome measure data was performed when a sufficient number of comparable studies was available. Meta-analyses were based on reported data at the end of the treatment period (EoT) and comparisons were between the CM intervention groups and the control groups at EoT. Dichotomous data are reported as a risk ratio (RR) with 95% confidence intervals (CI) while continuous data are reported as a mean difference (MD), or standardised mean difference (SMD), with 95% CIs. For dichotomous data, when the RR is greater than one and the upper and lower values of the 95% CI are both greater than one, this indicates that we can be 95% certain that there is a difference between the groups and the true effect lies within these CIs. The same is true for values less than one. In such cases, we say there is a 'significant difference' between the groups. For continuous data, when the MD is greater than zero and both the upper and lower values of the 95% CI are greater than zero, we say there is a 'significant difference' between the groups. The same is true on the negative side of the scale.[1]

Available case analysis with a random effects model was used in all analyses. This provides a conservative estimate of difference between groups and is applicable to data in which heterogeneity is present. Formal tests for heterogeneity were conducted using the I^2 statistic. An I^2 score greater than 50% was considered to indicate substantial heterogeneity.[1] Sensitivity analyses were undertaken to explore potential sources of heterogeneity based on 'low' risk of bias for the risk of bias domain sequence generation. Where possible and appropriate, planned subgroup analyses included type of control medication, duration of treatment, and/or CM formula.

Summary of Findings

Assessment Using GRADE

The Grading of Recommendations, Assessment, Development and Evaluation (GRADE) approach was used.[32] The GRADE approach summarises and rates the strength and quality ('certainty') of evidence in systematic reviews using a structured process for presenting evidence summaries. The results are presented in GRADE summary of findings tables. These provide an overview of the evidence for the main outcome measures.

A panel of experts was established to evaluate the certainty of evidence. The panel included the systematic review team, CM practitioners, integrative medicine experts, research methodologists, and conventional medicine physicians. The experts were asked to rate the clinical importance of key interventions from CHM, acupuncture therapies and other CM therapies, as well as comparators and outcomes. Results were collated, and based on the rating scores and subsequent discussion, a consensus on the content for the GRADE summary of findings (SoF) tables was achieved.

The certainty of evidence for each outcome was rated according to five factors outlined in the GRADE approach. The certainty of evidence might be rated down based on:

- Limitations in study design (risk of bias);
- Inconsistency of results (unexplained heterogeneity);
- Indirectness of evidence (interventions, populations, and outcomes important to the patients with the condition);
- Imprecision (uncertainty about the results);
- Publication bias (selective publication of studies).

These five factors are additive and a reduction in one or more factors will reduce the certainty of the evidence for that outcome.

The GRADE approach also includes methods for assessing observational studies. In this monograph GRADE summaries only include RCTs.

Treatment recommendations could also be assessed using the GRADE approach, but due to the diverse nature of CM practice, treatment recommendations were not included with the summary of findings. Therefore, the reader should interpret the evidence with reference to the local practice environment. It should also be noted that the GRADE approach requires judgments about the strength and quality of evidence and some subjective assessment. However, the experience of the panel members suggests the judgments are reliable and transparent representations of the certainty of evidence.

The GRADE levels of evidence[33] are grouped into four categories:

1. High certainty: We are very confident that the true effect lies close to that of the estimate of the effect;
2. Moderate certainty: We are moderately confident in the effect estimate: The true effect is likely to be close to the estimate of the effect, but there is a possibility that it is substantially different;

3. Low certainty: Our confidence in the effect estimate is limited: The true effect may be substantially different from the estimate of the effect;
4. Very low certainty: We have very little confidence in the effect estimate: The true effect is likely to be substantially different from the estimate of effect.

References

1. Higgins J, Green S, eds. (2011) Cochrane Handbook for Systematic Reviews of Interventions Version 5.1.0 The Cochrane Collaboration. Retrieved from http://www.cochrane- handbook.org.
2. Folstein MF, Folstein SE, McHugh PR. (1975) Mini-mental state. A practical method for grading the cognitive state of patients for the clinician. *J Psychiatr Res* **12**(3):189–198.
3. Crum RM, Anthony JC, Bassett SS, Folstein MF. (1993) Population-based norms for the Mini-Mental-State-Examination by age and educational level. *J Am Med Assoc* **269**(18):2386–2391.
4. Imai Y, Hasegawa K. (1994) The Revised Hasegawa Dementia Scale (HDS-R): Evaluation of its usefulness as a screening test for dementia. *J Hong Kong Coll Psychiatr* **4**(2):20–24.
5. Jeong JW, Kim KW, Lee DY, Lee SB, *et al.* (2007) A normative study of the Revised Hasegawa Dementia Scale: Comparison of demographic influences between the Revised Hasegawa Dementia Scale and the Mini-Mental Status Examination. *Dement Geriatr Cogn Disord* **24**(4):288–293.
6. Mohs RC, Rosen WG, Davis KL. (1983) The Alzheimer's disease assessment scale: An instrument for assessing treatment efficacy. *Psychopharmacol Bull* **19**(3):448–450.
7. Ylikoski R, Jokinen H, Andersen P, *et al.* (2007) Comparison of the Alzheimer's Disease Assessment Scale Cognitive Subscale and the Vascular Dementia Assessment Scale in Differentiating Elderly Individuals with Different Degrees of white Matter Changes. *Dement Geriatr Cogn Disord* **24**:73–81.
8. Nasreddine ZS, Phillips NA, Bedirian V, Charbonneau S, Whitehead V, Collin I, Cummings JL, Chertkow H. (2005) The Montreal Cognitive Assessment, MoCA: A brief screening tool for mild cognitive impairment. *J Am Geriatr Soc* **53**(4):695–699.

9. Kaufman DM, Weinberger M, Strain JJ, Jacobs JW. (1979) Detection of cognitive deficits by a brief mental status examination: The Cognitive Capacity Screening Examination, a reappraisal and a review. *Gen Hosp Psychiatr* **1**(3):247–255.
10. Lezak MD. (2012) *Neuropsychological Assessment.* Oxford University Press, Oxford.
11. Wechsler D. (1945) A standarized memory scale for clinical use. *J Psychol* **19**:87–95.
12. Dai XY, Gong YX, Zhong LP (1990). Factor analysis of the Mainland Chinese version of the Wechsler Adult Intelligence Scale. *Psychol Assess* **2**(1), 31–34.
13. Burns A, Lawlor B, Craig S. (2004) *Assessment Scales in Old Age Psychiatry*, 2nd ed. Martin Dunitz, London.
14. Reisberg B. (2007) Global measures: Utility in defining and measuring treatment response in dementia. *Int Psychogeriatr/IPA.* **19**(3):421–456.
15. Morris JC. (1993) The Clinical Dementia Rating (CDR): Current version and scoring rules. *Neurology* **43**(11):2412–2414.
16. Reisberg B, Ferris SH, de Leon MJ, Crook T. (1982) The global deterioration scale for assessment of primary degenerative dementia. *Am J Psychiatr* **139**:1136–1139.
17. Blessed G, Tomlinson BF, Roth M. (1968) The association between quantitative measures of dementia and of senile change in the cerebral grey matter of elderly subjects. *Br J Psychiatr* **114**:797–811.
18. Yang YH, Lai CL, Lin RT, Tai CT, *et al.* (2006) Cut-off values of Blessed Dementia Rating Scale and its clinical application in elderly Taiwanese. *Kaohsiung J Med Sci* **22**(8):377–384.
19. Mahoney F, Barthel D. (1965) Functional evaluation: The Barthel Index. *Md State Med J* **14**: 61–65.
20. Galasko D, Bennett D, Sano M, *et al.* (1997) An inventory to assess activities of daily living for clinical trials in Alzheimer's disease. The Alzheimer's disease cooperative study. *Alzheimer Dis Assoc Disord* **11** (Suppl) 2:S33–S39.
21. Lawton MP, Brody EM. (1969) Assessment of older people: Self-maintaining and instrumental activities of daily living. *Gerontologist* **9**(3):179–186.
22. Robert P, Ferris S, Gauthier S, Ihl R, *et al.* (2010) Review of Alzheimer's disease scales: Is there a need for a new multi-domain scale for therapy evaluation in medical practice? *Alzheimer Res Ther* **2**(4):24.

23. Pfeffer RI, Kurosaki TT, Harrah CH, Jr., Chance JM, *et al.* (1982) Measurement of functional activities in older adults in the community. *J Gerontol* **37**(3):323–329.
24. Cummings JL, Mega M, Gray K, Rosenbergthompson S, *et al.* (1994) The Neuropsychiatric Inventory: Comprehensive assessment of psychopathology in dementia. *Neurology* **44**(12):2308–2314.
25. Cummings JL. (1997) The Neuropsychiatric Inventory: Assessing psychopathology in dementia patients. *Neurology* **48**(5 Suppl 6):S10–S16.
26. Rush AJ, First MB, Blacker D. (2008) *Handbook of Psychiatric Measures,* 2nd ed. American Psychiatric Pub, Washington, DC.
27. Reisberg B, Borenstein J, Salob SP, Ferris SH, *et al.* (1987) Behavioral symptoms in Alzheimer's Disease: Phenomenology and treatment. *J Clin Psychiat* **48**:9–15.
28. Alexopoulos GS, Abrams RC, Young RC, Shamoian CA. (1988) Cornell scale for depression in dementia. *Biol Psychiatr* **23**(3):271–284.
29. Hamilton M. (1960) A rating scale for depression. *J Neurol Neurosurg Psychiatr* **23**:56–62.
30. Cohen-Mansfield J, Marx MS, Rosenthal AS. (1989) A description of agitation in a nursing home. *J Gerontol* **44**(3):M77–M84.
31. Tian JZ. (2012) *Chinese Guidelines for the Diagnosis and Treatment of Alzheimer's Disease and Other Dementias* [in Chinese: 中国痴呆诊疗指南]. People's Medical Publishing House, Beijing, People's Republic of China.
32. Schunemann H, Brozek J, Guyatt G, Oxman A, eds. (2013) GRADE handbook for grading quality of evidence and strength of recommendations (The GRADE Working Group). Retrieved from http://www.guidelinedevelopment.org/handbook/.
33. Schünemann HJ, Higgins JPT, Vist GE, *et al.* (2019) Chapter 14: Completing 'summary of findings' tables and grading the certainty of the evidence. In: Higgins JPT, Thomas J, Chandler J, Cumpston M, Li T, Page MJ, *et al.*, eds. Cochrane handbook for systematic reviews of interventions version 6.0 (updated July 2019). Retrieved from www.training.cochrane.org/handbook: Cochrane; 2019.

5

Clinical Evidence for Chinese Herbal Medicine

OVERVIEW

The efficacy of Chinese herbal medicines for vascular dementia has been investigated by numerous clinical studies that have been published in scientific journals in China and other countries. This chapter provides a synopsis and analysis of the clinical study literature and an assessment of the state of the evidence. Comprehensive searches of nine databases identified over 21,000 articles. After assessment with rigorous criteria, 221 clinical studies that investigated oral Chinese herbal medicines for vascular dementia were selected for inclusion in this chapter. A systematic review and a series of meta-analyses of the results of outcome measures were performed to determine the efficacy and safety of Chinese herbal medicine for vascular dementia.

Previous Systematic Reviews

Two systematic reviews were identified from the English-language database search while eight systematic reviews of Chinese herbal medicines (CHM) were identified from the Chinese literature through comprehensive searches up to May 2014. Five reviews evaluated the safety and efficacy of CHM for vascular dementia (VaD).[1–5] The meta-analyses in two systematic reviews found that CHM treatment groups were more effective than control interventions based on the total effective rate, the Mini-Mental State Examination (MMSE), and Hasegawa's Dementia Scale (HDS).[1,4] One systematic review reported that CHM was beneficial in improving Chinese medicine

(CM) syndrome scores and activities of daily living (ADL), but not MMSE scores.[2] Yi *et al.* found that CM treatment focusing on nourishing the Kidney for VaD had better effects than Western medicine/medication alone.[5] Another systematic review[3] did not conduct a meta-analysis as variation in outcome measures meant that the data were unsuitable for doing so. As such, a qualitative appraisal was conducted and it was concluded that CHM could be a safe and effective treatment for VaD, either alone or in conjunction with orthodox medications. *Chuan xiong* 川芎, *he shou wu* 何首乌, and *huang qi* 黄芪 were the most commonly used herbs in the studies included in this review. However, the included trials were generally 'low' in quality and the review authors concluded that further clinical trials were necessary.

In addition, a number of reviews have focused on specific CM formulae. One systematic review was conducted on the classical formula *Bu yang huang wu tang* 补阳还五汤 for VaD.[6] The results indicated that *Bu yang huang wu tang* 补阳还五汤 could improve scores on MMSE and HDS more than pharmacotherapy, but the small number of included studies and methodological shortcomings limit the certainty of the results. Two systematic reviews evaluated the efficacy and safety of *Bu chang nao xin tong jiao nang* 步长脑心通胶囊 for VaD.[7,8] Meta-analysis indicated that *Bu chang nao xin tong jiao nang* 步长脑心通胶囊 was more effective than pharmacotherapy in improving MMSE, HDS, and ADL. Another two systematic reviews focused on *Zhi ling tang* 智灵汤 and *Tian zhi ke li* 天智颗粒[9,10] and found that the currently available evidence was insufficient to make conclusions regarding their efficacy and safety in VaD.

This chapter includes orally administered traditional CHMs. No studies of topical CHMs for VaD were located. It also excludes injected products, plants not traditionally used in CM (such as brahmi), modified extracts of plants (such as EGb 761 from *Gingko biloba* L.), and plant-derived compounds (such as huperzine A). Therefore, systematic reviews on *Gingko biloba* extracts and huperzine A are not summarised here.

Identification of Clinical Studies

The database searches identified more than 21,000 potentially relevant citations and, following screening, more than 1,500 full-text articles were retrieved for detailed examination. After excluding studies that did not meet the selection criteria, 180 randomised controlled trials (RCTs) (H1–H180), 10 controlled clinical trials (CCTs) (H181–H190), and 31 non-controlled studies (H191–H221) remained, totalling 221 studies that tested the effects of orally administered CHMs and were included in this review (Figure 5.1).

Chinese Herbal Medicine

The 180 RCTs and 10 CCTs of orally administered CHMs included at least one internationally recognised evaluation scale that assessed one of the following aspects: cognitive function, ADL, behavioural and psychological symptoms of dementia (BPSD), or global evaluation (see Chapter 4, Table 4.2). The CHMs included single products and multi-ingredient formulae. These were administered orally in the form of decoctions, liquid extracts, granules, powders, capsules, or pills.

Randomised Controlled Trials of Oral Chinese Herbal Medicine

The 180 RCTs were conducted in China (n = 178) or Japan (n = 2) and a total of 14,834 participants were enrolled. The duration of the studies ranged from 14 days to 6 months. For convenience, study durations have been recorded in weeks in the following tables. Syndrome differentiation was used in 52 studies and the most frequently specified syndromes were *qi* deficiency with Blood stasis 气虚血瘀 (9 studies), deficiency of Kidney/Essence with Blood stasis 肾虚血瘀 (8 studies), and phlegm turbidity obstructing the Orifices 痰浊阻窍 (7 studies). 'Sea of Marrow' insufficiency 髓海不足 was mentioned in 6 studies, while Spleen and Kidney deficiency

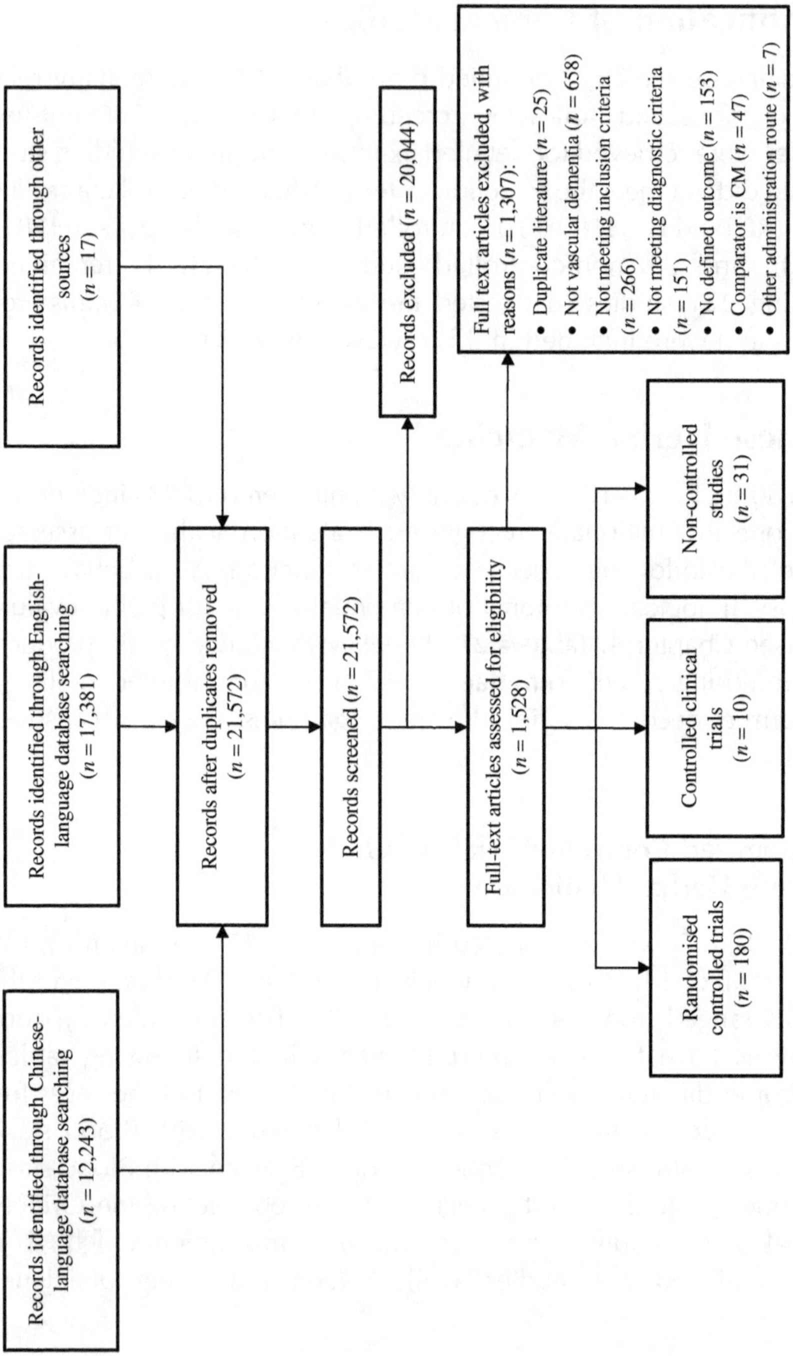

Figure 5.1 Flow Chart of Study Selection Process: Chinese Herbal Medicine

Table 5.1 Common Syndromes Reported in Randomised Controlled Trials

Most Common Syndromes	No. of Studies
Qi deficiency with Blood stasis 气虚血瘀	9
Deficiency of Kidney/Essence with Blood stasis 肾虚血瘀	8
Phlegm turbidity obstructing the Orifices 痰浊阻窍	7
'Sea of Marrow' insufficiency 髓海不足	6
Spleen and Kidney deficiency 脾肾两虚	5
Deficiency of Kidney Essence 肾精亏虚	5
Spleen and Kidney deficiency with phlegm turbidity and Blood stasis obstructing the collaterals 脾肾两虚, 痰瘀阻络	4
Liver and Kidney deficiency 肝肾亏虚	4
Phlegm turbidity and Blood stasis obstructing the collaterals 痰瘀阻络	3
Blood stasis obstructing the collaterals 瘀血阻络	3
Qi stagnation with Blood stasis 气滞血瘀	3

脾肾两虚 and deficiency of Kidney Essence 肾精亏虚 were each mentioned in 5 studies (Table 5.1).

The most commonly tested formulae in the RCTs are listed in Table 5.2. Fourteen of the 180 CHM interventions were unnamed formulae. The named formulae that were tested in the largest number of different clinical trials were modified *Bu yang huan wu tang* 补阳还五汤加减 (4 studies), which is a classical formula for stroke sequelae, and *Bu chang nao xin tong jiao nang* 步长脑心通胶囊 (4 studies), which is a commercial product manufactured in China. *Fu fang hai she jiao nang* 复方海蛇胶囊 (3 studies), *Cong sheng jiao nang* 聪圣胶囊 (3 studies), *Kang xin jiao nang* 康欣胶囊 (3 studies), and *Tian zhi ke li* 天智颗粒 (3 studies) were also commercial products manufactured in China that are used to treat VaD. *Di huang yin zi* 地黄饮子加减 (2 studies) is a classical formula that is used to treat a condition called *yin fei zheng* 喑痱证, the characteristics of which are dysfunction in speech and movement after stroke. In a number of studies, the formulae were modified by addition or subtraction of ingredients to suit individual patients.

Table 5.2 Frequently Used Formulae in Randomised Controlled Trials

Formula Name	Frequency of Use	Main Ingredients (Studies)
Modified *Bu yang huan wu tang* 补阳还五汤加减[1]	4	*Huang qi* 黄芪, *dang gui* 当归, *chuan xiong* 川芎, *chi shao* 赤芍, *hong hua* 红花, *tao ren* 桃仁, and *di long* 地龙 (H20, H160–H162)
Bu chang nao xin tong jiao nang 步长脑心通胶囊	4	*Huang qi* 黄芪, *dan shen* 丹参, *dang gui* 当归, *chuan xiong* 川芎, *chi shao* 赤芍, *hong hua* 红花, *ru xiang* 乳香, *mo yao* 没药, *tao ren* 桃仁, *gui zhi* 桂枝, *ji xue teng* 鸡血藤, *niu xi* 牛膝, *sang zhi* 桑枝, *quan xie* 全蝎, *di long* 地龙, *and shui zhi* 水蛭 (H23, H24, H99, H103)
Fu fang hai she jiao nang 复方海蛇胶囊	3	*Hai she* 海蛇, *hai shen*, 海参, *yuan zhi* 远志, and *shi chang pu* 石菖蒲 (H5, H64, H101)
Cong sheng jiao nang 聪圣胶囊	3	*Zhi he shou wu* 制何首乌, *he ye* 荷叶, *di long* 地龙, *rou cong rong* 肉苁蓉, and *lou lu* 漏芦 (H1, H26, H29)
Kang xin jiao nang 康欣胶囊	3	*Nv zhen zi* 女贞子, *tu si zi* 菟丝子, *gou qi zi* 枸杞子, *he shou wu* 何首乌, *huang jing* 黄精, *huang qi* 黄芪, *yin yang huo* 淫羊藿, *dang gui* 当归, *dan shen* 丹参, *dan pi* 丹皮, *ju hua* 菊花, *shan zha* 山楂, and *suan zao ren* 酸枣仁 (H25, H38, H69)
Tian zhi ke li 天智颗粒	3	*Tian ma* 天麻, *gou teng* 钩藤, *shi jue ming* 石决明, *du zhong* 杜仲, *sang ji sheng* 桑寄生, *fu shen* 茯神, *ji xue teng* 鸡血藤, *huai hua* 槐花, *zhi zi* 栀子, *huang qin* 黄芩, *chuan niu xi* 川牛膝, and *yi mu cao* 益母草 (H3, H94, H140)
Modified *Di huang yin zi* 地黄饮子加减[1]	2	*Di huang* 地黄, *ba ji tian* 巴戟天, *shan zhu yu* 山茱萸, *rou cong rong* 肉苁蓉, *shi hu* 石斛, *zhi fu zi* 制附子, *wu wei zi* 五味子, *rou gui* 肉桂, *fu ling* 茯苓, *mai dong* 麦冬, *shi chang pu* 石菖蒲, *yuan zhi* 远志, *sheng jiang* 生姜, *da zao* 大枣, and *bo he* 薄荷 (H136, H177)

Table 5.2 (*Continued*)

Formula Name	Frequency of Use	Main Ingredients (Studies)
Gou teng san 钩藤散	2	*Gou teng* 钩藤, *chen pi* 陈皮, *ban xia* 半夏, *mai dong* 麦冬, *fu ling* 茯苓, *ren shen* 人参, *ju hua* 菊花, *fang feng* 防风, *gan cao* 甘草, *shi gao* 石膏, and *sheng jiang* 生姜 (H122, H123)
Tong xin luo jiao nang 通心络胶囊	2	*Ren shen* 人参, *shui zhi* 水蛭, *quan xie* 全蝎, *tu bie chong* 土鳖虫, *wu gong* 蜈蚣, *chan tui* 蝉蜕, *chi shao* 赤芍, *bing pian* 冰片, *tan xiang* 檀香, *jiang xiang* 降香, *ru xiang* 乳香, and *suan zao ren* 酸枣仁 (H7, H63)
Yang xue qing nao ke li 养血清脑颗粒	2	*Dang gui* 当归, *chuan xiong* 川芎, *bai shao* 白芍, *shu di* 熟地, *gou teng* 钩藤, *ji xue teng* 鸡血藤, *zhen zhu mu* 珍珠母, *xia ku cao* 夏枯草, *yan hu suo* 延胡索, *jue ming zi* 决明子, and *xi xin* 细辛 (H76, H81)
Qi shen huan wu jiao nang 芪参还五胶囊	2	*Huang qi* 黄芪, *di long* 地龙, *bing pian* 冰片, *bai jiang can* 白僵蚕, *qin jiao* 秦艽, *cu da huang* 醋大黄, *shui zhi* 水蛭, *chuan xiong* 川芎, *dang gui* 当归, *gou teng* 钩藤, *yuan zhi* 远志, *zhi zi* 栀子, and *yu jin* 郁金 (H13, H56)

Notes: (1) Ingredients were sourced from *Zhong Yi Fang Ji Da Ci Dian* 中医方剂大辞典 and (2) the use of some herbs may be restricted in some countries. Readers are advised to comply with relevant regulations.

The herbs most frequently used as ingredients in the CHM interventions that were tested in the RCTs are listed in Table 5.3. *Acorus* species (*chang pu* 菖蒲) were used in 111 formulae, with 92 of these specifying *shi chang pu* 石菖蒲. *Ligusticum chuangxiong* Hort. (*chuan xiong* 川芎) was used in 91 formulae. *Polygonum multiflorum* Thunb. (*he shou wu* 何首乌) was used in 87 formulae. *Astragalus membranaceus* (Fisch.) Bge. (*huang qi* 黄芪) was used in 73 formulae. Other high frequency formulae ingredients included *dan shen* 丹参, *dang gui* 当归, *yuan zhi* 远志, and *shui zhi* 水蛭.

Table 5.3 Frequently Used Herbs in Randomised Controlled Trials

Herb Name	Scientific Name	Frequency of Use
Chang pu 菖蒲 (*shi chang pu* 石菖蒲)	*Acorus* spp. (*A. tatarinowii* Schott)	111 (92)
Chuan xiong 川芎	*Ligusticum chuangxiong* Hort.	91
He shou wu 何首乌	*Polygonum multiflorum* Thunb.	87
Huang qi 黄芪	*Astragalus membranaceus* (Fisch.) Bge.	73
Dan shen 丹参	*Salvia miltiorrhiza* Bge.	65
Dang gui 当归	*Angelica sinensis* (Oliv.) Diels	65
Yuan zhi 远志	*Polygala tenuifolia* Willd.	55
Shui zhi 水蛭	*Hirudo* or *Whitmania* spp.	50
Shu di huang 熟地黄	*Rehmannia glutinosa* Libosch.	49
Gou qi zi 枸杞子	*Lycium barbarum* L.	47
Ren shen 人参	*Panax ginseng* C. A. Mey.	38
Hong hua 红花	*Carthamus tinctorius* L.	37
Yu jin 郁金	*Curcuma wenyujin* Y. H. Chen et C. Ling	37
Di long 地龙	*Pheretima.*	36
Shan zhu yu 山茱萸	*Cornus officinalis* Sieb. et Zucc.	35
Chi shao 赤芍	*Paeonia lactiflora* Pall.	34
Tao ren 桃仁	*Prunus persica* (L.) Batsch.	33
Dan nan xing 胆南星	*Arisaema erubescens* (Wall.) Schott.	29
Fu ling 茯苓	*Poria cocos* (Schw.) Wolf	27
Ban xia 半夏	*Pinellia ternata* (Thunb.) Breit.	27

Note: The use of some herbs may be restricted in some countries. Readers are advised to comply with relevant regulations.

Risk of Bias

In general, the studies published in Chinese were more concise than those published in English and tended to provide less information on methodological aspects. Although all studies specified that 'randomisation' was used in the allocation of participants to CHM intervention and control groups, the majority of studies (77.2%) did not clearly specify the method of randomisation and a small percentage (6.1%) specified a method considered 'high' risk, such as allocation based on the

Table 5.4 Risk of Bias of Randomised Controlled Trials of Chinese Herbal Medicine

Risk of Bias Domain	Low Risk *n* (%)	Unclear Risk *n* (%)	High Risk *n* (%)
Sequence generation	30 (16.7)	139 (77.2)	11 (6.1)
Allocation concealment	0 (0)	180 (100)	0 (0)
Blinding of participants	15 (8.3)	2 (1.1)	163 (90.6)
Blinding of personnel	11 (6.1)	5 (2.8)	164 (91.1)
Blinding of outcome assessors	1 (0.5)	14 (7.8)	165 (91.7)
Incomplete outcome assessment	171 (95.0)	3 (1.7)	6 (3.3)
Selective outcome reporting	0 (0)	180 (100)	0 (0)

visiting order of the participants. No study described how allocation was concealed in detail. Only a few studies (8.3%) specified the use of blinding for participants and it appeared unlikely that the interventions in the other studies could have been blinded to participants, so the majority (90.6%) were considered 'high' risk for blinding of participants. The proportion was similar for blinding of personnel (91.1%) and outcome assessors (91.7%), since it was plausible that lack of blinding could have affected assessment of the neuropsychological scales. Incomplete outcome data was mostly judged as 'low' risk of bias. No protocols were identified for any of the studies (either in electronic databases or clinical trial registers), so all studies were assessed as 'unclear' risk of bias for selective reporting. Overall, the methodological quality was 'low' and results should be interpreted with caution as none of the studies were free from potential bias. See Table 5.4 for a summary.

Results of Meta-analyses of Outcome Measures

In the following section, the meta-analyses results are presented first for the RCTs and second for the CCTs. For the RCTs, results were available for the following outcome measures:

- Mini-Mental State Examination (MMSE)
- Hamilton Depression Scale (HDS)

- Alzheimer's Disease Assessment Scale — cognitive subscale (ADAS-cog)
- activities of daily living (ADL)
- Functional Activities Questionnaire (FAQ)
- Blessed Behavior Scale (BBS)
- Clock drawing test (CDT)
- Wechsler Memory Scale (WMS)
- Wechsler Adult Intelligence Scale (WAIS)
- Neuropsychiatric Inventory (NPI)
- Clinical Dementia Rating (CDR).

Within each outcome are groups for the type of comparison: oral CHM vs. inactive controls, oral CHM vs. pharmacotherapy, and integrative medicine (i.e., oral CHM plus pharmacotherapy vs. the same pharmacotherapy). In addition, the results from the meta-analyses are grouped according to the specific control intervention where possible.

Mini-Mental State Examination

MMSE is a commonly used outcome measure for problems with memory or other cognitive abilities. It can be used by clinicians to help diagnose dementia and to help assess its progression and severity. On this 30-point scale, higher scores indicate less cognitive impairment. Meta-analyses are reported in separate tables for comparisons between:

- Oral CHM vs. inactive controls (4 RCTs).
- Oral CHM alone vs. pharmacotherapy alone (106 RCTs).
- Integrative CHM (38 RCTs).

Chinese Herbal Medicine vs. Inactive Controls

For the three RCTs (H1, H2, H157) that compared oral CHMs (H1 *Cong sheng jiao nang* 聪圣胶囊, H2 *Bu shen yi zhi ke li* 补肾益智颗粒, and H157 *Jian nao yi zhi ke li* 健脑益智颗粒) with a placebo

Table 5.5 Chinese Herbal Medicine vs. Inactive Control: Mini-mental State Examination at the End of Treatment

Comparator	No. of Studies (Participants), Duration	Effect Size (MD [95% CI], I^2)	Included Studies
Placebo	3 (253), 8–12 wks	3.39 [1.77, 5.01]*, 59%	H1, H2, H157
No treatment	1 (113), 8 wks	2.58 [1.65, 3.51]*	H3

*Statistically significant. Abbreviations: CI, confidence interval; EoT, end of treatment; MD, mean difference; wks, weeks.

Note: H1 and H157 were three-group studies.

(n = 253), the meta-analysis of the mean difference (MD) showed that there was a significant difference between the oral CHM groups and the placebo groups at the end of treatment (EoT) (MD: 3.39 [1.77, 5.01], I^2 = 59%) (Table 5.5). In another study (H3), patients with VaD in the control group only received routine medications to treat vascular risk factors (e.g., anti-platelet aggregation drugs, anti-hypertensive drugs, hypoglycemic drugs, and anti-hyperlipidemic drugs). The intervention group added *Tian zhi ke li* 天智颗粒 to the routine medications. The result suggested that *Tian zhi ke li* 天智颗粒 was superior to routine supportive treatment alone (MD: 2.58 [1.65, 3.51]) (Table 5.5).

Chinese Herbal Medicine vs. Pharmacotherapy

Of the RCTs that used pharmacotherapy as controls, 106 met the inclusion criteria (H1, H4–H100, H142–H144, H157, H158, H171, H174, H179). A total of 8,644 people participated in these RCTs and their mean age ranged from 46 to 85 years. The main pharmacotherapy controls were as follows: (1) acetylcholinesterase inhibitors (AChEI) — Donepezil and huperzine A; (2) calcium channel antagonists — nimodipine and flunarizine; (3) ergot alkaloids — nicergoline, co-dergocrine mesylate (hydergine), and dihydroergotoxine injection; and (4) nootropics: Piracetam, aniracetam, and oxiracetam. The treatment duration of these studies ranged from three to 24 weeks. In addition, nine studies used multiple pharmacotherapies in their control groups. These studies (H16, H100, H142–H144, H158, H171, H174, H179) were not analysed separately and are thus included in the total pooled result.

The meta-analysis result for the total pool of 106 studies showed that the oral CHM groups had higher MMSE scores than control groups (MD: 1.76 [1.48, 2.04], $I^2 = 74\%$), but the heterogeneity was substantial. Subgroup analyses were conducted according to the different pharmacotherapy controls and the results are listed in Table 5.6. Sensitivity analysis was conducted for studies judged 'low' risk for sequence generation (SG).

Chinese Herbal Medicine vs. Donepezil

Five RCTs employed comparisons with the AChEI donepezil (H4–H8). Study durations ranged from eight to 24 weeks, with 358 participants enrolled in RCTs. At the EoT, there was no significant difference between the oral CHM and donepezil groups (MD: 0.14 [–0.85, 1.13], $I^2 = 0\%$).

Chinese Herbal Medicine vs. Huperzine A

Huperzine A can selectively inhibit acetylcholinesterase activity and facilitate the increase in acetylcholine levels in the brain, thereby improving cognitive function in patients with dementia.[11] Meta-analysis of eight studies (H9–H15, H17; $n = 796$ participants) showed that oral CHM therapy groups had significantly higher MMSE scores than the huperzine A groups, with considerable heterogeneity (MD: 1.81 [0.35, 3.28], $I^2 = 82\%$).

Chinese Herbal Medicine vs. Nimodipine

The six RCTs of oral CHM vs. nimodipine (H18–H23, $n = 455$ participants) had durations of eight to 12 weeks. The oral CHM groups were superior to the nimodipine groups at the EoT, with considerable heterogeneity (MD: 2.33 [0.39, 4.26], $I^2 = 93\%$).

Table 5.6 Chinese Herbal Medicine vs. Pharmacotherapy: Subgroup Analyses of Mini-mental State Examination at the End of Treatment

Comparator	No. of Studies (Participants), Duration	Effect Size (MD: [95% CI], I^2)	Included Studies
Donepezil	5 (358), 8–24 wks	0.14 [–0.85, 1.13], 0%	H4–H8
Huperzine A	8 (796), 4–24 wks	1.81 [0.35, 3.28]*, 82%	H9–H15, H17
Nimodipine	6 (455), 8–12 wks	2.33 [0.39, 4.26]*, 93%	H18–H23
Flunarizine	1 (60), 24 wks	2.65 [1.12, 4.18]*	H24
Co-dergocrine mesylate	29 (2,084), 4–24 wks	1.25 [0.83, 1.67]*, 53%	H1, H25–H51, H157
Dihydroergotoxine injection	1 (120), 6 wks	1.68 [0.59, 2.77]*	H52
Nicergoline	3 (185), 12 wks	2.84 [1.15, 4.54]*, 35%	H53–H55
Piracetam	38 (3,368), 4–24 wks	1.81 [1.45, 2.16]*, 52%	H56–H93
Oxiracetam	2 (125), 8–12 wks	–0.68 [–1.89, 0.52], 0%	H95
Aniracetam	4 (308), 8–24 wks	1.74 [0.64, 2.84]*, 20%	H96–H99
Total pool[1]	106 (8,844), 4–24 wks	1.76 [1.48, 2.04]*, $I^2 = 74\%$	H1, H4–H100, H142–H144, H157, H158, H171, H174, H179

*Statistically significant. Abbreviations: CI, confidence interval; MD, mean difference; wks, weeks.

Note: (1) Includes 9 studies of comparisons between CHMs and multiple pharmacotherapies.

Chinese Herbal Medicine vs. Flunarizine

One study (H24) showed that *Bu chang nao xin tong jiao nang* 步长脑心通胶囊 significantly improved scores on the MMSE compared with flunarizine at the EoT after 6 months of treatment (MD: 2.65 [1.12, 4.18], *n* = 60 participants).

Chinese Herbal Medicine vs. Co-dergocrine Mesylate

In the 29 RCTs (H1, H25–H51, H157; *n* = 2,084 participants) that compared oral CHM with co-dergocrine mesylate, the pooled result showed significantly higher MMSE scores in the oral CHM groups vs. the co-dergocrine mesylate groups at the EoT, with moderate heterogeneity (MD: 1.25 [0.83, 1.67], $I^2 = 53\%$).

Chinese Herbal Medicine vs. Dihydroergotoxine Injection

In one RCT (H52), a CHM decoction based on the herbs *shan zhu yu* 山茱萸, *he shou wu* 何首乌, *huang jing* 黄精, *yuan zhi* 远志, *shi chang pu* 石菖蒲, *jiang can* 僵蚕, *dan nan xing* 胆南星, *yu jin* 郁金, *dan shen* 丹参, and *chi shao* 赤芍 and was modified according to the syndrome was superior to dihydroergotoxine injection at the EoT (MD 1.68 [0.59, 2.77]).

Chinese Herbal Medicine vs. Nicergoline

Three RCTs (H53–H55, *n* = 185 participants) compared an oral CHM to nicergoline. The meta-analysis found that the oral CHM had higher MMSE scores than the nicergoline groups at the EoT (MD: 2.84 [1.15, 4.54], $I^2 = 35\%$).

Chinese Herbal Medicine vs. Piracetam

The 38 RCTs (H56–H93; *n* = 3,368 participants) of oral CHM vs. piracetam had durations of four to 24 weeks. The oral CHM groups were found to be superior to the piracetam groups at the EoT, with moderate heterogeneity (MD: 1.81 [1.45, 2.16], $I^2 = 52\%$).

Chinese Herbal Medicine vs. Oxiracetam

In the two RCTs (*n* = 125 participants) that compared oral CHM with oxiracetam (H94, H95), the pooled result showed no significant difference between oral CHM and oxiracetam at the EoT (MD: –0.68 [–1.89, 0.52], $I^2 = 0\%$).

Chinese Herbal Medicine vs. Aniracetam

Four studies (H96–H99) assessed the effects of oral CHM vs. aniracetam on cognition using the MMSE (*n* = 308 participants). The pooled result found greater benefits in the oral CHM intervention groups compared to the aniracetam groups at the EoT, without heterogeneity (MD: 1.74 [0.64, 2.84], I^2 = 20%).

Sensitivity Analysis

Eighteen studies that investigated the efficacy of oral CHM for VaD were judged as 'low' risk for sequence generation (H7, H13, H14, H20, H25, H31, H33, H34, H38, H45, H55, H59, H72, H82, H85, H87, H88, H100). The pooled result showed a significant benefit for the oral CHM groups compared to pharmacotherapy controls, with substantial heterogeneity (MD: 1.59 [0.83, 2.35], I^2 = 79%, *n* = 1,553 participants).

Integrative Chinese Herbal Medicine

A total of 38 RCTs (*n* = 2,765) investigated the effects of oral integrative CHM (H4, H5, H27, H101–H121, H145–H154, H165–H167, H176), which combined oral CHM with a pharmacotherapy, vs. the same pharmacotherapy without the CHM. The pharmacotherapies included donepezil, huperzine A, nimodipine, co-dergocrine mesylate, piracetam, oxiracetam, aniracetam, citicoline injection, sodium monosialotetrahexosylganglioside injection, and combinations of drugs used in VaD. The results of the meta-analysis of the total pool suggested that integrative CHM was superior to pharmacotherapy alone at the EoT, with moderate heterogeneity (MD: 1.99 [1.66, 2.32], I^2 = 42%).

Subgroup analyses of integrative CHM were conducted to evaluate the changes in MMSE scores at the EoT according to the different single pharmacotherapy controls. The results are listed in Table 5.7. Sensitivity analysis was conducted for studies judged as 'low' risk for SG.

Table 5.7 Integrative Chinese Herbal Medicine: Subgroup Analysis of Mini-mental State Examination at the End of Treatment

Comparator	No. of Studies (Participants), Duration	Effect Size (MD [95% CI], I^2)	Included Studies
Donepezil	5 (313), 8–24 wks	2.20 [1.18, 3.23]*, 0%	H4, H5, H101–H103
Huperzine A	2 (130), 4–12 wks	2.08 [0.38, 3.78]*, 68%	H104, H105
Nimodipine	3 (207), 8–12 wks	2.57 [1.49, 3.65]*, 43%	H106–H108
Co-dergocrine mesylate	4 (370), 4–12 wks	0.89 [–0.10, 1.88]*, 57%	H27, H109–H111
Aniracetam	3 (201), 4–12 wks	2.52 [1.00, 4.04]*, 56%	H112–H114
Piracetam	1 (77), 8 wks	2.57 [0.96, 4.18]*	H115
Oxiracetam	1 (60), 12 wks	1.20 [–0.53, 2.93]	H116
Citicoline injection	1 (98), 3 wks	2.01 [0.63, 3.39]*	H117
Sodium monosialotetra-hexosylganglioside injection	1 (46), 3 wks	5.41 [2.15, 8.67]*	H118
Total pool[1]	38 (2,765), 3–34 wks	1.99 [1.66, 2.32]*, I^2 = 42%	H4, H5, H27, H101–H121, H145–H154, H165–H167, H176

*Statistically significant. Abbreviations: CI, confidence interval; MD, mean difference; wks, weeks.

Note: (1) Includes 17 studies of comparisons between CHMs and multiple pharmacotherapies.

Chinese Herbal Medicine Plus Donepezil vs. Donepezil

Based on five RCTs (H4, H5, H101–H103; *n* = 313 participants) on integrative therapy using oral CHM plus donepezil compared to donepezil alone, there was a significant benefit of adding the oral CHM (MD: 2.20 [1.18, 3.23], I^2 = 0%).

Chinese Herbal Medicine Plus Huperzine A vs. Huperzine A

The two RCTs (H104, H105) of CHM plus huperzine A vs. huperzine A alone (*n* = 130 participants) both had durations of 12 weeks. The oral CHM plus huperzine A groups were superior to the control groups (huperzine A without CHM) at the EoT, with substantial heterogeneity (MD: 2.08 [0.38, 3.78], I^2 = 68%).

Chinese Herbal Medicine Plus Nimodipine vs. Nimodipine

The three RCTs (H106–H108) of CHM plus nimodipine vs. nimodipine (*n* = 207 huperzine A) had durations of 8 to 12 weeks. The integrative medicine groups were superior to the nimodipine without CHM groups at the EoT, with moderate heterogeneity (MD: 2.57 [1.49, 3.65], I^2 = 43%).

Chinese Herbal Medicine Plus Co-dergocrine Mesylate vs. Co-dergocrine Mesylate

Four RCTs with durations of four to 12 weeks (*n* = 370 participants) investigated comparisons between groups that received CHM plus co-dergocrine mesylate and groups that received co-dergocrine mesylate and no CHM (H27, H109–H111). The CHM plus co-dergocrine mesylate groups showed no significant increase in MMSE scores compared to the co-dergocrine mesylate-only groups, with moderate heterogeneity (MD: 0.89 [–0.10, 1.88], I^2 = 57%).

Chinese Herbal Medicine Plus Aniracetam vs. Aniracetam

The three RCTs (H112–H114) that compared oral CHM plus aniracetam to aniracetam alone (*n* = 201 participants) had durations of four to 12 weeks. The pooled result found oral CHM plus aniracetam groups to be superior to the aniracetam without CHM groups at the EoT, with moderate heterogeneity (MD: 2.52, [1.00, 4.04], I^2 = 56%).

Chinese Herbal Medicine Plus Other Pharmacotherapies

Four pharmacotherapies were investigated in one study each: piracetam (H115), oxiracetam (H116), citicoline injection (H117), and sodium monosialotetrahexosylganglioside injection (H118). For the single RCT that compared CHM plus oxiracetam vs. oxiracetam without the CHM, there was no significant difference between groups (MD: 1.20 [–0.53, 2.93]). However, the other three studies each showed a benefit in the integrative CHM groups (Table 5.7).

Sensitivity Analysis

In the nine studies of integrative CHM that were judged as 'low' risk for SG, there was a significant difference between groups (MD: 2.27 [1.63, 2.92], $I^2 = 16\%$, $n = 711$ participants), with reduced heterogeneity (H102, H104, H105, H110, H111, H112, H119–H121).

Summary for Mini-Mental State Examination

For the comparisons with placebo controls, the data suggests that the use of oral CHMs was associated with an improvement in MMSE scores based on two studies (H1, H2), with a similar result in the comparison with no treatment (H3). Considering the very small sample sizes and short durations of these RCTs, no firm conclusions regarding the efficacy of CHM are possible.

For the studies of oral CHM vs. pharmacotherapy, the pooled overall results showed a statistically significant increase in MMSE scores, with considerable heterogeneity. This suggests that it is more meaningful to consider the results for each of the comparisons separately. The subgroup analyses also suggested that oral CHMs might provide benefits when compared with a number of different pharmacotherapies at the EoT period, but CHMs were not found to be superior to donepezil or oxiracetam. Heterogeneity was also reduced in some of these subgroup analyses. The sensitivity analysis, according to 'low' risk of bias for SG, still showed a benefit for oral CHM, although substantial heterogeneity remained.

Used as integrative medicine, the addition of oral CHM increased the efficacy of the overall treatment. The meta-analysis results showed that there was a significant benefit of the integrative approach with 'moderate' heterogeneity. The subgroup analyses, according to the different controls, found that integrative CHM had an additional effect. Only one small study, which added a CHM to oxiracetam therapy, showed no statistical difference between the two groups. The benefit remained significant for the pool of nine studies judged as 'low' risk of bias for SG without important heterogeneity. Donepezil provides the most important comparison in these studies since this drug is recommended for dementia in international guidelines. The meta-analysis suggests that the effects of the oral CHMs used alone were not significantly different to the effect of donepezil, and combining oral CHMs with donepezil provided additional benefits compared to the use of donepezil alone, at least in the short-term (up to 24 weeks).

Hasegawa's Dementia Scale

HDS was used as an outcome measure in 90 RCTs. In three studies, the comparison was with a placebo and with pharmacotherapy in 64 RCTs. There were 23 studies of integrative medicine. On this 30-point scale, higher scores indicate less cognitive impairment.

Chinese Herbal Medicine vs. Placebo

Three RCTs (H122–H124) compared an oral CHM (*Choto san* 钩藤散 or *San bian wan* 三鞭丸) with a placebo (*n* = 235 participants). The results of the meta-analysis showed that there were significantly higher HDS scores in the oral CHM groups compared to the placebo groups at the EoT (Table 5.8).

Chinese Herbal Medicine vs. Pharmacotherapy

Sixty-four RCTs (*n* = 5,501 participants) that used HDS as an outcome measure had comparisons with a pharmacotherapy. Durations ranged from six to 24 weeks. Meta-analysis suggested that oral CHM and oral

Table 5.8 Chinese Herbal Medicine vs. Placebo: Hasegawa Dementia Scale at the End of Treatment

Intervention	No. of Studies (Participants), Duration	Effect Size (MD [95% CI], I^2)	Included Studies
Choto san 钩藤散	2 (176), 12 wks	2.26 [0.43, 4.08]*, 0%	H122, H123
San bian wan 三鞭丸	1 (59), 8 wks	4.69 [2.62, 6.76]*	H124
Total pool	3 (235), 8–12 wks	3.25 [1.47, 5.03]*, 38%	All above

*Statistically significant. Abbreviations: CI, confidence interval; MD, mean difference; wks, weeks.

CHM plus pharmacotherapy showed benefits to patients with VaD when compared to pharmacotherapy alone (MD: 3.08 [2.57, 3.59], I^2 = 93); however, the comparison showed considerable heterogeneity. Subgroup analyses were based on the comparator (Table 5.9) and a sensitivity analysis included studies judged as 'low' risk for SG.

Chinese Herbal Medicine vs. Huperzine A

Six RCTs (H9, H11–H14, H125) employed comparisons with huperzine A. Study durations ranged from eight to 24 weeks, with 642 participants enrolled in the RCTs. There was a significant increase in HDS scores in the oral CHM groups compared to the huperzine A groups at the EoT (MD: 3.06 [1.64, 4.48], I^2 = 82%) with considerable heterogeneity.

Chinese Herbal Medicine vs. Nimodipine

Meta-analysis of four studies (H18, H22, H126, H127) investigating oral CHM vs. nimodipine (n = 255 participants) showed that the oral CHM groups had significantly higher scores on the HDS than the nimodipine group, with low heterogeneity (MD: 3.41 [2.72, 4.11], I^2 = 21%).

Chinese Herbal Medicine vs. Co-dergocrine Mesylate

Ten studies (n = 592 participants) compared oral CHM with co-dergocrine mesylate (Table 5.9). The pooled result showed a significant difference

Table 5.9 Chinese Herbal Medicine vs. Pharmacotherapy: Subgroup Analysis of Hasegawa Dementia Scale at the End of Treatment

Comparator	No. of Studies (Participants), Duration	Effect Size (MD [95% CI], I^2)	Included Studies
Huperzine A	6 (642), 8–24 wks	3.06 [1.64, 4.48]*, 82%	H9, H11–H14, H125
Nimodipine	4 (255), 8–12 wks	3.41 [2.72, 4.11]*, 21%	H18, H22, H126, H127
Co-dergocrine mesylate	10 (592), 8–12 wks	1.28 [0.55, 2.02]*, 72%	H31, H33, H37, H42, H44, H46, H50, H51, H128, H129
Nicergoline	3 (185), 12 wks	4.42 [3.07, 5.77]*, 47%	H53–H55
Dihydroergotoxine	2 (172), 6–16 wks	4.63 [3.61, 5.64]*, 9%	H52, H130
Aniracetam	4 (341), 12–24 wks	4.41 [3.46, 5.37]*, 0%	H97, H99, H131, H132
Piracetam	21 (1,885), 4–24 wks	2.90 [1.89, 3.91]*, 91%	H67, H68, H72, H73, H75, H76, H79, H80, H83, H85, H87, H88, H90, H92, H93, H133–H138
Oxiracetam	1 (73), 8 wks	0.16 [–1.75, 2.07]	H95
Citicoline injection	1 (114), 8 wks	5.40 [3.44, 7.36]*	H168
Cerebroprotein hydrolysate injection	1 (142), 8 wks	3.11 [1.78, 4.44]*	H172
Total pool[1]	64 (5,501), 4–24 wks	3.08 [2.57, 3.59]*, 93%	H9, H11–14, H16, H18, H22, H31, H33, H37, H42, H44, H46, H50–55, H67, H68, H72, H73, H75, H76, H79, H80, H83, H85, H87, H88, H90, H92, H93, H95, H97, H99, H125–H139, H142, H144, H163, H168, H169, H171, H172, H175, H178–H180

*Statistically significant. Abbreviations: CI, confidence interval; MD, mean difference; wks, weeks.

Note: (1) Includes 11 studies of comparisons between CHMs and multiple pharmacotherapies.

in favour of oral CHMs at the EoT (MD: 1.28 [0.55, 2.02], $I^2 = 72\%$) with substantial heterogeneity.

Chinese Herbal Medicine vs. Nicergoline

Three RCTs (*n* = 185 participants) (H53–H55) compared oral CHMs to nicergoline and reported HDS scores as one of the outcomes. The results indicated that the oral CHM groups were superior to the nicergoline controls on HDS at the EoT (MD: 4.42 [3.07, 5.77], $I^2 = 47\%$) with moderate heterogeneity.

Chinese Herbal Medicine vs. Dihydroergotoxine

Two RCTs (*n* = 172 participants) (H52, H130) found that oral CHM decoctions were superior to dihydroergotoxine on HDS at the EoT (MD: 4.63 [3.61, 5.64], $I^2 = 9\%$).

Chinese Herbal Medicine vs. Aniracetam

Four studies (*n* = 341 participants) of oral CHM compared with aniracetam evaluated changes in HDS (H97, H99, H131, H132). The results indicated that oral CHM produced greater improvements in HDS scores than aniracetam at the EoT (MD: 4.41 [3.46, 5.37], $I^2 = 0\%$).

Chinese Herbal Medicine vs. Piracetam

Twenty-one oral CHM studies (*n* = 1,885 participants) used piracetam as a comparator and reported on HDS scores. Meta-analysis showed that the oral CHM groups were superior to the piracetam groups at the EoT (MD: 2.90, [1.89, 3.91], $I^2 = 91\%$), but the heterogeneity was considerable.

Chinese Herbal Medicine vs. Oxiracetam

In the single study (H95) that compared *Nao xue shu tong kou fu ye* 脑血疏通口服液 to oxiracetam capsules (*n* = 73 participants), the scores on the HDS showed no statistical difference between the two groups (MD: 0.16 [–1.75, 2.07]).

Sensitivity Analysis

Ten studies of oral CHM, compared with pharmacotherapy, were judged as 'low' risk of bias for SG (H13, H14, H31, H33, H55, H72, H85, H87, H88, H135). The pooled result showed a significant increase in HDS scores in the CHM groups (MD: 3.24 [1.87, 4.61], I^2 = 90%, *n* = 845 participants), albeit with considerable heterogeneity.

Integrative Chinese Herbal Medicine

Twenty-three RCTs (*n* = 1,922 participants) explored the efficacy and safety of integrative CHM (H102, H105, H107, H115, H117, H120, H130, H139–H141, H146–H148, H150, H153, H156, H160–H162, H164, H165, H173, H177) and reported results for HDS. The results of meta-analysis suggested that the HDS scores in the oral CHM plus pharmacotherapy groups were significantly higher compared with the pharmacotherapy alone groups at the EoT (MD: 3.15 [2.56, 3.74], I^2 = 89%), with considerable heterogeneity. Most of the studies used multiple drugs in combination as comparators. The subgroup analyses are limited to studies that included a single specific pharmacotherapy (Table 5.10).

One study of *Yin dan xin nao tong yuan jiao nang* 银丹心脑通软胶囊 (main ingredients: *yin xing ye* 银杏叶, *dan shen* 丹参, *deng zhan xi xin* 灯盏细辛, and *san qi* 三七) combined with donepezil (H102) found no significant difference between groups after 24 weeks. Another study of *Qing xin hua tan tang* 清心化痰汤 (main ingredients: *lian xin* 莲心, *huang lian* 黄连, *yuan zhi* 远志, *dan nan xing* 胆南星, and *shi chang pu* 石菖蒲) combined with huperzine A (H105) found a significant improvement in HDS scores after four weeks of treatment.

Sensitivity Analysis

The pooled HDS result for the three RCTs judged as 'low' risk of bias for SG (H102, H105, H120) that compared integrative CHM with pharmaceutical controls showed a significant increase in HDS scores in the CHM groups with reduced heterogeneity (MD: 2.22 [0.72, 3.72], I^2 = 63%, *n* = 209 participants).

Table 5.10 Integrative Chinese Herbal Medicine: Subgroup Analysis of Hasegawa Dementia Scale at the End of Treatment

Comparator	No. of Studies (Participants), Duration	Effect Size (MD [95% CI], I^2)	Included Studies
Donepezil	1 (79), 24 wks	1.83 [−1.21, 4.87]	H102
Huperzine A	1 (70), 4 wks	1.51 [1.19, 1.83]*	H105
Nimodipine	2 (140), 5–12 wks	1.00 [−0.02, 2.02], 75%	H107, H139
Co-dergocrine mesylate	1 (66), 8 wks	2.92 [0.52, 5.32]*	H140
Piracetam	1 (77), 8 wks	4.57 [3.15, 5.99]*	H115
Citicoline injection	2 (196), 3–6 wks	3.16 [1.71, 4.60]*, 15%	H117, H141
Total pool[1]	23 (1,922) 3–24 wks	3.15 [2.56, 3.74]*, 89%	H102, H105, H107, H115, H117, H120, H130, H139–H141, H146–H148, H150, H153, H156, H160–H162, H164, H165, H173, H177

*Statistically significant. Abbreviations: CI, confidence interval; MD, mean difference; wks, weeks.

Note: (1) Includes 15 studies of comparisons between CHMs and multiple pharmacotherapies.

Summary for Hasegawa's Dementia Scale

In the comparisons with placebo, oral CHM showed a significant short-term benefit for VaD patients. When oral CHMs were compared with all pharmacotherapies, it was found that oral CHMs were superior. In the comparisons with particular pharmacotherapies, only oral CHM vs. oxiracetam showed no significant difference, but this result was based on one study with a small sample size. No comparisons were conducted with donepezil.

Similarly, the results for integrative CHM showed an overall benefit at the EoT for adding CHMs to pharmacotherapies. Most of the integrative CHM studies that assessed outcomes with the HDS used different comparators. Only the comparisons with nimodipine and citicoline injection involved two studies. Subgroup meta-analysis suggested that oral CHM plus nimodipine was not significantly superior to nimodipine alone. A similar result was found in the single 24-week study which used donepezil as the comparator.

Alzheimer's Disease Assessment Scale — Cognitive Subscale

ADAS-cog is a 70-point scale in which lower scores indicate less cognitive impairment. Two three-armed studies (oral CHM vs. donepezil vs. oral CHM plus donepezil) were included in the meta-analyses. One study (n = 90 participants) compared *Huang pu tong qiao jiao nang* 黄蒲通窍胶囊 (main ingredients: *Shi chang pu* 石菖蒲, *yi zhi ren* 益智仁, *zhi he shou wu* 制何首乌, *chuan xiong* 川芎, *da huang* 大黄, and *ren shen* 人参) with donepezil (H4) for eight weeks. Compared to donepezil, there was no significant difference between groups at the end of eight weeks of treatment (MD: 0.54 [–5.43, 6.51], n = 60 participants) and there was a significant decrease in ADAS-cog scores in the integrative group (MD: –5.85 [–11.64, –0.06], n = 60 participants). The other study (H5), which had 63 participants, compared *Fu fang hai she jiao nang* 复方海蛇胶囊 (see Table 5.2 for ingredients) with donepezil for 24 weeks. There was no significant difference between groups for the CHM group compared with the donepezil group (MD: 1.30 [–3.13, 5.73], n = 40 participants) or in the comparison between the integrative group and donepezil (MD: –1.90 [–5.61, 1.81], n = 42 participants).

In the pooled results, there were no significant differences in ADAS-cog scores between groups for the comparison between CHM and donepezil. There was also no significant additional benefit from combining the CHMs with donepezil (Table 5.11).

Summary for Alzheimer's Disease Assessment Scale — Cognitive Subscale

No comparison with an inactive control was available. In the comparisons with active controls, only two studies comparing oral CHM with donepezil were included. The results suggested that use of oral CHM or oral CHM plus pharmacotherapy was not significantly different from

Table 5.11 Chinese Herbal Medicine vs. Donepezil: Alzheimer's Disease Assessment Scale — Cognitive Subscale at the End of Treatment

Intervention	No. of Studies (Participants), Duration	Effect Size (MD [95% CI], I^2)	Included Studies
Oral CHM	2 (100), 8–24 wks	1.03 [−2.53, 4.59], 0%	H4, H5
Oral CHM plus donepezil	2 (102), 8–24 wks	−3.23 [−6.88, 0.43], 21%	H4, H5

Abbreviations: CHM, Chinese herbal medicine; CI, confidence interval; MD, mean difference; wks, weeks.

donepezil alone, although the result for the integrative therapy group was suggestive of a trend. However, because these results were based on the same two RCTs, which had relatively small sample sizes, no conclusions could be drawn.

Activities of Daily Living

There were 83 studies that used ADL as an outcome. Three RCTs were three-armed studies. While there were several versions of ADL scales used, the specific version of the ADL scales for most of the studies could not be determined based on the information provided. In seven studies, versions of the Barthel Index (BI) were specified, and two studies mentioned the application of a 20-item version of ADL. We tried to contact the authors of the studies that had unclear sources of ADL scales through email, letter, or telephone, but replies were very few. In order to conduct meta-analysis, studies were grouped according to the direction of the ADL scale; that is, whether improvement was indicated by a lower score (i.e., 'lower is better') or a higher score (i.e., 'higher is better'). The MD was used to pool identical scales and the standardised mean difference (SMD) was used when the pool contained studies that may have employed different versions of ADL scales. Random effects models were used for MD and SMD. Meta-analyses are reported separately for comparisons between:

- Oral CHM vs. placebo (1 RCT).
- Oral CHM vs. pharmacotherapy (54 RCTs).
- Integrative CHM (31 RCTs) (Table 5.12).

Table 5.12 Chinese Herbal Medicine vs. Placebo or Pharmacotherapy: Activities of Daily Living at the End of Treatment

Comparison (ADL Scale)	No. of Studies (Participants) Duration	Effect Size (SMD [95% CI], I^2)	Included Studies
Oral CHM vs. placebo 'lower is better'	1 (70), 12 wks	−1.09 [−1.60, −0.58]*	H2
Oral CHM vs. pharmacotherapy 'lower is better'	44 (3,526), 4–24 wks	−0.66 [−0.88, −0.43]* 90%	H4–H6, H14, H17–H20, H24, H25, H27, H29, H34, H36, H38, H39, H41, H43, H45–H47, H50, H54, H56, H57 H62, H64–H67, H71, H75, H79, H81, H82, H89–H91, H94–H96, H133, H142, H143
Oral CHM vs. Pharmacotherapy (higher is better)	10 (759), 4–12 wks	0.80 [0.22, 1.38]* 93%	H7, H13, H21, H69, H52, H85, H87, H100, H128, H144

*Statistically significant. Abbreviations: ADL, activities of daily living; CHM, Chinese herbal medicine; CI, confidence interval; SMD, standardised mean difference.

Chinese Herbal Medicine vs. Placebo

One RCT ($n = 70$ participants) of 12 weeks duration (H2) compared *Bu shen yi zhi ke li* 补肾益智颗粒 (main ingredients: *Ying yang huo* 淫羊藿, *gou qi* 枸杞, *shou wu* 首乌, *huang qi* 黄芪, *huang jing* 黄精, *san qi* 三七, and *shi chang pu* 石菖蒲) with placebo and employed a 'lower is better' ADL scale. The result indicated that there was a significant improvement in ADL in the CHM group at the EoT (SMD: −1.09 [−1.60, −0.58]) (Table 5.12).

Chinese Herbal Medicine vs. Pharmacotherapy

Fourty-four studies ($n = 3{,}526$ participants) that compared oral CHM to a pharmacotherapy employed 'lower is better' ADL scales. The meta-analysis showed that the oral CHMs were superior to the pharmacotherapy controls (SMD: −0.66 [−0.88, −0.43], $I^2 = 90\%$), albeit with considerable heterogeneity (Table 5.12). In the 10 studies that used 'higher is better' ADL scales (*n* = 759 participants), the oral CHM groups had significantly higher scores (SMD: 0.80 [0.22, 1.38], I^2 = 93%) compared to the control groups at the EoT (Table 5.12).

Subgroup analyses were based on the comparator and type of ADL scale. Sensitivity analyses were based on 'low' risk of bias for SG.

Studies Using 'Lower is Better' Activities of Daily Living Scales

Three RCTs (H4–H6), which included 160 patients with VaD, compared oral CHM with a donepezil control (Table 5.13). There was an improvement based on 'lower is better' ADL scales within the oral CHM groups, but there was no difference between groups at the EoT (SMD: 0.15 [–0.35, 0.64], I^2 = 59%). Comparisons with huperzine A were conducted in two RCTs (H14, H17; *n* = 156 participants), which found no significant difference between groups at the EoT (SMD: –2.66 [–6.43, 1.11], I^2 = 98%). In the comparisons with nimodipine, the pooled result for three studies (H18–H20) showed a greater improvement in the CHM groups (MD: –1.02 [–1.98, –0.05], I^2 = 90%); however, heterogeneity was considerable.

Seven RCTs of oral CHM compared to pharmacotherapy were judged as having 'low' risk for SG (H14, H20, H25, H34, H38, H45, H82). The pooled result for 'lower is better' ADL scores was still significant between groups (SMD: –0.97 [–1.86, –0.09], I^2 = 96%, *n* = 652 participants); however, heterogeneity was not reduced.

Studies Using 'Higher is Better' Activities of Daily Living Scales

Of the 10 studies that compared oral CHMs with pharmacotherapies for VaD using 'higher is better' ADL scales, one study (H7) found that the effect of *Tong xin luo jiao nang* 通心络胶囊 (see Table 5.2 for ingredients) was not significantly different from that of donepezil (SMD: –0.26 [–0.63, 0.10]). Another study (H13) indicated that *Qi shen huan wu jiao nang* 芪参还五胶囊 (main ingredients: *Huang qi* 黄芪,

Table 5.13 Chinese Herbal Medicine vs. Pharmacotherapy: Subgroup Analysis of 'Lower is Better' Activities of Daily Living at the End of Treatment

Comparator	No. of Studies (Participants), Duration	Effect Size (SMD [95% CI], I²)	Included Studies
Donepezil	3 (160), 8–24 wks	0.15 [–0.35, 0.64], 59%	H4–H6
Huperzine A	2 (156), 4–8 wks	–2.66 [–6.43, 1.11], 98%	H14, H17
Nimodipine	3 (258), 8–12 wks	–1.02 [–1.98, –0.05]*, 90%	H18–H20
Flunarizine	1 (60), 24 wks	–2.12 [–2.76, –1.48]*	H24
Nicergoline	1 (65), 12 wks	–2.08 [–2.69, –1.47]*	H54
Co-dergocrine mesylate	13 (828), 4–24 wks	–0.20 [–0.41, 0.02], 64%	H25, H27, H29, H34, H36, H38, H39, H41, H43, H45–H47, H50
Piracetam	16 (1,462), 8–24 wks	–0.75 [–1.12, –0.39]*, 90%	H56, H57, H62, H64–H67, H71, H75, H79, H81, H82, H89–H91, H133
Oxiracetam	2 (125), 8–12 wks	–0.53 [–1.48, 0.43], 85%	H94, H95
Aniracetam	1 (68), 12 wks	–0.38 [–0.86, 0.10]	H96
Meclofenoxate	1 (80), 24 wks	–0.38 [–0.82, 0.06]	H143

*Statistically significant. Abbreviations: CI, confidence interval; SMD, standardised mean difference; wks, weeks.

di long 地龙, *bing pian* 冰片, *bai jiang can* 白僵蚕, *qin jiao* 秦艽, *cu da huang* 醋大黄, *shui zhi* 水蛭, *chuan xiong* 川芎, *dang gui* 当归, *gou teng* 钩藤, *yuan zhi* 远志, *zhi zi* 栀子, and *yu jin* 郁金) was superior to huperzine A (SMD: 1.88 [1.26, 2.49]). In a comparison with nimodipine, one 12-week RCT (H21; *n* = 80 participants) reported superiority for a CHM decoction containing *zhi shou wu* 制首乌, *sang shen* 桑椹, *gou qi zi* 枸杞子, *dan shen* 丹参, *san qi* 三七, *tian ma* 天麻, and *bai shao* 白芍 at the EoT (SMD: 1.83 [1.30, 2.35]) (Table 5.14).

The pooled 'higher is better' ADL result for 4 RCTs that were judged as 'low' risk of bias for SG (H7, H85, H87, H100) showed no

Table 5.14 Chinese Herbal Medicine vs. Pharmacotherapy: Subgroup Analysis of 'Higher is Better' Activities of Daily Living at the End of Treatment

Comparator	No. of Studies (Participants), Duration	Effect Size (SMD [95% CI], I^2)	Included Studies
Donepezil	1 (118), 12 wks	–0.26 [–0.63, 0.10]	H7
Huperzine A	1 (60), 8 wks	1.88 [1.26, 2.49]*	H13
Nimodipine	1 (80), 12 wks	1.83 [1.30, 2.35]*	H21
Dihydroergotoxine injection	1 (120), 6 wks	0.48 [0.12, 0.84]*	H52
Co-dergocrine mesylate	1 (60), 12 wks	0.00 [–0.51, 0.51]	H128
Piracetam	3 (182), 4–12 wks	0.21 [–0.30, 0.72], 64%	H69, H85, H87

*Statistically significant. Abbreviations: CI, confidence interval; SMD, standardised mean difference; wks, weeks.

significant difference when oral CHM was compared with pharmacotherapy (SMD: 0.86 [–0.33, 2.05], $I^2 = 96\%$, $n = 320$ participants); however, heterogeneity was considerable.

Integrative Chinese Herbal Medicine

Integrative CHM improved the scores of 'lower is better' ADL in people with VaD compared to pharmacotherapy alone (SMD: –1.52 [–2.04, –1.01], $I^2 = 95\%$) based on 22 studies ($n = 1{,}688$ participants). However, heterogeneity was considerable in this pool (Table 5.15). In the comparisons for 'higher is better' ADL scores, the pooled result for nine studies ($n = 658$ participants) of oral CHM combined with pharmacotherapy showed a significant increase in scores (SMD: 0.85 [0.61, 1.10], $I^2 = 55\%$) compared to the pharmacotherapy-alone control groups at the EoT (Table 5.15).

Subgroup analyses were based on the specific pharmacotherapy combined with CHM and on the type of ADL scale. Sensitivity analyses were based on 'low' risk of bias for SG.

Table 5.15 Integrative Chinese Herbal Medicine: Activities of Daily Living at the End of Treatment

Comparison (ADL Scale)	No. of Studies (Participants), Duration	Effect Size (SMD [95% CI], I^2)	Included Studies
Oral CHM plus pharmacotherapy vs. pharmacotherapy alone 'lower is better'	22 (1,688), 3–24 wks	–1.52 [–2.04, –1.01]*, 95%	H4, H5, H17, H27, H102–H105, H108, H110, H112, H116–H118, H120, H145–H151
Oral CHM plus pharmacotherapy vs. pharmacotherapy alone 'higher is better'	9 (658), 5–12 wks	0.85 [0.61, 1.10]*, 55%	H106, H111, H113, H119, H121, H152–H155

*Statistically significant. Abbreviations: ADL, activities of daily living; CHM, Chinese herbal medicine; CI, confidence interval; SMD, standardised mean difference; wks, weeks.

Studies Using 'Lower is Better' Activities of Daily Living Scales

Five studies (H4, H5, H101–H103) of eight to 24 weeks in duration compared oral CHM plus donepezil with donepezil alone (n = 313 participants). The pooled result revealed that the integrative CHM groups were superior to the donepezil-alone groups (SMD: –0.49 [–0.86, –0.11], $I^2 = 63\%$); however, moderate heterogeneity remained. There was no additional benefit observed for CHM combined with huperzine A compared to huperzine A alone with considerable heterogeneity (SMD: –4.86 [–13.45, 3.74], $I^2 = 99\%$) based on 2 studies (H104, H105; n = 130 participants). For the two RCTs (H27, H110) of CHM combined with co-dergocrine mesylate (n = 250 participants), there was no significant difference between groups (SMD: –0.46 [–1.15, 0.22], $I^2 = 86\%$). Single studies investigated comparisions with nimodipine (H108), aniracetam (H112), oxiracetam (H116), citicoline injection (H117), and monosialotetrahexosylganglioside injection (H118). These reported significant improvements in the integrative CHM groups except for the comparison with oxiracetam (Table 5.16).

Table 5.16 Integrative Chinese Herbal Medicine: Subgroup Analysis of 'Lower is Better' Activities of Daily Living at the End of Treatment

Comparator	No. of Studies (Participants), Duration	Effect Size (SMD [95% CI], I^2)	Included Studies
Donepezil	5 (313), 6–12 wks	–0.49 [–0.86, –0.11]*, 63%	H4, H5, H101–H103
Huperzine A	2 (130), 4–12 wks	–4.86 [–13.45, 3.74], 99%	H104, H105
Nimodipine	1 (83), 8 wks	–1.88 [–2.41, –1.34]*	H108
Co-dergocrine mesylate	2 (250), 4–8 wks	–0.46 [–1.15, 0.22], 86%	H27, H110
Aniracetam	1 (66), 4 wks	–0.76 [–1.26, –0.26]*	H112
Oxiracetam	1 (60), 12 wks	–0.49 [–1.00, 0.02]	H116
Citicoline injection	1 (98), 3 wks	–0.42 [–0.82, –0.02]*	H117
Monosialotetra-hexosylganglioside injection	1 (46), 3 wks	–2.45 [–3.23, –1.67]*	H118

*Statistically significant. Abbreviations: CI, confidence interval; SMD, standardised mean difference; wks, weeks.

Studies Using 'Higher is Better' Activities of Daily Living Scales

Based on two studies (H106, H155; n = 144 participants), there was no significant benefit of combining oral CHM with nimodipine compared to nimodipine alone after 5–12 weeks of treatment (SMD: 0.52 [–0.27, 1.31], I^2 = 82%); however, heterogeneity was considerable (Table 5.17). In addition, one study (n = 68 participants) compared an oral CHM plus co-dergocrine mesylate with co-dergocrine mesylate alone (H111). The main herbs were *tai zi shen* 太子参, *mai dong* 麦冬, *wu wei zi* 五味子, *shan zhu yu* 山茱萸, *gou qi zi* 枸杞子, *yin yang huo* 淫羊藿, *huang qi* 黄芪, *chi shao* 赤芍, *di long* 地龙, *ge gen* 葛根, *dan shen* 丹参, *shu di huang* 熟地黄, and *zhi he shou wu*

Table 5.17 Integrative Chinese Herbal Medicine: Subgroup Analysis of 'Higher is Better' Activities of Daily Living at the End of Treatment

Comparator	No. of Studies (Participants), Duration	Effect Size (SMD [95% CI], I^2)	Included Studies
Nimodipine	2 (144), 5–12 wks	0.52 [–0.27, 1.31], 82%	H106, H155
Co-dergocrine mesylate	1 (68), 12 wks	1.31 [0.78, 1.84]*	H111
Aniracetam	1 (75), 12 wks	1.33 [0.82, 1.83]*	H113

*Statistically significant. Abbreviations: CI, confidence interval; SMD, standardised mean difference; wks, weeks.

制何首乌, with additions of *quan chong* 全虫 and *tao ren* 桃仁 for Blood stagnation (*yu xue* 瘀血); *tian ma* 天麻 and *gou teng* 钩藤 for dizziness and tinnitus; or *fa ban xia* 法半夏, *dan nan xing* 胆南星, and *chen pi* 陈皮 for excessive phlegm, bloating, and poor appetite. The result showed that the integrative CHM group was superior to the control group (SMD: 1.31 [0.78, 1.84]) after 12 weeks. Another study (H113) comparing oral CHM (based on *zhi shou wu* 制首乌, *gou qi zi* 枸杞子, *yin yang huo* 淫羊藿, *mai dong* 麦冬, *shu di huang* 熟地黄, *shan yu rou* 山萸肉, *ge gen* 葛根, *dan shen* 丹参, *di long* 地龙, and *chuan xiong* 川芎 with additions based on symptoms or syndrome) plus aniracetam to aniracetam alone found a similar result (SMD: 1.33 [0.82, 1.83]) after 12 weeks.

Sensitivity Analysis

For integrative CHM, six RCTs that used 'lower is better' ADL scales as one of the outcomes were judged as 'low' risk of bias for SG (H102, H104, H105, H110, H112, H120). At the EoT, there was a significant difference between groups based on 'lower is better' ADL scores in favor of CHM treatments (SMD: –1.44 [–2.47, –0.42], I^2 = 96%, n = 465 participants). However, heterogeneity was still considerable. For the three studies that were judged as 'low' risk of bias for SG (H111, H119, H121) and used 'higher is better' ADL scores, the results were still significant (SMD: 0.89 [0.53, 1.24], I^2 = 45%, n = 254 participants) with moderate heterogeneity.

Summary for Activities of Daily Living Scales

In comparison with placebo, only one study (H2) was included and the result indicated that oral CHM produced a significant improvement in ADL. As the sample size of this study was relatively small, firm conclusions could not be drawn. For the pooled meta-analyses, oral CHM alone or combined with pharmacotherapy appeared to improve ADL scores compared to pharmacotherapy alone in people with VaD and on both 'lower is better' and 'higher is better' ADL scales. But there was considerable heterogeneity in the results.

Compared to specific pharmacotherapies, the oral CHMs were not superior to donepezil on both kinds of ADL scales. However, the CHMs were significantly better than nimodipine on both types of ADL scales. Among the studies of integrative medicine, the five studies that combined CHM with donepezil showed superiority compared to donepezil alone on 'lower is better' ADL scales, but no data was available for 'higher is better' ADL scales. For CHM combined with nimodipine, there was an apparent benefit based on 'lower is better' ADL scales in one study, but not on 'higher is better' ADL scales based on two studies.

Although the sample sizes of the main pools were large, there was considerable diversity in the comparators and the scales which reduced the size of the subgroup pools. This combined with the considerable heterogeneity in some of the subgroups made it difficult to draw conclusions. Also, the clinical significance of these results is difficult to interpret since multiple scales were combined into an SMD analysis.

Functional Activities Questionnaire

FAQ is a standardised assessment of instrumental ADL. It is a commonly used social function scale measuring the current level of performance on 10 daily tasks. There were 13 RCTs that used FAQ as one of the outcomes to assess the efficacy of oral CHM in VaD. All comparisons were made with pharmacotherapies.

Twelve RCTs (n = 1,188 participants) compared oral CHM with a pharmacotherapy (Table 5.18). Durations ranged from eight to 24 weeks. The total pooled result showed that the oral CHMs were

Table 5.18 Chinese Herbal Medicine: Functional Activities Questionnaire at the End of Treatment

Comparator	No. of Studies (Participants), Duration	Effect Size (MD [95% CI], I^2)	Included Studies
Oral CHM vs. Pharmacotherapy			
All types of pharmacotherapy	12 (1,188), 8–24 wks	−1.41 [−2.26, −0.56]*, 74%	H11, H12, H18, H33, H72, H88, H99, H129, H131, H134, H135, H138
Huperzine A	2 (300), 24 wks	−0.22 [−0.91, 0.48], 0%	H11, H12
Nimodipine	1 (36), 8 wks	−0.71 [−3.91, 2.49]	H18
Co-dergocrine mesylate	2 (114), 8–12 wks	−2.99 [−8.35, 2.36], 85%	H33, H129
Piracetam	5 (518), 8–12 wks	−1.53 [−2.40, −0.67]*, 44%	H72, H88, H134, H135, H138
Aniracetam	2 (220), 12–24 wks	−1.76 [−2.93, −0.60]*, 95%	H99, H131
Oral CHM Plus Pharmacotherapy vs. Pharmacotherapy			
Piracetam	1 (96), 12wks	−4.60 [−6.90, −2.30]*	H156

*Statistically significant. Abbreviations: CHM, Chinese herbal medicine; CI, confidence interval; MD, mean difference; wks, weeks.

superior to pharmacotherapies (MD: −1.41 [−2.26, −0.56], $I^2 = 74\%$) at the EoT. Subgroup meta-analyses suggested that oral CHM showed greater benefit for patients with VaD than did piracetam or aniracetam, but there was no difference between groups for comparisons with huperzine, nimodipine, or co-dergocrine mesylate. The single study (H156) of integrative medicine found that a CHM decoction made by the authors (composed of: *Huang qi* 黄芪, *huang jing* 黄精, *shu di* 熟地, *shan yao* 山药, *gou qi zi* 枸杞子, *shui zhi* 水蛭, *shi chang pu* 石菖蒲, *yu jin* 郁金, *yi zhi ren* 益智仁, *tao ren* 桃仁, *hong hua* 红花, *di long* 地龙, and *sha ren* 砂仁) combined with piracetam was superior to piracetam alone after 12 weeks of treatment.

In the oral CHM groups, four studies were judged as 'low' risk for SG (H33, H72, H88, H135). The pooled result was significant in favour of oral CHMs (MD: –1.22 [–2.15, –0.29], $I^2 = 59\%$, $n = 443$ participants) compared to pharmacoptherapies, but with heterogeneity was still substantial.

Summary for Functional Activities Questionnaire

When oral CHM was compared with pharmacotherapy, the total pool found that oral CHM was superior to pharmacotherapy based on FAQ scores with substantial heterogeneity. However, significant differences were found only for the comparisons with piracetam and aniracetam, whereas in the comparisons with huperzine, nimodipine, and co-dergocrine mesylate, there were no significant differences between oral CHMs and pharmacotherapies. The single study that tested integrative CHM as the intervention (H156) reported a significant benefit for oral CHM plus piracetam. While the total pool was relatively large, the results for the subgroups were based on small numbers of studies and there were no comparisons done with donepezil, so the results are difficult to interpret.

Blessed Behaviour Scale

The BBS is a clinical rating scale derived from the Blessed Dementia Scale[13] that measures changes in performance on everyday activities, self-care habits, and changes in personality, interests, and drives. A close friend or relative is asked to provide behaviour ratings of the examinee during the preceding six months,[12] with lower scores indicating more improvement. The BBS was revised to 19 items and there are a total of 50 points in the Chinese version.[14] Fifteen RCTs evaluated the efficacy of oral CHMs compared to pharmacotherapies using the BBS. Three RCTs were three-armed studies and twelve were two-armed studies. Meta-analyses are reported separately for comparisons between:

- Oral CHM vs. placebo (2 RCTs).
- Oral CHM vs. pharmacotherapy (14 RCTs).
- Integrative CHM (2 RCTs).

Chinese Herbal Medicine vs. Placebo

Two RCTs (H1, H157; *n* = 183 participants) compared oral CHM with placebo. The result of the meta-analysis showed that there was no significant difference between the oral CHM groups and the placebo groups based on the BBS at the EoT (MD: –1.82 [–5.25, 1.60], I^2 = 86%); however, heterogeneity was considerable (Table 5.19).

Chinese Herbal Medicine vs. Pharmacotherapy

Fourteen RCTs (*n* = 1,293 participants) compared an oral CHM to pharmacotherapy and reported scores for the BBS. Meta-analysis found a significant overall reduction in the scores on the BBS for the oral CHM groups compared to pharmacotherapy (MD: –2.02 [–2.64, –1.41], I^2 = 84%). In the subgroup analyses, oral CHM showed superior effects compared to co-dergocrine mesylate, piracetam, and the

Table 5.19 Chinese Herbal Medicine: Blessed Behavior Scale at the End of Treatment

Comparator	No. of Studies (Participants), Duration	Effect Size (MD [95% CI], I^2)	Included Studies
Placebo	2 (183), 8 wks	–1.82 [–5.25, 1.60], 86%	H1, H157
All types of pharmacotherapy	14 (1,293), 4–24 wks	–2.02 [–2.64, –1.41]*, 84%	H1, H26, H27, H29, H30, H40, H43, H45, H49, H56, H59, H84, H157, H158
Co-dergocrine mesylate	10 (937), 4–24 wks	–2.03 [–2.83, –1.23]*, 84%	H1, H26, H27, H29, H30, H40, H43, H45, H49, H157
Piracetam	3 (278), 8–12 wks	–1.88 [–3.54, –0.23]*, 74%	H56, H59, H84
Piracetam plus nimodipine	1 (78), 12 wks	–2.12 [–3.09, –1.15]*	H158

*Statistically significant. Abbreviations: CI, confidence interval; MD, mean difference; wks, weeks.

combination of piracetam plus nimodipine (Table 5.19), but heterogeneity was considerable. For oral CHM vs. pharmacotherapy, only two studies (H45, H59) were judged as 'low' risk for SG. The pooled result of these two studies showed no significant difference between groups, with reduced heterogeneity (MD: –0.86 [–1.96, 0.24], $I^2 = 43\%$, $n = 324$ participants).

Integrative Chinese Herbal Medicine

As integrative therapy, the combination of oral CHM plus pharmacotherapy was more effective than pharmacotherapy alone (MD: –4.60 [–6.90, –2.30], $I^2 = 0\%$, $n = 220$ participants). However, there were only two studies included in the pool. One study (H27), which had three arms, found that CHM combined with co-dergocrine mesylate was better than co-dergocrine mesylate alone (MD: –3.63 [–5.70, –1.56], $n = 120$ participants) after four weeks. The CHM had the principal ingredients of *shi chang pu* 石菖蒲, *yu jin* 郁金, *yuan zhi* 远志, *shu di* 熟地, *chuan xiong* 川芎, *lu jiao jiao* 鹿角胶, and *he shou wu* 何首乌, with the addition of *huang qi* 黄芪, *bai zhu* 白术, and *fu ling* 茯苓 for Spleen deficiency (*pi xu* 脾虚); *gui ban* 龟版 and *e jiao* 阿胶 for Kidney deficiency (*shen xu* 肾虚); *tao ren* 桃仁 and *hong hua* 红花 for Blood stagnation (*yu xue* 瘀血); and *zhi ban xia* 制半夏 and *zhi nan xing* 制南星 for excessive phlegm (*tan sheng* 痰盛). The other study (H151) found that another CHM decoction (*bie jia* 鳖甲, *she gan* 射干, *huang qin* 黄芩, *chai hu* 柴胡, *shu fu* 鼠妇, *gan jiang* 干姜, *da huang* 大黄, *shao yao* 芍药, *gui zhi* 桂枝, *ting li* 葶苈, *shi wei* 石韦, *hou po* 厚朴, *dan pi* 丹皮, *qu mai* 瞿麦, *zi wei* 紫葳, *ban xia* 半夏, *ren shen* 人参, *jin chong* 䗪虫, *e jiao* 阿胶, *feng wo* 蜂窝, *chi xiao* 赤硝, *jiang lan* 蜣螂, and *tao ren* 桃仁) combined with piracetam, nimodipine, and aspirin enteric-coated tablets appeared superior to this combination of drugs without the CHM after 8 weeks of treatment (MD: –2.75 [–4.73, –0.77], $n = 100$ participants).

Summary for the Blessed Behaviour Scale

Meta-analysis found that oral CHMs were superior to pharmacotherapy but not to placebo, with considerable heterogeneity in both pools. The results of the subgroup meta-analyses were consistent with the overall meta-analysis of comparisons with pharmacotherapy. In the sensitivity analysis, there was no significant difference between groups in the two studies judged as 'low' risk of bias for SG. Integrative medicine appeared to be more beneficial compared with pharmacotherapy alone, but this was based on only two studies.

Other Outcome Measures Reported in Randomised Controlled Trials

Small numbers of RCTs reported data for the following outcome measures:

- CDT: 1 study
- WMS: 6 studies
- WAIS: 3 studies
- NPI: 2 studies
- CDR: 2 studies

Clock Drawing Test

One study (H19; *n* = 160 participants) reported data for this four-point scale in which higher scores indicate better cognition. It found a significant increase in CDT when oral CHM with the principal ingredients of *huang qi* 黄芪, *xi yang shen* 西洋参, *ge gen* 葛根, *tian ma* 天麻, and *shui zhi* 水蛭 was compared to nimodipine (MD: 0.38 [0.22, 0.54]).

Wechsler Memory Scale

Five studies (H7, H67, H68, H93, H98; *n* = 384 participants) compared oral CHMs with pharmacotherapy and found a significant difference between groups on the WMS at the EoT (MD: 2.90 [0.52, 5.28], I^2 = 0%). One study (H117) compared the combination of an oral CHM and citicoline injection vs. citicoline injection alone. The CHM was a manufactured product called *Xin ke shu pian* 心可舒片 with the main ingredients of *dan shen* 丹参, *san qi* 三七, *ge gen* 葛根, *shan zha* 山楂, and *mu xiang* 木香. The result showed a significant increase in the WMS for the combination of the CHM plus citicoline injection (MD: 10.94 [2.85, 19.03]).

Wechsler Adult Intelligence Scale

Two studies (H68, H135) used the WAIS as an outcome and both compared oral CHMs with piracetam. In the pooled result, there was no significant difference between groups at the EoT (MD: 8.10 [–5.32, 21.53], I^2 = 84%, *n* = 144 participants). One study (H135) found a significant increase in total IQ (intelligence quotient) in the group that used *Yi zhi jiao nang* 益智胶囊 (*ren shen* 人参, *huang qi* 黄芪, *zhi shou wu* 制首乌, *shi chang pu* 石菖蒲, *yuan zhi* 远志, *san qi* 三七, *chuan bei mu* 川贝母, and *dong chong xia cao* 冬虫夏草) after treatment for three months (MD: 15.21 [6.78, 23.64], *n* = 100 participants). However, the other study (H68), which used *Gai liang san jia san* 改良三甲散 (*gui jia* 龟甲, *bie jia* 鳖甲, *jin chong* 䗪虫, *di long* 地龙, *shi chang pu* 石菖蒲, and *he shou wu* 何首乌), showed no significant difference between groups after three months of treatment (MD: 1.50 [–5.18, 8.18], *n* = 44 participants).

Neuropsychiatric Inventory

Two studies (H63, H143; *n* = 180 participants) reported data for NPI, which evaluated the BPSD in VaD patients. The pooled result showed that oral CHM interventions were superior to pharmacotherapies at the EoT (MD: –6.68 [–9.03, –4.32], I^2 = 77%). One study (H63) compared the CHM *Tong xin luo jiao nang* 通心络胶囊 (*ren shen* 人参, *shui zhi* 水蛭, *quan xie* 全蝎, *tu bie chong* 土鳖虫, *wu gong* 蜈蚣, *chan tui* 蝉蜕, *chi shao* 赤芍, *bing pian* 冰片, *tan xiang* 檀香, *jiang xiang* 降香, *ru xiang* 乳香, and *suan zao ren* 酸枣仁) with piracetam (*n* = 100 participants) for six months and found a significant reduction in NPI scores (MD: –7.89 [–9.52, –6.26], *n* = 100 participants). The other study (H143), which compared *Yi zhi xing nao tang* 益智醒脑汤 (*gou qi zi* 枸杞子, *shan yao* 山药, *huai niu qi* 怀牛膝, *shi chang pu* 石菖蒲, *chuan shan long* 穿山龙, *shui zhi* 水蛭, and *dan nan xing* 胆南星) with meclofenoxate, also reported a significant reduction in NPI scores (MD: –5.49 [–7.04, –3.94], *n* = 80 participants) in the CHM group compared to the control after six months of treatment.

Clinical Dementia Rating

Reduction in CDR scores indicates an improvement. In a comparison with placebo, one study (H2) reported improved CDR scores (MD: –0.60 [–0.72, –0.48], *n* = 70 participants) after 12 weeks of treatment with *Bu shen yi zhi ke li* 补肾益智颗粒. Another study (H116) compared *San qi shu tong jiao nang* 三七通舒胶囊 (an extract of *san qi* 三七) plus oxiracetam capsule vs. oxiracetam capsule alone. The result showed a significant benefit over oxiracetam capsule alone (MD: –0.65 [–0.76, –0.54], *n* = 60 participants) after 12 weeks.

GRADE for Main Chinese Herbal Medicine Comparisons

An assessment of the certainty of the evidence was made for a number of the above outcomes and comparisons using the Grading of Recommendations Assessment, Development and Evaluation (GRADE). The interventions, comparators, and outcomes to be included were selected based on the consensus process described in Chapter 4. The outcome measures MMSE, HDS, ADAS-cog, 'lower is better' ADL, 'higher is better' ADL, and FAQ were selected. Comparisons were CHM vs. inactive control, CHM vs. donepezil, and CHM plus donepezil vs. donepezil alone.

Oral Chinese Herbal Medicine vs. Placebo

Evidence for oral CHM vs. placebo control was of 'moderate' to 'low' certainty (Table 5.20). Oral CHM improved the scores on MMSE, HDS, and 'lower is better' ADL. However, no studies reported on ADAS-cog, 'higher is better' ADL, or FAQ.

Oral Chinese Herbal Medicine vs. Donepezil

Evidence for oral CHM vs. donepezil was of 'low' to 'very low' certainty (Table 5.21). There were no significant differences in MMSE, ADAS-cog, 'lower is better' ADL, and 'higher is better' ADL between oral CHM and donepezil. No studies reported on HDS or FAQ.

Table 5.20 GRADE: Oral Chinese Herbal Medicine vs. Placebo

Outcomes (Treatment Duration)	No of Participants (Studies)	Certainty of Evidence	Anticipated Absolute Effects	
			Risk with Inactive Control	**Risk Difference with CHM[3]**
MMSE (mean 9.3 weeks)	253 (3 RCTs)	⊕⊕◯◯ LOW[1,2]	Mean MMSE in control group = **17.86**	MD **3.39 higher** (1.77 higher to 5.01 higher)
HDS (mean 10.7 weeks)	235 (3 RCTs)	⊕⊕⊕◯ MODERATE[2]	Mean HDS in control group = **17.00**	MD **3.25 higher** (1.47 higher to 5.03 higher)
'Lower is better' ADL (12 weeks)	70 (1 RCT)	⊕⊕⊕◯ MODERATE[2]	Mean 'lower is better' ADL in control group = **48.10**	SMD **1.09 SD lower** (1.60 lower to 0.58 lower)

Notes: (1) Considerable statistical heterogeneity; (2) small sample size limits certainty of results and (3) the risk in the intervention group (and its 95% confidence interval) is based on the assumed risk in the comparison group and the relative effect of the intervention (and its 95% CI).

Abbreviations: ADL, activities of daily living; CHM, Chinese herbal medicine; HDS, Hasegawa Dementia Scale; MD, mean difference; MMSE, Mini-mental State Examination; SMD, standardised mean difference; SD, standard deviation; RCT, randomised controlled trial.

Adverse events: Adverse events (AEs) were reported in four studies. One study reported five cases with AEs in the intervention group: urticaria, diarrhea, appetite loss, heartburn, hypertension; and two cases in the control group: oral bitterness and liver dysfunction. Another study reported two cases of AEs in the intervention group: one case suffered elevated liver enzyme AST and ALT levels during treatment but these returned to normal after discontinuation; one case suffered mild hypokalemia, but medication was continued. The other two studies reported that no AEs occurred during the treatments.

Study References: MMSE: H1, H2, H157; HDS: H122, H123, H124; 'lower is better' ADL: H2.

Integrative Medicine: Oral Chinese Herbal Medicine Combined with Donepezil vs. Donepezil Alone

Evidence for oral CHM combined with donepezil vs. donepezil with CHM was of 'low' to 'very low' certainty (Table 5.22). Oral CHM increased the scores on the MMSE and decreased scores on 'lower is better' ADL. However, it did not improve the scores on ADAS-cog or the HDS. No studies reported on 'higher is better' ADL or FAQ.

Table 5.21 GRADE: Oral Chinese Herbal Medicine vs. Donepezil

Outcomes (Treatment Duration)	No of Participants (Studies)	Certainty of Evidence	Anticipated Absolute Effects	
			Risk with Donepezil	Risk Difference with CHM[4]
MMSE (mean 11.6 weeks)	358 (5 RCTs)	⊕⊕◯◯ LOW[1,2]	Mean MMSE in control group = **19.92**	MD **0.14 higher** (0.85 lower to 1.13 higher)
ADAS-cog (mean 16.0 weeks)	100 (2 RCTs)	⊕⊕◯◯ LOW[1,2]	Mean ADAS-cog in control group = **21.34**	MD **1.03 higher** (2.53 lower to 4.59 higher)
'Lower is better' ADL (mean 14.7 weeks)	160 (3 RCTs)	⊕◯◯◯ VERY LOW[1,2,3]	Mean 'lower is better' ADL in control group = **37.77**	SMD **0.15 SD higher** (0.35 lower to 0.64 higher)
'Higher is better' ADL (12 weeks)	118 (1 RCT)	⊕⊕◯◯ LOW[1,2]	Mean 'higher is better' ADL in control group = **76.00**	SMD **0.26 SD lower** (0.63 lower to 0.10 higher)

Notes: (1) Lack of blinding of participants and personnel; (2) considerable statistical heterogeneity; (3) small sample size limits certainty of results and (4) the risk in the intervention group (and its 95% confidence interval) is based on the assumed risk in the comparison group and the relative effect of the intervention (and its 95% CI).

Abbreviations: ADAS-cog, Alzheimer's Disease Assessment Scale — cognitive subscale; ADL, activities of daily living; CHM, Chinese herbal medicine; HDS, Hasegawa Dementia Scale; MD, mean difference; MMSE, Mini-mental State Examination; SMD, standardised mean difference; SD, standard deviation; RCT, randomised controlled trial.

Adverse events: Five studies reported on AEs. Two studies reported that no AEs occurred during the treatment. The other three studies reported that there were no AEs in the CHM intervention groups; and the following AEs in the control groups: Two cases of dizziness, headache, and mild diarrhea, two cases of nausea, three cases of nausea and vomiting.

Study References: MMSE: H4–H8; ADAS-cog: H4, H5; 'lower is better' ADL: H4–H6; 'higher is better' ADL: H7.

Randomised Controlled Trial Evidence for Individual Oral Chinese Herbal Medicine Formulae

The most commonly reported formulae from Chapter 2 tested in the included RCTs were modified *Bu yang huan wu tang* 补阳还五汤加减 (4 studies) and the closely related formula *Bu chang nao xin tong jiao nang* 步长脑心通胶囊 which was equally common in the RCTs (4 studies).

Table 5.22 GRADE: Oral Chinese Herbal Medicine Plus Donepezil vs. Donepezil

Outcomes (Treatment Duration)	No of Participants (Studies)	Certainty of Evidence	Anticipated Absolute Effects	
			Risk with Donepezil	Risk Difference with CHM[4]
MMSE (mean 15.2 weeks)	313 (5 RCTs)	⊕⊕◯◯ LOW[1,2]	Mean MMSE in control group = **19.29**	MD **2.20 higher** (1.18 higher to 3.23 higher)
ADAS-cog (mean 24.0 weeks)	102 (2 RCTs)	⊕⊕◯◯ LOW[1,2]	Mean ADAS-cog in control group = **21.34**	MD 3.23 lower (6.88 lower to 0.43 higher)
HDS (24.0 weeks)	79 (1 RCT)	⊕⊕◯◯ LOW[1,2]	Mean HDS in control group = **18.53**	MD **1.83 higher** (1.21 lower to 4.87 higher)
'Lower is better' ADL (mean 15.2 weeks)	313 (5 RCTs)	⊕◯◯◯ VERY LOW[1,2,3]	Mean 'lower is better' ADL in control group = **29.13**	SMD **0.49 SD lower** (0.86 lower to 0.11 lower)

Notes: (1) Lack of blinding of participants and personnel; (2) Considerable statistical heterogeneity; (3) small sample size limits certainty of results and (4) The risk in the intervention group (and its 95% confidence interval) is based on the assumed risk in the comparison group and the relative effect of the intervention (and its 95% CI).

Abbreviations: ADAS-cog, Alzheimer's Disease Assessment Scale — cognitive subscale; ADL, activities of daily living; CHM, Chinese herbal medicine; HDS, Hasegawa Dementia Scale; MD, mean difference; MMSE, Mini-Mental State Examination; SMD, standardised mean difference; SD, standard deviation; RCT, randomised controlled trial.

Adverse events: Five studies reported on AEs. One study reported two cases of diarrhea, constipation, fatigue, and agitation in the intervention group; two cases of diarrhea, constipation, fatigue, and agitation occurred in each group. Another study reported three cases of nausea and vomiting and one case of loss of appetite and general malaise in the intervention group; three cases suffered nausea and vomiting in the control group. The other three studies reported that no AEs occurred during the treatments.

Study References: MMSE: H4, H5, H101–H103; ADAS-cog: H4, H5; HDS: H102; 'lower is better' ADL: H4, H5, H101–H103.

Modified *Bu yang huan wu tang* 补阳还五汤加减 was created by *Wang qing ren* 王清任, a famous medical expert in the Qing dynasty, and was recorded in the book *Yi Lin Gai Cuo* 医林改错 (c. 1830). The main ingredients are *huang qi* 黄芪, *dang gui* 当归, *chuan xiong* 川芎, *chi shao* 赤芍, *tao ren* 桃仁, *hong hua* 红花, and *di long* 地龙. It is a classical formula for the treatment of stroke sequelae and its main actions are tonifying *qi* and activating Blood 益气活血. The main ingredients of *Bu chang nao xin tong jiao nang* 步长脑心通胶囊, which is a modern manufactured Chinese medicine based on *Bu yang huan wu tang* 补阳还五汤,[15] are *huang qi* 黄芪, *dang gui* 当归, *chuan xiong* 川芎, *chi shao* 赤芍, *tao ren* 桃仁, *hong hua* 红花, *di long* 地龙, *dan shen* 丹参, *ru xiang* 乳香, *mo yao* 没药, *ji xue teng* 鸡血藤, *niu xi* 牛膝, *gui zhi* 桂枝, *sang zhi* 桑枝, *quan xie* 全蝎, and *shui zhi* 水蛭.

In total, modified *Bu yang huan wu tang* 补阳还五汤加减 was used in four RCTs. One of these used the decoction in comparison to nimodipine (H20). The intervention in the other three RCTs was integrative medicine (H160–H162). The results showed that the groups that received modified *Bu yang huan wu tang* 补阳还五汤加减 had larger improvements in the scores on the MMSE and 'lower is better' ADL than the nimodipine-alone groups (Table 5.23). Based on three RCTs, modified *Bu yang huan wu tang* 补阳还五汤加减 plus pharmacotherapy improved HDS scores compared to pharmacotherapy alone (Table 5.23).

Bu chang nao xin tong jiao nang 步长脑心通胶囊 was compared with a pharmacotherapy in three RCTs (H23, H24, H99). In the pooled analyses, there were significant improvements in the MMSE, HDS, and 'lower is better' ADL scores in the CHM groups, but no difference between groups on the FAQ (Table 5.23). Only one study compared *Bu chang nao xin tong jiao nang* 步长脑心通胶囊 plus donepezil to donepezil alone (H103). There was an improvement in the integrative CHM group compared to the donepezil-alone group based on 'lower is better' ADL at the EoT, but there was no significant difference in terms of the MMSE (Table 5.23).

GRADE for Individual Formulae

A GRADE assessment of the certainty of evidence for the formulae tested in multiple RCTs was made for modified *Bu yang huan wu tang* 补阳还五汤加减 and *Bu chang nao xin tong jiao nang* 步长脑心通胶囊, which were used in four RCTs each. The selected outcome measures were MMSE, HDS, ADAS-cog, 'lower is better' ADL, 'higher is better' ADL and FAQ.

Table 5.23 Chinese Herbal Medicine Formulae vs. Pharmacotherapy

Chinese Herbal Medicine Intervention	Comparator	Outcome	No. of Studies (Participants)	Effect Size ([95% CI], I^2)	Included Studies
Modified *Bu yang huan wu tang*	Nimodipine	MMSE	1 (62)	MD: 3.33 [0.73, 5.93]*	H20
		'Lower is better' ADL	1 (62)	SMD: –1.83 [–2.43, –1.23]*	H20
Modified *Bu yang huan wu tang* plus pharmacotherapy	Pharmacotherapy	HDS	3 (242)	MD: 4.73 [2.98, 6.49]* 52%	H160–H162
Bu chang nao xin tong jiao nang	Pharmacotherapy	MMSE	3 (233)	MD: 1.84 [0.95, 2.73]*, 2%	H23, H24, H99
		HDS	1 (120)	MD: 4.01 [2.07, 5.95]*	H99
		'Lower is better' ADL	1 (60)	SMD: –2.12 [–2.76, –1.48]*	H24
		FAQ	1 (120)	MD: 0.05 [–1.09, 1.19]	H99
Bu chang nao xin tong jiao nang plus donepezil	Donepezil	MMSE	1 (64)	MD: 1.87 [–0.05, 3.79]	H103
		'Lower is better' ADL	1 (64)	SMD: –0.66 [–1.16, –0.15]*	H103

*Statistically significant. Abbreviations: ADL, activities of daily living; CI, confidence interval; FAQ, Functional Activities Questionnaire; HDS, Hasegawa Dementia Scale; MD, mean difference; MMSE, Mini-Mental State Examination; SMD, standardised mean difference.

Modified Bu yang huan wu tang vs. Pharmacotherapy

Evidence for modified *Bu yang huan wu tang* 补阳还五汤加减 vs. pharmacotherapy (nimodipine) was of 'low' certainty (Table 5.24) and only one study was included (H20). The result suggested that modified *Bu yang huan wu tang* 补阳还五汤加减 was superior to nimodipine based on MMSE and 'lower is better' ADL scores. The other outcomes were not reported.

Table 5.24 GRADE: Modified *Bu yang huan wu tang* vs. Nimodipine

Outcomes (Treatment Duration)	No of Participants (Studies)	Certainty of Evidence	Anticipated Absolute Effects	
			Risk with Nimodipine	Risk Difference with CHM[3]
MMSE (mean 8.0 weeks)	62 (1 RCT)	⊕⊕◯◯ LOW[1,2]	Mean MMSE in control group = **16.71**	MD **3.33 higher** (0.73 higher to 5.93 higher)
'Lower is better' ADL (8.0 weeks)	62 (1 RCT)	⊕⊕◯◯ LOW[1,2]	Mean 'lower is better' ADL in control group = **19.28**	SMD **1.83 SD lower** (2.43 lower to 1.23 lower)

Notes: (1) Lack of blinding of participants and personnel; (2) small sample size limits certainty of results and (3) the risk in the intervention group (and its 95% confidence interval) is based on the assumed risk in the comparison group and the relative effect of the intervention (and its 95% CI).

Abbreviations: ADL, activities of daily living; CHM, Chinese herbal medicine; MD, mean difference; MMSE, Mini-Mental State Examination; SMD, standardised mean difference; SD, standard deviation; RCT, randomised controlled trial.

Adverse events: The study reported that no adverse events occurred during the treatment.

Study References: MMSE: H20; 'lower is better' ADL: H20.

Modified Bu yang huan wu tang Combined with Pharmacotherapy vs. Pharmacotherapy

Evidence for modified *Bu yang huan wu tang* 补阳还五汤加减 combined with pharmacotherapy vs. the same pharmacotherapy alone was of 'very low' certainty (Table 5.25). The pooled results based on three RCTs (H160–H162) showed that modified *Bu yang huan wu tang* 补阳还五汤加减 plus pharmacotherapy significantly improved the

Table 5.25 GRADE: Modified *Bu yang huan wu tang* Plus Pharmacotherapy vs. Pharmacotherapy

Outcomes (Treatment Duration)	No of Participants (Studies)	Certainty of Evidence	Anticipated Absolute Effects	
			Risk with Pharmacotherapy	Risk difference with CHM[4]
HDS (mean 6.0 weeks)	242 (3 RCTs)	⊕○○○ VERY LOW[1,2,3]	Mean HDS in control group = **17.67**	MD **4.73 higher** (2.98 higher to 6.49 higher)

Notes: (1) Lack of blinding of participants and personnel; (2) Considerable statistical heterogeneity and (3) Small sample size limits certainty of results and (4) The risk in the intervention group (and its 95% confidence interval) is based on the assumed risk in the comparison group and the relative effect of the intervention (and its 95% CI).

Abbreviations: CHM, Chinese herbal medicine; HDS, Hasegawa Dementia Scale; MD, mean difference, SMD: standardised mean difference, SD: standard deviation; RCT, randomised controlled trial.

Adverse events: The three studies reported no adverse events occurred during the treatment period.

Study References: HDS: H160–H162.

scores on the HDS compared with pharmacotherapy alone. Other outcomes were not reported.

Bu chang nao xin tong jiao nang vs. Pharmacotherapy

Evidence for *Bu chang nao xin tong jiao nang* 步长脑心通胶囊 vs. pharmacotherapy was of 'low' certainty (Table 5.26). There were significant improvements in outcomes based on the MMSE in three studies (H23, H24, H99), HDS in one study (H99) and 'lower is better' ADL in one study (H24), but CHM was not superior to the control group based on the FAQ in one study (H99). The other outcomes were not reported.

Bu chang nao xin tong jiao nang Combined with Pharmacotherapy vs. Pharmacotherapy

Only one study (H103) that tested *Bu chang nao xin tong jiao nang* 步长脑心通胶囊 combined with donepezil compared to donepezil alone was included. The result showed that *Bu chang nao xin tong jiao nang* 步长脑心通胶囊 combined with donepezil significantly

Table 5.26 GRADE: *Bu chang nao xin tong jiao nang* vs. Pharmacotherapy

Outcomes (Treatment Duration)	No of Participants (Studies)	Certainty of Evidence	Anticipated Absolute Effects	
			Risk with Pharmacotherapy	Risk Difference with CHM[3]
MMSE (mean 20.0 weeks)	233 (3 RCTs)	⊕⊕◯◯ LOW[1,2]	Mean MMSE in control group = **17.79**	MD **1.84 higher** (0.95 higher to 2.73 higher)
HDS (24.0 weeks)	120 (1 RCT)	⊕⊕◯◯ LOW[1,2]	Mean HDS in control group = **16.73**	MD **4.01 higher** (2.07 higher to 5.95 higher)
'Lower is better' ADL (mean 24.0 weeks)	60 (1 RCT)	⊕⊕◯◯ LOW[1,2]	Mean 'lower is better' ADL in control group = **24.11**	SMD **2.12 SD lower** (2.76 lower to 1.48 lower)
FAQ (24.0 weeks)	120 (1 RCT)	⊕⊕◯◯ LOW[1,2]	Mean FAQ in control group = **11.28**	MD **0.05 higher** (1.09 lower to 1.19 higher)

Notes: (1) Lack of blinding of participants and personnel; (2) small sample size limits certainty of results and (3) The risk in the intervention group (and its 95% confidence interval) is based on the assumed risk in the comparison group and the relative effect of the intervention (and its 95% CI).

Abbreviations: MD, mean difference, SMD: standardised mean difference, SD: standard deviation.

Abbreviations: ADL, activities of daily living; CHM, Chinese herbal medicine; FAQ, Functional Activities Questionnaire; HDS, Hasegawa Dementia Scale; MD, mean difference; MMSE, Mini-Mental State Examination; SMD, standardised mean difference; SD, standard deviation; RCT, randomised controlled trial.

Adverse events: One study reported nine cases of stomach discomfort, nausea, or loss of appetite in the intervention group, and 12 cases of loss of appetite or nausea in the control group. The other two studies did not report adverse events.

Study References: MMSE: H23, H24, H99; HDS: H99; 'lower is better' ADL: H24; FAQ: H99.

reduced 'lower is better' ADL scores, but scores based on the MMSE were not significantly different. The certainty of the evidence is 'low' and other outcomes were not reported (Table 5.27).

Frequently Reported Herbs in Meta-analyses Showing Favourable Effects

Cognitive impairment is a major issue in VaD. In order to identify herbs that may have effects on cognition, the most frequently used

Table 5.27 GRADE: *Bu chang nao xin tong jiao nang* Plus Donepezil vs. Donepezil

Outcomes (Treatment Duration)	No of Participants (Studies)	Certainty of Evidence	Anticipated Absolute Effects	
			Risk with Pharmacotherapy	**Risk Difference with CHM[3]**
MMSE (8.0 weeks)	64 (1 RCT)	⊕⊕◯◯ LOW[1,2]	Mean MMSE in control group = **18.78**	MD **1.87 higher** (0.05 lower to 3.79 higher)
'Lower is better' ADL (8.0 weeks)	64 (1 RCT)	⊕⊕◯◯ LOW[1,2]	Mean 'lower is better' ADL in control group = **19.28**	SMD **0.66 SD lower** (1.16 lower to 0.15 lower)

Notes: (1) Lack of blinding of participants and personnel; (2) Small sample size limits certainty of results and (3) The risk in the intervention group (and its 95% confidence interval) is based on the assumed risk in the comparison group and the relative effect of the intervention (and its 95% CI).

Abbreviations: ADL, activities of daily living; CHM, Chinese herbal medicine; MD, mean difference; MMSE, Mini-Mental State Examination; SMD, standardised mean difference; SD, standard deviation; RCT, randomised controlled trial.

Adverse events: The study reported no adverse events occurred during the treatment.

Study References: MMSE: H103; 'lower is better' ADL: H103.

herbs in meta-analyses of cognitive outcome measures showing favourable effects were examined. As there were too few studies of comparisons with placebo, the comparator used was a specific pharmacotherapy. The cognitive outcome measures included MMSE, ADAS-cog, HDS, and CDT.

Chinese Herbal Medicine vs. Specific Pharmacotherapy for Cognitive Outcome Measures

Data were available for oral CHM vs. specific pharmacotherapy based on MMSE, HDS, and/or CDT as cognitive outcome measures. Each of the 15 meta-analyses found that oral CHMs were superior to controls in terms of these measures of cognition. No data was available for ADAS-cog. In total, 103 RCTs were included in these pools. The most frequently used herbs are presented in Table 5.28.

Table 5.28 Frequently Used Herbs in Meta-analyses of Oral Chinese Herbal Medicine vs. Specific Pharmacotherapy with Cognitive Outcomes

15 Meta-analyses (MMSE, HDS and CDT); 103 RCTs[1]

Herbs	Scientific Name	Frequency of Use
Chang pu 菖蒲 (*shi chang pu* 石菖蒲)	*Acorus* spp. (*A. tatarinowii* Schott)	60 (47)
He shou wu 何首乌	*Polygonum multiflorum* Thunb.	52
Chuan xiong 川芎	*Ligusticum chuanxiong* Hort.	49
Huang qi 黄芪	*Astragalus membranaceus* (Fisch.) Bge.	47
Dang gui 当归	*Angelica sinensis* (Oliv.) Diels	38
Dan shen 丹参	*Salvia miltiorrhiza* Bge.	37
Yuan zhi 远志	*Polygala tenuifolia* Willd.	28
Shui zhi 水蛭	*Hirudo* or *Whitmania* spp.	27
Shu di huang 熟地黄	*Rehmannia glutinosa* Libosch.	26
Gou qi zi 枸杞子	*Lycium barbarum* L.	22
Ren shen 人参	*Panax ginseng* C. A. Mey.	22

Notes: (1) See Tables 5.6 and 5.9, section on CDT for included studies and (2) The use of some herbs may be restricted in some countries. Readers are advised to comply with relevant regulations.

Abbreviations: CDT: Clock drawing test; HDS, Hasegawa Dementia Scale; MMSE, Mini-Mental State Examination; RCT, randomised controlled trial.

Integrative Chinese Herbal Medicine vs. the Same Pharmacotherapy for Cognitive Outcome Measures

For integrative CHM (oral CHM plus specific pharmacotherapy) vs. the same pharmacotherapy alone, data were available for cognitive outcomes based on the MMSE and HDS. No data were available for ADAS-cog and CDT. These 12 meta-analyses found that integrative CHM produced significant cognitive benefits. There were 22 RCTs included in the meta-analysis pools and the most frequently used herbs are listed in Table 5.29.

Overall, the most frequent herbs for the two sections above are also herbs that appear generally frequently in the RCTs (Table 5.3). This indicates that the meta-analyses of these cognitive outcomes

Table 5.29 Frequently Used Herbs in Meta-analyses of Integrative Oral Chinese Herbal Medicine vs. the Same Pharmacotherapy with Cognitive Outcomes

12 Meta-Analyses (MMSE and HDS; 22 RCTs)[1]		
Herbs	**Scientific Name**	**Frequency of Use**
Shi chang pu 石菖蒲	*Acorus tatarinowii* Schott	14
Chuan xiong 川芎	*Ligusticum chuanxiong* Hort.	12
Dan shen 丹参	*Salvia miltiorrhiza* Bge.	9
Shu di huang 熟地黄	*Rehmannia glutinosa* Libosch.	9
He shou wu 何首乌	*Polygonum multiflorum* Thunb.	8
Yuan zhi 远志	*Polygala tenuifolia* Willd.	7
Dan nan xing 胆南星	*Arisaema erubescens* (Wall.) Schott.	6
Fu ling 茯苓	*Poria cocos* (Schw.) Wolf	6
Ge gen 葛根	*Pueraria lobata* (Willd.) Ohwi	6
Yu jin 郁金	*Curcuma wenyujin* Y. H. Chen et C. Ling	6

Notes: (1) See Tables 5.7 and 5.10 for included studies and (2) the use of some herbs may be restricted in some countries. Readers are advised to comply with relevant regulations.

Abbreviations: HDS, Hasegawa Dementia Scale; MMSE, Mini-Mental State Examination; RCT, randomised controlled trial.

were based on CHM interventions that were typical of the formulae used more broadly in the clinical trials for VaD.

Controlled Clinical Trials of Oral Chinese Herbal Medicine

Chinese herbal medicine was evaluated in 10 non-randomised CCTs (H181–H190) with durations ranging from four to 24 weeks. The 10 CCTs were all conducted in China. The CCTs enrolled 720 participants with one three-armed study that tested two CHMs and nine two-armed studies. Five studies reported syndromes and two studies modified treatment based on syndrome differentiation (H189, H190). The most commonly mentioned syndromes were as follows:

- 'Sea of Marrow' insufficiency 髓海不足/脑髓不充: 3 studies.
- Phlegm turbidity obstructing the Orifices 痰浊阻窍/痰浊闭窍: 3 studies.
- Blood stasis 血瘀/气虚血瘀: 2 studies.
- Liver and Kidney deficiency 肝肾亏虚: 2 studies.

In some studies, these syndromes were combined to form complex syndrome descriptions.

All studies tested oral CHM interventions, including manufactured products and multi-ingredient decoctions. Different CHMs were used in each study and some of the formulae used frequently in the RCTs were also tested in these CCTs, including *Bu yang huan wu tang* 补阳还五汤, *Tian zhi ke li* 天智颗粒, and *Kang xin jiao nang* 康欣胶囊. The herb frequency analysis is based on only nine studies since one study did not specify formula ingredients (Table 5.30). The most commonly used herbs were similar to those in the RCT pool.

Table 5.30 Frequently Used Herbs in Controlled Clinical Trials

Herb Name	Scientific Name	Frequency of Use
Chang pu 菖蒲 (*shi chang pu* 石菖蒲)	*Acorus* spp. (*A. tatarinowii* Schott)	6 (5)
Chuan xiong 川芎	*Ligusticum chuangxiong* Hort.	6
He shou wu 何首乌	*Polygonum multiflorum* Thunb.	5
Huang qi 黄芪	*Astragalus membranaceus* (Fisch.) Bge.	5
Dan shen 丹参	*Salvia miltiorrhiza* Bge.	4
Dang gui 当归	*Angelica sinensis* (Oliv.) Diels	4
Yu jin 郁金	*Curcuma wenyujin* Y. H. Chen et C. Ling	4
Gou qi zi 枸杞子	*Lycium barbarum* L.	4
Chi shao 赤芍	*Paeonia lactiflora* Pall.	3
Chuan niu xi 川牛膝	*Cyathula officinalis* Kuan	3
Dan nan xing 胆南星	*Arisaema erubescens* (Wall.) Schott.	3
Dang shen 党参	*Codonopsis pilosula* (Franch.) Nannf.	3
Hong hua 红花	*Carthamus tinctorius* L.	3
Tian ma 天麻	*Gastrodia elata* Bl.	3
Yi zhi ren 益智仁	*Alpinia oxyphylla* Miq.	3
Yuan zhi 远志	*Polygala tenuifolia* Willd.	3
Ban xia 半夏	*Pinellia ternata* (Thunb.) Breit.	2
Chai hu 柴胡	*Bupleurum chinense* DC.	2
Di long 地龙	*Pheretima*.	2
Tao ren 桃仁	*Prunus persica* (L.) Batsch.	2

Note: The use of some herbs may be restricted in some countries. Readers are advised to comply with relevant regulations.

Mini-Mental State Examination

In four CCTs (*n* = 269 participants) that compared oral CHM with pharmacotherapy alone, the meta-analysis showed improved scores on the MMSE at the EoT (MD: 1.58 [0.22, 2.94]) (Table 5.31). For oral CHM plus pharmacotherapy compared with pharmacotherapy alone, two studies were included (*n* = 120 participants) and the result showed that there was a significant improvement in the integrative groups (MD: 5.69 [4.33, 7.06]) (Table 5.31).

Table 5.31 Chinese Herbal Medicine vs. Controls: Mini-Mental State Examination at the End of Treatment

Comparator	No. of Studies (Participants), Duration	Effect Size (RR [95% CI], I^2)	Included Studies
CHM vs. pharmacotherapy	4 (269), 8–12 wks	1.58 [0.22, 2.94]*, 40%	H182, H184, H188, H189
CHM plus pharmacotherapy vs. pharmacotherapy alone	2 (120), 4–24 wks	5.69 [4.33, 7.06]*, 5%	H187, H190

*Statistically significant. Abbreviations: CHM: Chinese herbal medicine; RR: risk ratio; CI, confidence interval; wks, weeks.

Hasegawa's Dementia Scale

HDS was used in three CCTs (*n* = 219 participants) that compared oral CHM with pharmacotherapy (H183, H185, H189). The oral CHM groups were not significantly different from the pharmacotherapy groups based on HDS scores at the EoT (MD: 3.32 [–1.12, 7.75], I^2 = 83%). One CCT (H181) with 4 weeks of treatment (*n* = 49 participants) compared *Yi zhi tong luo tang* 益智通络汤 (*he shou wu* 何首乌, *gou qi zi* 枸杞子, *shu di* 熟地, *bai shao* 白芍, *ren shen* 人参, *chuan xiong* 川芎, *shi chang pu* 石菖蒲, *chai hu* 柴胡, *yu jin* 郁金, *mu li* 牡蛎, and *ji nei jin* 鸡内金) plus pharmacotherapy using co-dergocrine mesylate, citicoline, and piracetam vs. the same pharmacotherapies alone and the result showed a significant improvement in HDS scores in the integrative CHM group at the EoT (MD: 3.00 [0.40, 5.60]).

'Lower is Better' Activities of Daily Living

There were three CCTs (H186, H188, H189) (n = 237 participants) that compared oral CHM with pharmacotherapy using 'lower is better' ADL. One was a three-armed study and two were two-armed studies. The pooled result showed that groups did not differ significantly in terms of 'lower is better' ADL outcomes at the EoT (SMD: −0.11 [–0.66, 0.44], I^2 = 80%). In the single study (H187) that compared modified *Xue fu zhu yu tang* 血府逐瘀汤 (*tao ren* 桃仁, *hong hua* 红花, *dang gui* 当归, *chuan xiong* 川芎, *chi shao* 赤芍, *chuan niu xi* 川牛膝, *zhi qiao* 枳壳, *jie geng* 桔梗, *chai hu* 柴胡, and *zhi gan cao* 炙甘草) plus donepezil with donepezil-alone (n = 48 participants) using 'higher is better' ADL, there was a significant improvement in the integrative medicine group (SMD: 0.78 [0.19, 1.37]) after 6 months.

Non-controlled Studies of Oral Chinese Herbal Medicine

In total, 31 non-controlled studies (H191–H221; n = 1,396 participants) investigated an oral CHM intervention for VaD and each of these studies applied a different CHM intervention. Two of the CHM interventions were unnamed. Two studies (H218, H221) used single herb extracts (*Cistanche deserticola* Y. C. Ma, *Rou cong rong* 肉苁蓉 and *Polygonum multiflorum* Thunb, *He shou wu* 何首乌) while the others were multi-ingredient oral CHMs. Six studies used syndrome differentiation. The most common syndromes were as follows:

- 'Sea of Marrow' insufficiency 髓海不足: 3 studies.
- Kidney deficiency with phlegm stagnation blocking the Orifices 肾虚痰瘀阻窍: 2 studies.

- Effulgent Heart-Liver fire 心肝火旺: 2 studies.
- Liver and Kidney deficiency 肝肾亏虚: 2 studies.

The list of most frequently included herbs in the oral CHM interventions shows distinct similarities with the lists for the RCTs and CCTs. (Table 5.32).

Table 5.32 Frequently Used Herbs in Non-controlled Studies

Herb Name	Scientific Name	Frequency of Use
Chang pu 菖蒲 (*shi chang pu* 石菖蒲)	*Acorus* spp. (*A. tatarinowii* Schott)	17 (15)
Chuan xiong 川芎	*Ligusticum chuangxiong* Hort.	16
Yuan zhi 远志	*Polygala tenuifolia* Willd.	14
Dan shen 丹参	*Salvia miltiorrhiza* Bge.	11
Dang gui 当归	*Angelica sinensis* (Oliv.) Diels	11
Di long 地龙	*Pheretima spp.*	9
Chi shao 赤芍	*Paeonia lactiflora* Pall.	8
Shui zhi 水蛭	*Hirudo* or *Whitmania* spp.	8
Yu jin 郁金	*Curcuma wenyujin* Y. H. Chen et C. Ling	8
Hong hua 红花	*Carthamus tinctorius* L.	7
Ren shen 人参	*Panax ginseng* C. A. Mey.	7
Dan nan xing 胆南星	*Arisaema erubescens* (Wall.) Schott.	6
Fu ling 茯苓	*Poria cocos* (Schw.) Wolf	6
Tao ren 桃仁	*Prunus persica* (L.) Batsch.	6
He shou wu 何首乌	*Polygonum multiflorum* Thunb.	6
Gou qi zi 枸杞子	*Lycium barbarum* L.	5
Huang qi 黄芪	*Astragalus membranaceus* (Fisch.) Bge.	5
Shan zhu yu 山茱萸	*Cornus officinalis* Sieb. et Zucc.	5
Ban xia 半夏	*Pinellia ternata* (Thunb.) Breit.	4
Huang jing 黄精	*Polygonatum kingianum* Coll. et Hemsl.	4

Note: The use of some herbs may be restricted in some countries. Readers are advised to comply with relevant regulations.

Safety of Chinese Herbal Medicine for Vascular Dementia

In the 180 RCTs, 30 mentioned there were no adverse events (AEs) in both the intervention and control groups, while 19 studies provided specific AEs for the oral CHM and control groups. Overall, gastro-intestinal symptoms including nausea/vomiting, loss of appetite, constipation, and diarrhea were the most common AEs in both the oral CHM groups (62 cases) and control groups (50 cases), followed by insomnia which was reported in eight cases in the control groups and two cases in the oral CHM groups. Five cases of dizziness/headache were reported in the control groups, but no similar AEs were reported in the intervention groups. Other mild AEs were reported in the oral CHM groups, including dry mouth ($n = 2$) and rash ($n = 3$). Only one study reported a case of elevated liver enzymes, which normalized after the treatment stopped. The RCTs also reported the following AEs in the control groups: dry mouth ($n = 3$), oral bitterness ($n = 2$), and hot feeling ($n = 6$). It was not possible to calculate AE incidence since it was not always clear whether data indicated the number of participants who experienced the AEs or number of AE reports.

In the CCTs, two studies (H182, H185) mentioned that there were no AEs reported and one study (H188) reported mild diarrhea (1 case) in the CHM group. In the non-controlled studies, 5 studies mentioned that there were no AEs reported (H193, H195, H209, H210, H221) while 3 studies, which included 160 participants, reported 13 cases of AEs including stomach discomfort, dizziness, nausea, insomnia, fatigue, constipation, drowsiness, and proteinuria (H194, H218, H220). In addition, one participant had a recurrence of diabetes and was hospitalized (H218). This was the only serious AE reported and the cause was unclear. Overall, oral CHM appeared to be well-tolerated in people with VaD.

Clinical Evidence for Commonly Used Oral Formulae

Of the seven orally administered formulae discussed in Chapter 2 for the syndromes associated with VaD, four were tested in at least one of the included RCTs, none were included in the CCTs, and one was in a non-controlled study. These formulae were modified in some studies.

- Modified *Bu yang huan wu tang* 补阳还五汤加减 was used in four RCTs (H20, H160–H162) and one non-controlled study (H213).
- *Tong qiao huo xue tang* 通窍活血汤 was used in one RCT (H15) and one non-controlled study (H214).
- *Qi fu yin* 七福饮 (H107) and *Huan shao dan* 还少丹 (H22) were each used in one RCT.
- *Tian ma gou teng yin* 天麻钩藤饮, *Xi xin tang* 洗心汤, *Gui pi tang* 归脾汤, and *Huang lian jie du tang* 黄连解毒汤 were not tested in any of the included clinical trials.

In the case of modified *Bu yang huan wu tang* 补阳还五汤加减, the meta-analysis based on one small RCT (H20; *n* = 62 participants) showed that modified *Bu yang huan wu tang* 补阳还五汤加减 significantly improved outcomes compared to nimodipine based on the MMSE (MD: 3.33 [0.73, 5.93]) and 'lower is better' ADL (SMD: –1.83 [–2.43, –1.23]). Modified *Bu yang huan wu tang* 补阳还五汤加减 combined with pharmacotherapy in three studies (H160, H161, H162; *n* = 242 participants) led to improved HDS scores when compared to the same pharmacotherapies alone (MD: 4.73 [2.98, 6.49], I^2 = 52%).

One study (H15; *n* = 160 participants) found that *Tong qiao huo xue tang* 通窍活血汤 was not superior to huperzine A after 4 weeks (MMSE, MD: –1.04 [–1.98, –0.10]). Another study (H107; *n* = 60 participants) found that *Qi fu yin* 七福饮 led to significant improvements on the MMSE (MD: 2.14 [1.12, 3.16]) and HDS (MD: 1.44 [1.02, 1.86]) when compared to nimodipine alone after 12 weeks of treatment. *Huan shao dan* 还少丹 was found to be neither superior nor inferior to nimodipine based on the MMSE (MD: 0.27 [–0.69, 1.23]) after 8 weeks of treatment (H22); however, it showed a significant benefit based on HDS scores (MD: 3.13 [2.75, 3.51]). Overall, the assessable data for the formulae from Chapter 2 indicate that they appear beneficial for VaD patients; however, the evidence was mainly based on single studies.

heterogeneity. It should be noted that most studies specified that participants in both groups received supportive treatment for their various health conditions during the trials.

When a CHM was combined with a pharmacotherapy as an integrative medicine treatment, the combination tended to be superior to the same pharmacotherapy used alone for the meta-analyses of MMSE, HDS, ADL, and BBS. However, the heterogeneity in these results ranged from 'moderate' to 'considerable'. The subgroup analyses tended to reduce heterogeneity. For CHM combined with donepezil (Table 5.7), there was a significant improvement of MD 2.20 points on the MMSE (5 RCTs, n = 313 participants) with zero heterogeneity, while for CHM plus nimodipine, the improvement on the MMSE was MD 2.57 points (3 RCTs, n = 207 participants) with moderate (43%) heterogeneity. For ADAS-cog (Table 5.11), the meta-analysis of CHM plus donepezil showed no significant difference with 21% heterogeneity, but there were only two studies (n = 102 participants) in the pool and the MD [95% CI] was 3.23 [–6.88, 0.43], suggesting a trend that was consistent with the MMSE results. However, there was insufficient power to detect a significant difference in ADAS-cog. Taken together, the meta-analysis results suggest that combining CHM with donepezil or nimodipine appears to provide additional cognitive benefits compared to monotherapy with donepezil or nimodipine alone.

Most of the formulae used in the studies were designed by the investigators or were commercially manufactured products without a classical name. Of the classical formulae, *Bu yang huan wu tang* 补阳还五汤 was the most commonly used and the related formula, *Bu chang nao xin tong jiao nang* 步长脑心通胶囊, was the most common commercial product. Meta-analysis found that modified *Bu yang huan wu tang* 补阳还五汤 was more effective than pharmacotherapy in terms of the MMSE and 'lower is better' ADL based on a single study. Based on three RCTs (n = 242 participants), *Bu yang huan wu tang* 补阳还五汤 plus pharmacotherapy was also found to be beneficial in terms of the HDS when compared to pharmacotherapy alone (Table 5.23).

Bu chang nao xin tong jiao nang 步长脑心通胶囊 was derived from *Bu yang huan wu tang* 补阳还五汤, so both formulae have many ingredients in common.[15] Meta-analysis results indicated that *Bu chang nao xin tong jiao nang* 步长脑心通胶囊 compared to pharmacotherapy alone showed improved scores on the MMSE based on three RCTs (*n* = 233 participants). Single studies showed improvements based on HDS and 'lower is better' ADL scores, but no difference was found based on the FAQ. One study tested integrative treatment with *Bu chang nao xin tong jiao nang* 步长脑心通胶囊 and found the combination to be superior to donepezil alone on 'lower is better' ADL outcomes, but not for the MMSE.

The results of the studies on the two similar formulae above suggest that they are beneficial for VaD when used singly or in combination with pharmacotherapies, but there were too few studies available to make strong conclusions. Due to differences in the inclusion and exclusion criteria used in this chapter, there were fewer studies of these formulae included in our meta-analyses compared to some previous systematic reviews.[6–8] However, the overall results and conclusions are similar.

Overall, the methodological reporting quality of the studies was not adequate and most studies were not blinded, so there remains a strong potential for bias due to methodological weaknesses. In the sensitivity analyses that focused on RCTs judged as having 'low' risk for randomisation sequence generation (SG), the results tended to reflect those of the total meta-analysis pools with some reductions in the degree of heterogeneity, but this was not always the case. Unfortunately, there were too few studies that employed blinding for additional sensitivity analyses to be generally applied.

AE reporting was not adequate in many of the RCTs, so it was not possible to provide a comprehensive assessment of the safety of the interventions. Based on the available data, AEs were mostly mild and similar in type and incidence between the intervention and control groups. They mainly included dizziness, headache, and gastro-intestinal symptoms.

In conclusion, the results from the meta-analyses suggest that oral CHM was beneficial when used alone or in combination with pharmacotherapy based on MMSE, HDS, ADL, BBS, and FAQ outcomes. However, there was risk of bias due to lack of blinding and other methodological shortcomings leading to potential overestimation of effects. Further RCTs with large sample sizes employing rigorous methodology are needed to investigate the effects of CHM treatment for VaD.

References

1. Wang X, Zhu YY, Hu LS. (2006) A meta-analysis of Chinese herbal medicines for vascular dementia. *J Nanjing Tradit Chin Med Uni* **22**(3):181–182, cover 3.
2. Niu YL, Liang WX. (2007) Systemic evaluation in treating vascular dementia with TCM. *Tianjin J Tradit Chin Med* **24**(3):190–194.
3. Man SC, Chan KW, Lu JH, Durairajan SS, *et al.* (2012) Systematic review on the efficacy and safety of herbal medicines for vascular dementia. *Evid Based Complement Alternat Med* **2012**:426215. doi: 10.1155/2012/426215.
4. Qin XD, Liu Y, Wu YQ, Wang S, *et al.* (2013) A meta-analysis of Chinese herbal medicines for vascular dementia. *Neural Regen Res* **8**(18): 1685–1692.
5. Yi YQ, Ge JW, Deng YH, Yu R, *et al.* (2013) Meta-analysis of the clinical effects of Chinese Medicine treatment by kidney on vascular dementia. *J Hunan Uni Chin Med* **33**(11):93–97.
6. Shu JZ. (2010) Meta-analysis of Bu yang huang wu decoction in treating vascular dementia. *Gansu J TCM* **23**(8):14–16.
7. Liu W, Xiao JX, Fang J, Ye RP, *et al.* (2011) A meta-analysis of Bu chang nao xin tong capsule for vascular dementia. *Med Inf* **24**(1): 43–244.
8. Li M, Hu B, Xiong GR, Tan XM. (2012) Meta analysis on curative effects of naoxintong capsules in treatment of vascular dementia. *Chin J Evid Based Cardiovasc Med* **4**(1):6–12.
9. Yue YR, Wu TX, Dong BR. (2005) Zhiling decoction for vascular dementia: A systematic review. *Chin J Evid Based Med* **5**(9):692–695.

10. Li YF, Li L, Peng XX. (2011) Efficacy and safety evaluation of Tian zhi granule treatment for vascular dementia. *Beijing J Tradit Chin Med* **30**(5):333–337.
11. Xing SH, Zhu CX, Zhang R, *et al.* (2014) Huperzine A in the treatment of Alzheimer's disease and vascular dementia: A meta-analysis. *Evid Based Complement Alternat Med* **2014**:363985.
12. Blessed G, Tomlinson BE, Roth M. (1968) The association between quantitative measure of dementia and of senile change in the cerebral gray matter of elderly subjects. *Br J Psychiat* **114**: 797–811.
13. Kurita A, Blass JP, Nolan KA, Black RS, *et al.* (1993) Relationship between cognitive status and behavioral symptoms in Alzheimer's disease and mixed dementia. *J Am Geriatr Soc* **41**(7):732–736.
14. Gao SR, Yuan JM. (1998) The diagnosis and treatment of dementia. Science and technology of China Press, Beijing. [高素荣, 袁锦楣. (1998) 痴呆诊疗学. 北京: 科学技术出版社.]
15. Zhao T. 赵涛, 薛人珲, 刘娜, 赵步长, *et al.* (2012) 脑心通胶囊的组方分析. 光明中医. **27**(12):2576–2578.

List of Clinical Studies Included in Chapter 5

Study Number	References
H1	邹忆怀, 谢颖桢, 高颖, 孟繁星, *et al.* (2001) 聪圣胶囊治疗血管性痴呆 30 例临床研究. 北京中医药大学学报. **24**(6):54–57.
H2	杨东东. (2006) 补肾益智颗粒治疗轻中度血管性痴呆的有效性的临床研究. 成都中医药大学学报. **29**(2):6–7.
H3	李建波, 张殿印, 侯玉琴. (2012) 天智颗粒治疗血管性痴呆 59 例疗效观察. 中国实用神经疾病杂志. **15**(3):84–85.
H4	陈永华, 江停战, 张波, 黄为, *et al.* (2012) 黄蒲通窍胶囊治疗血管性痴呆的临床观察. 中西医结合心脑血管病杂志. **8**(1):41–43.
H5	严永兴, 梁丽贞, 周智林. (2007) 复方海蛇胶囊及盐酸多奈哌齐联合治疗血管性痴呆的临床研究. 中国中西医结合杂志. **27**(10):887–890.
H6	李璟怡, 黄俊山, 张作丹, 林坚, *et al.* (2009) 软脉灵口服液治疗血管性痴呆的临床研究. 中西医结合心脑血管病杂志. **7**(9):1032–1034.
H7	陈春雷, 邱智辉, 苏世鑫, 郑忠诚. (2009) 通心络治疗血管性痴呆的疗效观察. 疑难病杂志. **8**(5):272–274.

(Continued)

Study Number	References
H8	程传浩, 马云枝, 马龙. (2007) 复智胶囊治疗血管性痴呆40例. 中医研究. **20**(4):42–43.
H9	吴宏生, 单亚利, 刘景. (2008) 补肾活血汤治疗血管性痴呆临床观察. 北京中医药. **27**(3):192–194.
H10	董宏利. (2012) 桃红四物汤加味治疗血管性痴呆30例临床观察. 江苏中医药. **44**(11):38–39.
H11	沈世豪, 王玲琳, 张莉. (2012) 益气活血醒脑方治疗血管性痴呆临床疗效观察. 上海中医药杂志. **44**(5):63–64.
H12	施荣康, 王玲琳, 蔡新荣. (2008) 中药方剂与哈伯因对比治疗血管性痴呆患者的临床疗效观察. 社区卫生保健. **7**(5):324–326,332.
H13	祁建平, 王利春, 刘国华. (2008) 芪参还五胶囊治疗瘀血阻络型血管性痴呆临床对照研究. 中国中医药信息杂志. **15**(5):81–82.
H14	郭一多. (2009) 祛浊增智汤联合西药治疗血管性痴呆48例. 河南中医. **29**(7):695–696.
H15	卢昌均, 安红伟, 刘国成, 鹿俊磊. (2012) 通窍活血汤治疗血管性痴呆的临床研究. 河北中医. **34**(2):171–173.
H16	张维颖, 卢致鹏 (2006). 补肾健脑汤治疗血管性痴呆的临床研究. 中西医结合心脑血管病杂志. **4**(8):680–681.
H17	王彦华 (2007). 益髓增智汤治疗血管性痴呆. 医药论坛杂志. **28**(20):118,121.
H18	程为平, 马莉, 原田俊英, 王庆武. (2004) 脑智通胶囊治疗血管性痴呆18例疗效观察. 新中医. **36**(1):16–18.
H19	姜海鹏, 况时祥. (2012) 脑通胶囊治疗血管性痴呆早期疗效观察. 中国中医急症. **19**(10):1669–1670,1678.
H20	孙丽芳, 张丽欣, 王志刚. (2013) 补阳还五汤加减治疗血管性痴呆32例. 河北中医药学报. **28**(3):11–12.
H21	孙小平. (2012) 益气补肾活血化瘀方治疗血管性痴呆的临床观察. 临床合理用药杂志. **5**(14):67.
H22	吴天晨, 许若晴. (2012) 还少丹加减治疗血管性痴呆32例临床观察. 湖南中医杂志. **28**(5):43–44.
H23	郑德俊, 徐俊, 方穗雄, 潘锦瑶, *et al.* (2009) 步长脑心通对血管性痴呆患者行为学障碍影响. 中医药信息. **26**(4):75–76.
H24	余德海, 李玮, 李林. (2012) 步长脑心通胶囊治疗血管性痴呆30例疗效观察. 云南中医中药杂志. **33**(6):42–43.

(*Continued*)

(**Continued**)

Study Number	References
H25	蔡晶, 杜建, 黄俊山, 林求诚, *et al.* (2003) 康欣胶囊对血管性痴呆影响的临床观察. 中国老年学杂志. **23**(8):482–484.
H26	曹晓岚, 宋旭霞, 胡志强, 梅彤, *et al.* (2002) 聪圣胶囊治疗老年期血管性痴呆临床研究. 中国中医急症. **11**(2):80–81.
H27	崔应麟, 张志鑫, 常通玮. (2009) "通窍益智汤" 治疗血管性痴呆临床研究. 江苏中医药. **41**(6):26–27.
H28	黄晓明, 张丽萍. (2009) 益气活血补肾法治疗血管性痴呆的临床研究. 浙江中医杂志. **44**(11):791–792.
H29	贾绍燕, 史咏梅, 高颖 (指导). (2004) 益肾化浊法治疗血管性痴呆 48 例临床观察. 中国中医药信息杂志. **11**(4):338–339.
H30	李世够. (2012) 益智汤治疗血管性痴呆 30 例. 河南中医. **32**(3):322–323.
H31	廖晓岚, 陈康远, 郑泽荣, 刘晖, *et al.* (2004) 首灵健脑胶囊改善血管性痴呆患者脑功能的效果分析. 中国临床康复. **8**(1):112–114.
H32	罗增刚, 周文泉, 高普, 崔玲. (2001) 参麻益智胶囊治疗老年血管性痴呆的临床研究. 中医杂志. **42**(8):470–473.
H33	彭伟, 邓华亮. (2007) 活血化瘀、补肾益智法治疗血管性痴呆的临床效应比较研究. 长春中医药大学学报. **23**(6):29–30.
H34	乔之龙, 张昱, 王玉璧. (2011) 补肾益智汤治疗老年血管性痴呆肾虚髓减证临床研究. 光明中医. **26**(10):1990–1991.
H35	邵义泽. (2003) 醒脑复苏汤治疗中、轻度老年血管性痴呆的临床观察. 河北中医. **25**(4):253–255.
H36	沈双宏, 杜建. (2004) 补肾健脾养血活血方治疗血管性痴呆肾虚血瘀型的临床研究.湖南中医学院学报. **24**(4):41–43, 50.
H37	孙文燕, 傅仁杰, 孙建宁. (2010) 启神胶囊治疗血管性痴呆的临床疗效初步观察. 中药药理与临床. **26**(5):141–142.
H38	王谨敏, 王梅平, 杜建, 蔡晶, *et al.* (2007) 针灸结合康欣胶囊治疗肾虚血瘀型血管性痴呆的临床研究. 中西医结合心脑血管病杂志. **5**(5):398–400.
H39	王小青. (2012) 补肾益气法治疗肾精亏虚证血管性痴呆临床分析. 光明中医. **27**(1):78–79.
H40	王炎焱, 路辉, 陈馥, 吴英, *et al.* (2002) 神通胶囊治疗脑血管性痴呆临床与实验研究. 中医杂志. **43**(6):437–439.
H41	魏孟玲. (2013) 补脾益心汤加减治疗老年血管性痴呆心脾两虚证疗效研究. 中西医结合心脑血管病杂志. **11**(6):703–704.

(*Continued*)

Study Number	References
H42	文天保, 高丽霞. (2013) 健脑益智汤治疗血管性痴呆 30 例临床观察. 山西中医学院学报. **14**(2):51–52.
H43	吴松鹰, 方素钦, 梁晖. (2004) 苁蓉总甙胶囊治疗髓海不足型血管性痴呆的随机双盲对照研究. 福建中医药. **35**(4):3–4.
H44	吴晓红. (2005) 益气活血法治疗多发性梗死性痴呆 30 例临床研究. 中医杂志. **46**(4):267–269.
H45	徐鸿雁, 李婧辉, 綦宏伶, 吴松柏, *et al.* (2011) 脑复聪胶囊治疗多梗死性痴呆 256 例临床观察. 医学信息. **24**(4):181,183.
H46	杨文明, 户文娟, 韩明向, 周宜轩, *et al.* (2002) 智脑胶囊治疗血管性痴呆 60 例临床研究. 中国实验方剂学杂志. **8**(6):48–51.
H47	张弛, 梅建伟, 张新芳, 张英强. (2010) 脑力苏汤剂治疗血管性痴呆临床疗效观察:附 60 例病例报告.成都中医药大学学报. **33**(4):21–24.
H48	张连城, 张权. (2011) 补肾中药治疗血管性痴呆 32 例临床研究. 国医论坛. **26**(1):22–23.
H49	张云岭, 梅建勋, 张伯礼, 王永炎. (1998) 健脑益智冲剂治疗多发梗塞性痴呆轻中度的临床观察. 北京中医药大学学报. **21**(5):42–44.
H50	赵学军, 樊莉, 陈建宗, 张发荣, *et al.* (1997) 脑力康口服液治疗血管性痴呆患者神经心理障碍 47 例临床观察. 新中医. **29**(11):15–16.
H51	赵琰, 周文泉, 高普, 崔玲. (1999) 仙龙胶囊治疗血管性痴呆的临床研究. 中国中西医结合杂志. **19**(10):585–588.
H52	利春红. (2007) 自拟中药补肾涤痰化瘀汤治疗血管性痴呆 60 例临床观察. 内科. **2**(3):370–371.
H53	丁旸. (2005) 脑脉泰胶囊治疗老年血管性痴呆临床观察. 中国中医药信息杂志. **12**(3):60.
H54	张利平. (2009) 通窍健脑汤治疗血管性痴呆 35 例. 中医研究. **22**(4):23–24.
H55	石宝连. (2008) 补肾活血化痰法治疗血管性痴呆 30 例临床观察. 中国中医药信息杂志. **15**(2):76–77.
H56	白晶, 李宝栋, 王利春, 段洪波. (2013) 芪参还五胶囊对轻度血管性痴呆认知功能的影响. 中国中医药信息杂志. **20**(4):65–66.
H57	曹利民, 胡志诚. (2009) 益肾通络化瘀汤治疗血管性痴呆 45 例. 浙江中医杂志. **44**(1):33.
H58	常增义, 乔钦才, 张永红, 乔钦增. (2008) 芪红口服液改善老年血管性痴呆患者智能的临床研究. 中国药物与临床. **8**(3):240–241.

(*Continued*)

(***Continued***)

Study Number	References
H59	陈利平, 王发渭, 贾建军, 郝爱真. (2007) 参龙汤治疗老年血管性痴呆的临床研究. 解放军医学杂志. **32**(8):866–868.
H60	戴飞跃, 黄保民, 肖辉. (2006) 益脑灵治疗血管性痴呆疗效观察. 辽宁中医杂志. **33**(7):826–827.
H61	龚振岭, 龚志刚, 靳国春, 杨建忠, *et al.* (2004) 痴呆康胶囊治疗血管性痴呆 128 例疗效观察. 中国医药学报. **19**(4):253–254.
H62	郭明冬, 周文泉, 李贻奎, 安玉凤, *et al.* (2012) 参芎补肾胶囊对轻度血管性痴呆患者的疗效及对脑神经递质的影响. 中医杂志. **53**(2):126–128, 32.
H63	郝伟平, 叶锋华, 李丽珠. (2006) 通心络胶囊治疗血管性痴呆患者临床观察. 临床心身疾病杂志. **12**(6):424–425.
H64	何宇平, 杨越, 张伟萍, 吕海琼. (2006) 复方海蛇胶囊治疗血管性痴呆的疗效观察. 中国实用神经疾病杂志. **9**(2):66–67.
H65	洪茂林, 侯国典, 洪利生, 皮兴文, *et al.* (2002) 寿星胶囊治疗血管性痴呆的临床研究. 湖北中医杂志. **24**(4):3–5.
H66	黄启辉, 谭朝晖, 李庆明. (2002) 脑还丹胶囊治疗轻中度血管性痴呆临床观察. 广州中医药大学学报. **19**(3):169–171.
H67	李长生, 李军, 关新华, 王荣霞, *et al.* (2008) 首乌益智胶囊治疗血管性痴呆 80 例临床研究. 中国老年学杂志. **28**(4):369–371.
H68	刘涛, 王灿晖, 杨进, 吴瑞枝, *et al.* (2005) 改良三甲散对血管性痴呆病患者智能状态的调节作用. 中国中西医结合杂志. **25**(6):492–495.
H69	Liu XF, Du J, Cai J, Liu XF, *et al.* (2007) Clinical systematic observation of Kangxin capsule curing vascular dementia of senile kidney deficiency and blood stagnation type. *J Ethnopharm.* **112**(2):350–355.
H70	沈志芳, 乔钦增, 曹桂山. (2012) 红灯散瘀汤改善老年血管性痴呆患者智能研究. 中西医结合心脑血管病杂志. **10**(7):816–817.
H71	舒宏, 丁春, 周毅, 邓志洪. (2013) 圣济二精颗粒治疗血管性痴呆临床疗效观察. 湖北中医杂志. **35**(2):9–10.
H72	陶根鱼. (2004) 醒脑丸治疗血管性痴呆临床研究. 陕西中医学院学报. **27**(1):5–7.
H73	万毅, 王汝丰. (1998) 复聪汤治疗血管性痴呆临床研究. 河北医学. **4**(11):24–27.

(*Continued*)

Study Number	References
H74	王兵. (2010) 益肾通窍汤治疗血管性痴呆 40 例临床观察.内蒙古中医药. **29**(23):18–19.
H75	王凤菊, 吕士君, 董征. (2002) 益智通络胶囊治疗血管性痴呆的临床研究. 现代中西医结合杂志. **11**(4):295–297.
H76	王国华, 陈治林. (2012) 养血清脑颗粒治疗血管性痴呆 48 例. 内蒙古中医药. **31**(16):9.
H77	王健, 陈其维, 海英, 白丽, *et al.* (2004) 回天片治疗血管性痴呆的临床研究. 中医药学刊. **22**(9):1691–1694.
H78	王健, 陈其维, 白丽. (2005) 健脑聪明口服液治疗血管性痴呆的临床研究. 辽宁中医杂志. 32(1):3–5.
H79	王金桥, 李福田, 王树林, 赵东升, *et al.* (2000) 补肺复聪汤治疗多发梗死性痴呆临床研究. 山东中医杂志. **19**(11):649–652.
H80	王志宏, 刘素梅, 于文涛. (2005) 补肾活血法治疗血管性痴呆患者 86 例临床观察. 中华实用中西医杂志. **18**(19):1115–1116.
H81	武红斌, 许海宁, 贺会刚. (2007) 养血清脑颗粒治疗血管性痴呆病人临床观察. 中西医结合心脑血管病杂志. **5**(11):1069–1070.
H82	夏翔, 沈小珩, 柳玉瑾, 郃杏芳, *et al.* (2001) 百岁方口服液治疗血管性痴呆的临床观察. 中国中西医结合杂志. **21**(8):569–572.
H83	许凤华, 张洪斌. (2002) 血管性痴呆血瘀证的研究. 山东中医药大学学报. **26**(3):210–213.
H84	徐因, 张子明, 李子印, 杨泉鱼, *et al.* (2000) 益智丸治疗老年期血管性痴呆临床观察. 河北中医. **22**(11):821 822.
H85	杨东威, 王熙, 叶志峰. (2007) 首乌延寿丹治疗血管性痴呆 40 例. 中医杂志. **48**(9):823–824.
H86	翟广琪. (2013) 益气聪明汤治疗血管性痴呆 30 例. 河南中医. **33**(11):1890–1891.
H87	占戈, 满伟. (2007) 益肾醒脑汤治疗血管性痴呆疗效观察. 北京中医药大学学报·中医临床版. **14**(5):13–16.
H88	张法荣, 张洪斌. (2002) 中药康脑灵治疗血管性痴呆临床观察. 山东中医药大学学报. **26**(3):197–198.
H89	张玉金, 张文芝. (2002) 脑安胶囊治疗脑血管性痴呆疗效观察. 实用中医药杂志. **18**(12):32.
H90	赵玉娟. (2007) 补肾益智汤治疗血管性痴呆 33 例临床观察. 中国中医药科技. **14**(2):129–130.

(*Continued*)

(*Continued*)

Study Number	References
H91	赵志坤, 贾凤新, 李桂, 李兰者, *et al.* (2009) 益智聪明方治疗血管性痴呆 51 例临床观察. 河北中医. **31**(4):493–496.
H92	周海哲, 袁普卫, 李军. (2007) 脑泰通颗粒治疗血管性痴呆的临床观察. 辽宁中医杂志. **34**(2):176–177.
H93	周建英, 孙长春, 顾月星. (2005) 益气复智颗粒对血管性痴呆患者精神量表评定的影响. 医学研究生学报. **18**(5):415–416.
H94	武继涛. (2011) 天智颗粒治疗轻、中度血管性痴呆27例. 中国实验方剂学杂志. **17**(17):272–273.
H95	张志刚, 项宝玉, 刘晴. (2012) 脑血疏通口服液治疗轻中度血管性痴呆的临床研究. 中西医结合心脑血管病杂志. **10**(4):438–439.
H96	李跃华. (2011) 培元通脑胶囊治疗老年血管性痴呆的临床观察. 求医问药. **9**(6):143,110.
H97	王尊钙, 温小芬. (2011) 醒脑汤治疗血管性痴呆临床观察. 中国中医急症. **20**(1):47–49.
H98	张玉麟, 王义方, 高之旭. (2001) 中药"菖术汤"治疗血管性痴呆的临床研究. 上海精神医学. **13**(3):146–148.
H99	周伟, 吴永斌, 许贤瑞. (2009) 脑心通胶囊治疗血管性痴呆患者临床观察. 山东医药. **49**(8):99–100.
H100	黄琍琳. (2007) 健脑益智汤治疗血管性痴呆疗效观察. 中医药临床杂志. **19**(4):366–367.
H101	王轶虎. (2011) 多奈哌齐联合复方海蛇胶囊治疗血管性痴呆 68 例. 浙江中西医结合杂志. **21**(7):488–489.
H102	许珂, 王克非. (2011) 盐酸多奈哌齐联合银丹心脑通软胶囊对血管性痴呆患者认知功能的影响. 中西医结合心脑血管病杂志. **9**(10):1213–1215.
H103	黄根宪, 陆建兵. (2013) 脑心通胶囊联合多奈哌齐治疗血管性痴呆 32 例. 浙江中医杂志. **48**(10):775–776.
H104	黄漫, 吴远华, 曹丽平, 绍勇(指导). (2012) 补肾通髓醒脑方治疗卒中后血管性痴呆的临床观察. 贵阳中医学院学报. **34**(3):174–175.
H105	徐新春, 张亚敏, 张慧. (2008) 清心化痰汤结合西药治疗血管性痴呆 36 例临床观察. 上海中医药杂志. **42**(2):35–37.
H106	周嘉澄, 刘刚, 梁迪赛, 关浩峰. (2012) 补虚通窍汤治疗血管性痴呆的疗效观察. 中医临床研究. **4**(9):21–23.
H107	祝华君. (2009) 七福饮加减治疗血管性痴呆 30 例. 浙江中医杂志. **44**(2):128.

(Continued)

Study Number	References
H108	朱江. (2005) 尼莫地平结合醒脑胶囊治疗血管性痴呆 54 例临床观察. 广东医学院学报. **23**(2):152–154.
H109	杜庆娟, 闫伟, 张哲一. (2009) 益脑增智胶囊治疗血管性痴呆的临床研究. 吉林医学. **30**(24):3129–3130.
H110	段保亮. (2010) 自拟醒脑汤治疗血管性痴呆 80 例. 光明中医. **25**(8): 1386–1387.
H111	余天智. (2011) 益气养阴活血补肾法治疗血管性痴呆 34 例临床观察. 广西医学. **33**(2):248–250.
H112	曹玮, 李金伟. (2010) 增智通窍汤联合茴拉西坦治疗血管性痴呆疗效观察. 中医药临床杂志. **22**(11):979–980.
H113	冯莹莹. (2013) 补肾活血健脑汤治疗血管性痴呆 38 例. 中国中医药科技. **20**(4):431–432.
H114	杨华, 潘智琴, 张江涛, 王翰. (2012) 温胆汤联合茴拉西坦治疗痰浊阻窍型血管性痴呆 30 例观察. 浙江中医杂志. **47**(5):326.
H115	戚传远. (2009) 自拟乌黄益智汤治疗血管性痴呆. 光明中医. **24**(2):287–288.
H116	李伟伟, 王鸣池, 于盼盼, 王悦. (2013) 奥拉西坦联合三七通舒治疗血管性痴呆的临床疗效观察. 西部中医药. **26**(2):81–83.
H117	张经华. (2008) 中西医结合治疗血管性痴呆的临床研究. 中国中医药现代远程教育. **6**(12):1487–1488.
H118	李敬会, 夏忠诚, 桂程丽. (2013) 补肾益智汤联合神经节苷酯治疗血管性痴呆. 辽宁中医杂志. **40**(3):481–483.
H119	师会, 王惠明. (2006) 补肾活血法治疗血管性痴呆临床疗效观察. 天津中医药. **23**(3):200–202.
H120	徐莹, 吴限. (2013) 心脑通络液治疗血管性痴呆的临床观察. 天津中医药大学学报. **32**(2):84–86.
H121	钟炳武, 何明大. (2007) 益智健脑汤治疗血管性痴呆 55 例. 上海中医药杂志. **41**(4):34–36.
H122	Shimada Y, Terasawa K, Yamamoto T, Maruyama I, *et al.* (1995) A well-controlled study of Choto-san and placebo in the treatment of vascular dementia. *J Tradit Med* **11**:246–255.
H123	Terasawa K, Shimada Y, Kita T, Yamamoto T, *et al.* (1997) Choto-san in the treatment of vascular dementia: A double-blind, placebo-controlled study. *Phytomedicine* **4**(1):15–22.

(*Continued*)

(*Continued*)

Study Number	References
H124	王东明, 李爱敏, 原永贵, 王莉, *et al.* (2003) 三鞭丸治疗血管性痴呆对事件相关电位影响的研究. 中华临床医药杂志. **4**(7):30–31.
H125	张瑞彬, 武宏. (2012) 健脑汤治疗血管性痴呆 76 例临床观察. 中医临床研究. **4**(7):91–92.
H126	卢瑞丽. (2011) 通窍化浊汤治疗血管性痴呆 30 例疗效观察. 新中医. **43**(7):42–43.
H127	苏春芝, 李静君, 杜英, 赵瑞芹, *et al.* (2005) 益智金丹治疗老年期血管性痴呆 50 例疗效观察. 新中医. **37**(8):42–44.
H128	单丽华, 孙英健, 王媛媛. (2008) 九味增智饮治疗血管性痴呆病气虚血瘀证30例临床观察. 新中医. **40**(9):59–60.
H129	傅仁杰, 吴继全, 章少华, 郭改惠, *et al.* (1998) 启神胶囊治疗血管性痴呆的临床观察. 中国医药学报. **13**(1):39–40.
H130	张跃林. (2007) 祛湿化痰除瘀方治疗血管性痴呆 43 例的临床观察. 中国医学杂志. **5**(11):7–8.
H131	曹云. (2010) 益肾通络醒神法治疗多发梗塞性痴呆 50 例.陕西中医. **31**(2):153–155.
H132	张崇泉, 金幼兰, 赵李剑. (2001) 健脑通络胶囊治疗血管性痴呆的临床研究. 中国中医药信息杂志. **8**(4):51–52.
H133	包祖晓, 胡灵敏, 陈存国. (2005) 益气活血醒脑颗粒治疗血管性痴呆临床观察. 中国中医药信息杂志. **12**(1):72–73.
H134	樊学忠, 杨保林. (2004) 水蛭通胶囊治疗老年脑血管性痴呆的临床研究. 中国中西医结合杂志. **24**(8):694–697.
H135	纪立金, 张美增. (2004) 强脾补精化瘀益智胶囊治疗多发梗塞性痴呆的疗效及对智商的影响. 福建中医学院学报. **14**(1):1–3.
H136	吴俊喜, 李国卿, 李静君, 贾艳萍, *et al.* (2001) 地黄饮子加减胶囊治疗老年期血管性痴呆 68 例疗效观察. 河北中医. **23**(2):88–89.
H137	吴力萍, 陶连方. (2009) 补肾益气化瘀胶囊治疗血管性痴呆临床研究. 医学研究杂志. **38**(1):100–102.
H138	周广萍, 魏霞. (2001) 益脑灵口服液治疗血管性痴呆的临床研究. 山东中医杂志. **20**(1):14–15.
H139	张燕. (2003) 增智汤治疗血管性痴呆 76 例临床观察. 光明中医. **18**(3):50.
H140	施海婷. (2011) 天智颗粒治疗血管性痴呆疗效观察. 中西医结合心脑血管病杂志. **9**(8):955–956.

(*Continued*)

Study Number	References
H141	王来群. (2008) 益气补肾活血化痰开窍法治疗血管性痴呆临床观察. 辽宁中医药大学学报. **10**(9): 96–97.
H142	刘德桓, 周文强, 许真真, 郭伟聪, *et al.* (2002) 健脑合剂治疗老年血管性痴呆的临床研究. 福建中医学院学报. **12**(2):4–7.
H143	牛敬宪, 李咏梅. (2008) 益智醒脑汤对血管性痴呆患者认识功能障碍的影响. 中西医结合心脑血管病杂志. **6**(11):1288–1289.
H144	田军彪, 杨倩, 王艳君, 蔡月花. (2003) 强力增智饮治疗血管性痴呆 42 例临床观察. 中华实用中西医杂志. **16**(1):10.
H145	郜海生. (2008) 自拟补肾逐瘀汤辅助治疗老年血管性痴呆 48 例疗效观察. 山东医药. **48**(48):117.
H146	芦凤琴, 闫伟. (2011) 加味二陈汤治疗脑卒中后血管性痴呆 40 例. 中国中医急症. **20**(4):641–642.
H147	蒙坚. (2010) 化痰复智汤治疗血管性痴呆 48 例观察. 浙江中医杂志. **45**(12): 882.
H148	韦华军. (2011) 加服自拟益肾健脑通络汤治疗血管性痴呆 24 例. 广西中医药. **34**(4):14–15.
H149	张朝贵. (2010) 中西医结合治疗血管性痴呆 76 例临床观察. 四川中医. **28**(12):83–84.
H150	张振强. (2006) 健脑益智汤加味治疗血管性痴呆的临床观察. 河南大学学报·医学版. **25**(3):43–44.
H151	赵勇军, 薛秀荣. (2010) 鳖甲煎丸治疗血管性痴呆 50 例. 中国中医急症. **19**(10):1782–1783.
H152	李贤, 封桂宇. (2008) 益肾活血法结合西药治疗血管性痴呆 35 例. 广西中医学院学报. **11**(1):13–15.
H153	马琳, 孙莉. (2009) 疏肝解郁法治疗血管性痴呆 30 例临床观察. 中国现代医生. **47**(21): 114–118.
H154	马瑞莲, 王静, 许东, 马风琴. (2007) 中西医结合治疗血管性痴呆病临床研究. 宁夏医学杂志. **29**(4):321–322.
H155	周正国, 曲芳, 单丽华, 孙英健. (2010) 益气化痰法治疗血管性痴呆(痰浊阻窍证)的临床研究. 实用中医内科杂志. **24**(2):86–87.
H156	王光明, 吴俊贞, 靳建鸣. (2002) 中西医结合治疗血管性痴呆临床观察. 天津中医. **19**(1):27.
H157	张伯礼, 王永炎, 陈汝兴, 王荫华, *et al.* (2002) 健脑益智颗粒治疗血管性痴呆的随机双盲临床研究. 中国中西医结合杂志. **22**(8):577–580.

(*Continued*)

(*Continued*)

Study Number	References
H158	刘永辉, 戚慧敏. (2014) 补肾安神益智汤治疗血管性痴呆疗效观察. 中医临床研究. **6**(4):17–19.
H159	张美增, 董芝欣, 毛拥军, 杜芳. (2005) 益智胶囊对多发梗死性痴呆患者智力的影响. 中国临床康复. **9**(36):155–157.
H160	杜秦川, 马瑞莲, 王静. (1997) 中西医结合治疗老年血管性痴呆 45 例疗效观察. 山西中医. **13**(6):23–24.
H161	王震宇. (2005) 补阳还五汤治疗血管性痴呆 39 例.陕西中医. **26**(8):781–782.
H162	阎奇. (2007) 中西医结合治疗血管性痴呆 43 例疗效观察. 四川中医. **25**(5):41–42.
H163	陈德仁. (2005) 益肾活血化痰开窍法治疗多梗死性痴呆 30 例临床观察. 江苏中医药. **26**(4):16–17.
H164	陈改花, 郝丽霞. (2005) 中西医结合治疗血管性痴呆 42 例临床观察. 山西中医学院学报. **6**(1):33–34.
H165	陈绍辉, 祝淑贞. (2011) 中西医结合治疗血管性痴呆. 新乡医学院学报. **28**(4):483–484,487.
H166	陈威, 江钢辉, 杨磊, 蒋红玉. (2012) 益气养阴法对血管性痴呆高同型半胱氨酸血症的影响. 新中医. **44**(8):56–57.
H167	崔杰强, 丁红梅. (2006) 胶蒲益智方治疗血管性痴呆临床观察. 中华现代医学与临床. **4**(8):49–50.
H168	冯红岩. (2006) 增智通窍汤治疗血管性痴呆 76 例. 河南中医. **26**(9):37–38.
H169	韩桂华, 常明华. (2005) 涤痰化瘀填精益髓法治疗血管性痴呆疗效观察. 辽宁中医杂志. **32**(1):45.
H170	侯刚. (1999) 健脾活血开窍益智法治疗老年脑血管性痴呆 52 例临床观察. 新中医. **31**(6):57–58.
H171	厉秀云, 贾杰, 李振民, 刘素珍, 刘玉洁 (指导). (2008) 复聪饮治疗多发梗死性痴呆 125 例临床观察. 河北中医. **30**(3):244–245.
H172	刘光亭. (2005) 血管性痴呆患者智力状态、血液流变学和血脂变化及补肾益脑胶囊的干预作用. 中国临床康复. **9**(20):50–51.
H173	宋丽, 李喜红. (2011) 自拟健智方 I 号治疗血管性痴呆病 105 例. 中国社区医师·医学专业. **19**:208.
H174	童丽, 吴萍, 李福安, 魏全嘉. (2006) 益痴胶囊治疗老年期血管性痴呆 24 例临床观察. 江苏中医药. **27**(8):31–32.

(Continued)

Study Number	References
H175	王兴柱. (2008) 益气补肾、活血开窍法治疗血管性痴呆 65 例临床研究. 四川中医. **26**(11):71–73.
H176	项颗, 孙莉. (2005) 填精益智活血方治疗血管性痴呆的临床观察. 中国医药研究. **3**(2):135.
H177	谢静红. (2006) 地黄饮子治疗血管性痴呆 39 例. 福建中医药. **37**(1):38.
H178	杨传印, 李富旺. (2005) 通窍益智汤治疗血管性痴呆 80 例临床观察. 中国中医基础医学杂志. **11**(10):790.
H179	袁兵. (2012) 降脂复聪丸治疗血管性痴呆 35 例. 中国中医药现代远程教育. **10**(11):109–110.
H180	刘锁超, 张文学. (2002) 益智汤治疗血管性痴呆 82 例临床观察. 四川中医. **20**(9):27–28.
H181	丁占勤. (2003) 中西医结合治疗血管性痴呆 31 例临床观察. 山东医药. **43**(16):54.
H182	罗康. (2000) 扶正涤痰化瘀法治疗血管性痴呆 68 例临床观察. 广西中医药. **23**(3):1–3.
H183	马瑞莲, 王静. (1998) 补阳还五汤治疗血管性痴呆 60 例. 陕西中医. **19**(9):408.
H184	毛敬洁, 王宏, 蔡晶, 沈双宏, *et al.* (2010) 康欣胶囊对血管性痴呆患者脑血流灌注的影响. 福建中医药大学学报. **20**(6):23–25.
H185	乔钦增, 郭全合, 刘和荣, 侯津杰, *et al.* (2002) 复神益智胶囊改善老年血管性痴呆患者记忆、判断功能的研究. 中国临床康复. **6**(1):55–56.
H186	田立, 宋立公. (2007) 虚实分型辨治血管性痴呆 80 例临床观察. 中西医结合心脑血管病杂志. **5**(11):1072–1073.
H187	王玉宇. (2013) 血府逐瘀汤合安理申治疗血管性痴呆 24 例疗效观察. 浙江中医杂志. **48**(10):730–731.
H188	吴斌, 徐清, 顾君, 董爱国. (2013) 天智颗粒治疗轻、中度血管性痴呆疗效观察. 中国健康心理学杂志. **21**(12):1774–1776.
H189	张志真, 周德安, 盛丽, 刘慧林, *et al.* (2000) 疏调益智方治疗血管性痴呆的临床研究. 北京中医. **19**(4):11–14.
H190	赵卫东, 左新芳, 程桂林, 魏琴. (2000) "生髓散" 加用尼莫地平治疗中老年血管性痴呆 40 例临床观察. 湖北民族学院学报·医学版. **17**(3):30.
H191	曹建恒. (2009) 涤痰化瘀宣窍方治疗血管性痴呆 55 例. 中医研究. **22**(5):38–39.

(Continued)

(Continued)

Study Number	References
H192	陈光. (2002) 补肾化痰通络法治疗血管性痴呆 32 例临床观察. 北京中医. **21**(1):7–9.
H193	贵友, 陈楷, 周文全, 赵雍, *et al.* (1998) 天麻促智冲剂治疗老年血管性痴呆临床观察. 中国中药杂志. **23**(11):695–698.
H194	方传刚. (1999) 益脑聪明汤治疗血管性痴呆 68 例疗效分析. 现代中医. **12**(4):17–18.
H195	葛近峰, 何爱芳, 宁子秀. (2010) 步长脑心通胶囊合高压氧治疗血管性痴呆 36 例. 辽宁中医杂志. **37**(6):1050–1051.
H196	郭增元, 段迎喜. (2006) 启智汤治疗血管性痴呆 77 例. 中国中医药信息杂志. **13**(7):75.
H197	惠振亮, 刘淑雅. (2008) 益智聪明汤配合心理疏导智力训练治疗血管性痴呆 42 例. 陕西中医. **29**(2):172–174.
H198	厉秀云, 贾杰, 李立军, 李振民. (2008) 复聪饮合醒脑静治疗血管性痴呆 60 例. 四川中医. **26**(5):71.
H199	刘华, 周君富. (1994) 补肾活血化痰法治疗脑血管性痴呆的临床研究. 浙江中医杂志. **29**(12):530–532.
H200	刘俊峰, 张建伟. (2007) 桃仁红花煎加减治疗血管性痴呆 20 例. 新中医. **39**(1):50.
H201	骆凯, 苗绿, 史洪亮, 薛薇. (2006) 增智益脑汤治疗中风后痴呆112例. 辽宁中医杂志. **33**(2):196–197.
H202	苗雪梅, 冯周琴, 李蕴琛. (1995) 青龙胶丸治疗血管性痴呆的临床研究. 中国蛇志杂志. **7**(1):13–15.
H203	缪峰, 周海哲, 杨秀清. (2003) 地黄饮子加减治疗中风痴呆 30 例. 陕西中医. **24**(2):132–134.
H204	孙培军, 司国民. (2006) 益智通脉汤治疗血管性痴呆 32 例临床观察. 贵阳中医学院学报. **28**(3):30–31.
H205	滕晶, 张洪斌. (2000) 康脑灵 II 号治疗血管性痴呆实验与临床研究. 山东中医药大学学报. **24**(1):48–51.
H206	田丁军, 芮小江, 李建军. (2003) 复方蛭龙制剂治疗血管性痴呆 72 例. 中国临床康复. **7**(31):4290.
H207	田军彪, 王艳君, 王石红, 蔡月花. (2004) 强力增智饮对血管性痴呆患者血脂及血液流变学的影响. 河北中医药学报. **19**(2):3–4.

(*Continued*)

Study Number	References
H208	王灿晖, 刘涛, 杨进, 吴瑞枝, *et al*. (1999) 滋肾通窍法对血管性痴呆患者精神量表评定的观察. 中国中西医结合杂志. **19**(7):405–406.
H209	王健, 王中男. (1998) 颐神养脑胶囊对 30 例血管性痴呆患者作用的临床观察. 长春中医学院学报. **14**(1):18–19.
H210	王树国. (2007) 填髓祛邪合剂治疗血管性痴呆 54 例. 山西中医. **23**(4): 19–20.
H211	王香存. (2004) 醒脑益智汤加减治疗血管性痴呆 68 例. 河南中医. **24**(12):28.
H212	王宗源. (1999) 地黄饮子化裁治疗脑血管性痴呆 34 例. 南京中医药大学学报. **15**(3):146–147.
H213	温秦庆. (2013) 补阳还五汤加味治疗脑血管性痴呆疗效观察. 陕西中医. **33**(12):1614–1615.
H214	武宏. (2006) 通窍活血汤加减治疗血管性痴呆 40 例. 陕西中医. **27**(11):1337–1338.
H215	谢广平, 陈泽文. (2009) 加味孔圣枕中丹治疗中风后痴呆 52 例. 中国中医急症. **18**(9):1511.
H216	于杰, 李桂清, 王鹏琴, 张明波, *et al*. (1998) 通脉益智丹治疗脑血管性痴呆 50 例临床观察. 实用中西医结合杂志. **11**(8):707.
H217	张冰, 刘颖, 徐秋萍, 张丰硕, *et al*. (1999) 益脑颗粒治疗血管性痴呆 32 例疗效分析. 北京中医药大学学报. **22**(4):53–55.
H218	张彦红, 朱磊, 梁伟雄. (2012) 苁蓉总苷胶囊治疗髓海不足型轻中度血管性痴呆 40 例. 中医研究. **25**(6):41–44.
H219	赵美玲, 仝战旗. (1997) 参仙汤对脑血管性痴呆智能障碍影响的临床研究. 军医进修学院学报. **18**(4):283–284.
H220	周强, 蔡军, 庄玉兰. (2006) 中西医结合治疗血管性痴呆临床观察. 中医药学刊. **24**(12):2347–2348.
H221	谭佩珍, 杨期东, 谭兴林, 徐东华, *et al*. (2002) 何首乌治疗血管性痴呆的疗效观察. 河南医药信息. **10**(12):7–9.

6

Pharmacological Actions of the Common Herbs

OVERVIEW

The therapeutic effects of Chinese herbal medicines for vascular dementia are due to the activities of the chemical compounds they contain. This section reviews the available experimental evidence for the ten Chinese herbs most frequently used in the formulae listed in the randomised clinical trials in Chapter 5 and identifies the biological activities relevant to dementia and cerebrovascular injury.

Introduction

Chinese herbal formulae exert their actions through the active constituent compounds in the herbs used. Although clinical trials can assess the efficacy and safety of formulae and herbs, the mechanisms of action of the herbs are not usually investigated during clinical trials. Experimental studies, both *in vitro* and *in vivo,* have investigated herb extracts and their constituent compounds in a range of experimental models with the aim of identifying their actions and potential mechanisms of action. These may explain some of the reported therapeutic benefits of Chinese herbs for vascular dementia (VaD).

This chapter reviews evidence from animal models, cell lines, and other experimental studies of relevance to dementia, ageing, and ischemia for the ten herbs identified as the most frequently used ingredients in the herbal interventions tested in the randomised controlled trials (RCTs) in Chapter 5. The commonly used herbs include *shi chang pu* 石菖蒲, *chuan xiong* 川芎, *dang gui* 当归, *he shou wu* 何首乌, *huang qi* 黄芪, *dan shen* 丹参, *yuan zhi* 远志, *shui zhi* 水蛭, *di huang* 地黄, and *gou qi zi* 枸杞子.

Abbreviations Used in this Chapter

6-OHDA: 6-hydroxydopamine; 6-OHDA: oxidopamine; Abeta: beta-amyloid; Ach: acetylcholine; AChE: acetylcholinesterase; ADSC: adipose-derived stem cells; AGEs: advanced glycation end products; AKT: RAC-alpha serine/threonine-protein kinase; APP/PS1 double transgenic mouse model; APP: amyloid precursor protein; AQP4: aquaporin 4; AST: astragaloside; BACE1: beta-secretase 1; Bax: bcl-2-like protein 4; BDNF: brain-derived neurotrophic factor; BP: 3-butylidenephthalide; COX-2: cyclooxygenase-2; DJ-1: deglycase (DJ-1) gene; ER: endoplasmic reticulum; FDA: Food and Drug Administration; *Fmr1*: Fragile X mental retardation gene; GABA: gamma-aminobutyric acid; GAD65: glutamic acid decarboxylase; GFAP: glial-fibrillary-acid protein; GluR1: glutamate receptor 1; GSH: glutathione; GSH-Px: GSH peroxidase; GST: glutathione S transferase; HDL: high-density lipo-proteins; HMGB1: high-mobility group box1 (HMGB1); HMG-CoA: 3-hydroxy-3-methyl-glutaryl-coenzyme A reductase; i.p.: intraperitoneal; IL-1β: interleukin-1beta; IL-6: interleukin-6; iNOS: inducible nitric oxide synthase; JNK: c-Jun N-terminal Kinase; KO: knockout; LDH: lactate dehydrogenase; LDL: low-density lipoprotein; L-NBP: L-3-n-butyl-phthalide; LPS: lipopolysaccharide; MDA: malondialdehyde; MMP: matrix metallopeptidase; MMP-9: matrix metallopeptidase 9; MPO: myeloperoxidase; N2a-SweAPP: Swedish amyloid precursor protein; NF-κB: nuclear factor kappa-B; NGF: nerve growth factor; NSC: neural stem cell; PD: Parkinson's disease; PGE2: prostaglandin E2; PTZ: pentylenetetrazole; RANTES: regulated on activation, normal T cell expressed and secreted; ROS: reactive oxygen species; SOD: superoxide dismutase; STZ: streptozotocin; sVCAM-1: soluble vascular cell adhesion molecule-1; SYP: synaptophysin; TMP: tetra methyl pyrazine; TNF-α: tumour necrosis factor alpha; TSG: 2,3,5,4′-tetrahydroxystilbene-2-O-beta-D-glucoside; TST: tail suspension test; XIAP: X-linked inhibitor of apoptosis protein.

Experimental Studies on *shi chang pu* 石菖蒲

Shi chang pu 石菖蒲 is sourced from *Acorus tatarinowii* Schott and *Acorus gramineus* Sol. Aiton. It predominantly contains flavonoid glycosides, phenylpropanoid and phenylpropane derivatives (α-asarone, β-asarone), amides, and lignans (eudesmin, tatarinowin, acortatarinowin).[1–3]

Much of the research on *Acorus* species has focused on neuroprotection in Alzheimer's disease (AD), but neuroprotection is also of relevance to VaD.

Extracts

In an APP/PS1 double transgenic mouse model of AD where the mice show excessive formation of beta-amyloid (Abeta) plaques, daily treatment with *A. gramineus* extracts showed dose-dependent improvements in tests of memory and learning in a Morris water maze. In rat brains, expression of synaptophysin (SYP) and glutamate receptor 1 (GluR1) in the hippocampus were found to be higher in treated animals.[4] An aqueous extract of *A. tatarinowii* protected rat pheochromocytoma cells (PC12), which differentiate into neurons, against cell death induced by Abeta(25-35) via reductions in DNA damage, release of reactive oxygen species (ROS), and inhibition of caspase-3 activation.[5] In a forced treadmill running test, rats treated with an aqueous extract of *A. tatarinowii* showed prolonged time to exhaustion that was dose-dependent for 10 mg/kg and 100 mg/kg. Inhibition of exercise-induced increase in serotonin (5-HT) in the dorsal raphe may have accounted for the anti-fatigue effects.[6]

Asarones

Both β- and α-asarone can cross the blood-brain barrier. These two compounds have received considerable attention in models of neurological disorders.[7,8]

β-asarone

Animal studies have shown that β-asarone improved cognitive function and attenuated neural damage. Following intra-hippocampal injection of Abeta(1-42) to induce an AD model in rats, intra-gastric β-asarone attenuated neuronal apoptosis and suppressed the effect of Abeta on the expression of multiple markers of neuronal apoptosis including caspase-9, bcl-2-like protein 4 (Bax), and Bcl2-associated agonist of cell death (Bad).[9] In a rat AD model induced by D-galactose and aluminium chloride, injection of β-asarone (25 mg/kg, 50 mg/kg or 100 mg/kg) improved performance in a Morris water maze, but there was no clear dose-related effect. There was also improved cerebral blood flow in the β-asarone high-dose group.[10]

In animal models of Parkinson's disease (PD), β-asarone has shown neuroprotective effects. In mice that were administered the neurotoxin 6-hydroxydopamine (6-OHDA) unilaterally to induce a model of PD, intra-gastric administration of β-asarone improved performance on open field behavioural and rotarod tests, suggesting improved recovery. Immuno-staining indicated reduced loss of dopaminergic neurons and nerve fibres.[11] In a similar model in rats, 15 mg/kg of β-asarone administered intra-gastrically per day reduced markers of endoplasmic reticulum (ER) stress, suggesting a possible mechanism for β-asarone's neuroprotective activity.[12] In the same rat model, co-administration of β-asarone and levodopa (L-dopa) enhanced the blood-brain barrier permeability of levodopa and increased the level of dopamine in the striatum.[13]

α-asarone

In mice with cognitive deficits induced by scopolamine, pre-administration of α-asarone (at 10 and 30 mg/kg, but not 3 mg/kg) improved performance in Y maze passive avoidance tests. In mouse brains, α-asarone attenuated increased levels of acetylcholinesterase (AChE), malondialdehyde (MDA) and superoxide dismutase (SOD) activity in the hippocampus and cerebral cortex, suggesting that α-asarone may restore acetylcholine activity and reduce the levels of free radicals.[14]

In rats with memory impairment induced by noise stress, pre-treatment with α-asarone and *A. calamus* extract improved performance in an eight-arm radial maze over 30 days compared to normal Wistar rats administered vehicle only. Hippocampal analysis revealed that α-asarone and the extract reduced SOD and AChE activity.[15]

In Abeta(23-35) injected rats, pre-administration of α-asarone demonstrated neuroprotective effects as well as improved spatial memory and learning, reduced nitrite production, and reduced elevation of glial-fibrillary-acid protein (GFAP), indicating a reduction in Abeta-induced neurotoxicity.[16]

In BV2 microglia stimulated with lipopolysaccharide (LPS) to induce an acute inflammatory response and up-regulation of the inflammatory factors, tumour necrosis factor alpha (TNF-α), interleukin-1beta (IL-1β), and interleukin-6 (IL-6), pre-treatment with α-asarone (10, 50 and 250 mM) prevented expression of these cytokines, blocked translocation of the nuclear factor kappa-B (NF-κB) p65 subunit to the nucleus, and reduced levels of both inducible nitric oxide synthase (iNOS) and cyclooxygenase-2 (COX-2).[17]

In rats that have been fed a hypercholesterolemic diet for eight days, co-administration of α-asarone reduced serum low-density lipoprotein (LDL) while not affecting high-density lipoproteins (HDL); it had no effect on normolipemic rats and stimulated bile flow and bile salt secretion in both groups of rats, with greater increases in hypercholesterolemic rats. These effects appear to emerge via inhibition of 3-hydroxy-3-methyl-glutaryl-coenzyme A reductase (HMG-CoA) activity and stimulation of bile flow.[18]

Fragile X mental retardation gene (*Fmr1*) knockout (KO) mice, which demonstrate locomotor hyperactivity similar to that found in a number of neurological/psychiatric disorders, were administered saline, α-asarone, or galantamine (positive control). In an open-field test, hyperactivity was reduced in both the α-asarone and galantamine groups. Levels of acetylcholine (ACh) in the striatum were increased and α-asarone attenuated the increased AChE activity of the *Fmr1* KO mice.[19]

In a tail suspension test (TST) in mice, which is used to test anti-depressant activity, intraperitoneal (i.p.) α-asarone was shown to have antidepressant-like effects at lower doses (20 mg/kg, i.p.) and depressant-like effects at higher doses (50 and 100 mg/kg, i.p.). The antidepressant-like effects were mediated via noradrenergic and serotonergic systems.[20]

Epileptic seizures are more prevalent in the dementia population.[21] The anticonvulsant activity of α-asarone has been investigated in a number of studies. In mice with seizures induced by pentylenetetrazole and kainite, α-asarone prolonged latency to clonic and tonic seizures and reduced mortality. It also appeared to inhibit hippocampal neuron activity and enhance tonic gamma-aminobutyric acid (GABA)ergic inhibition.[22] Moreover, α-asarone has been shown to blockade voltage-gated sodium channels and activate $GABA_A$ receptors present on mitral cell dendrites.[23]

In a rat model of anxiety induced by the stress hormone corticosterone, α-asarone improved performance on an elevated plus maze test and other tests of exploratory behaviours, indicating an anxiolytic-like effect. It appeared to modify the central noradrenergic system and decrease the mRNA expression of brain-derived neurotrophic factor (BDNF).[24]

Both α- and β-asarone have shown weak carcinogenic effects in studies of pre-weanling mice that received a series of injections. Concerns about genotoxic potential led to restrictions on the β-asarone content in foods in Europe[25,26] and to the prohibition of *A. calamus* and its derivatives by the Food and Drug Administration (FDA) of the United States.[27,28]

Eudesmin

A number of lignins derived from *A. tatarinowii* have shown antioxidant properties[2] and the lignin eudesmin has shown anti-inflammatory, antihypertensive, and anticonvulsant activities that may be relevant to VaD. In LPS-stimulated murine macrophage cells, eudesmin inhibited TNF-α without evidence of toxicity and attenuated T-cell proliferation induced by concanavilin A.[29] In thoracic rat aorta stimulated by phenylephrine, eudesmin (10–35 μg/ml) had a relaxant effect that was dependent on the endothelium-derived relaxant factor nitric oxide (NO) via activation of histamine H1 receptors.[30] In mouse seizure models employing maximal electroshock test and pentylenetetrazole (PTZ), administration of eudesmin (5, 10, and 20 mg/kg, i.p.) showed reductions in tonic seizures as well as sedative effects. After treatment, GABA levels increased while glutamic acid (Glu) decreased. These effects were mediated by up-regulation of glutamic acid decarboxylase (GAD65) and $GABA_A$ receptor expression. In addition, eudesmin produced an increase in the apoptosis regulator Bcl-2 and down-regulated caspase-3, indicating protective anti-apoptotic effects on neurones.[31]

Experimental Studies on *chuan xiong* 川芎

In the marketplace, the botanical source of *chuan xiong* 川芎 is *Ligusticum chuanxiong* Hort. (LC) (also known as *L. wallichii* Franch). Analyses have identified the main constituent compounds to include ferulic acid, caffeic acid, senkyunolide A, senkyunolide I, senkyunolide H, Z-ligustilide, tetramethylpyrazine (TMP), 3-butylidenephthalide (BP), 3-n-butylphthalide, riligustilide, levistolide A, vanillin, chrysophanol, and β-sitosterol.[32–39] A number of the same compounds are found in *dang gui* 当归, including ferulic acid and Z-ligustilide, so these two compounds are discussed in the section on *dang gui* 当归 below.

Research indicates that some phytochemicals found in *chuan xiong* show protective effects in models of ischemia, are neuroprotective, and can promote neurogenesis. Such activities may benefit cognitive function and cell regeneration in VaD.

Tetramethylpyrazine

Tetramethylpyrazine has been shown to inhibit platelet aggregation in rats[40] and in human platelet suspensions.[41] It has also shown antithrombotic effects in mice[42] and inhibited platelet thrombus formation in human blood in a high shear rate model.[43] In a rat model of ischemic brain injury, pre-treatment with TMP reduced inflammation, infarction volume, and brain oedema, and showed neuroprotective effects.[44] In cerebral ischemic/reperfusion injury in rats induced by middle cerebral artery occlusion, pre-treatment with TMP resulted in concentration-dependent neuroprotective effects and reductions in behavioural disturbances.[45] It is likely that TMP acts by suppressing inflammatory responses, has antioxidant actions, and reduces neuronal apoptosis.[45–47]

In addition to its protective effects, TMP promoted cell proliferation and differentiation following ischemic injury[48] in a rat model of cerebral ischemia and has also been shown to promote SH-SY5Y neural stem cell (NSC) differentiation into neurons.[49] In mouse brain endothelial cells, TMP at low concentrations promoted proliferation and cell migration.[50] In a neurogenesis model, TMP was also found to promote the migration of neural progenitor/precursor cells to ischemic regions.[51]

L-3-n-butyl-phthalide

The compound L-3-n-butyl-phthalide (L-NBP), which is found in the seeds of *Apium graveolens* L. and in *chuan xiong*, has been shown to pass from serum to the brains of mice.[38] A synthetic derivative of L-NBP, known as DL-3-n-butylphthalide, was approved by the State Food and Drug Administration of China in 2002 for clinical use in stroke patients.[52] In rats with memory impairment induced by chronic cerebral hypoperfusion, post-surgery administration of L-NBP improved performance in a Morris water maze.[53] In rat hippocampal neurons and human neuroblastoma SH-SY5Y cells, pre-treatment with L-NBP reduced Abeta(25-35)-induced neurotoxicity and inhibited hyperphosphorylation of Tau protein.[54] In rats that received intra-cerebroventricular infusion of synthetic human Abeta(1-40) for 17 days, gastric administration of L-NBP attenuated performance impairments in a Morris water maze, decreased Abeta-induced oxidative stress, and reduced abnormal phosphorylation of Tau protein.[55] In human neuroblastoma SK-N-SH cells treated with hydrogen peroxide (H_2O_2) to induce apoptosis, pre-incubation with L-NBP improved cell viability and modulated the expression of markers of apoptosis induced by H_2O_2.[56] In memory impaired APP/PS1 double transgenic mice and normal mice, treatment with L-NBP resulted in improvement in learning and memory in a Morris water maze for both groups of L-NBP-treated mice.[52]

Butylidenephthalide

Butylidenephthalide, also found in dang gui 当归, has been shown to inhibit platelet aggregation in plasma from rabbits and humans.[57] In LPS-induced inflammation in rat brain microglia, pre-treatment with butylidenephthalide inhibited production of NO, TNF-α, and IL-1β and reduced cell death in hippocampal slice cultures, indicating neuroprotective effects.[58]

Other Compounds

Rats with aluminium chloride-induced dementia treated with caffeic acid or rivastigmine (positive control) both performed better in Morris water maze tests. Caffeic acid inhibited AChE in the rat brains, although the effect was considerably less compared to that for rivastigmine. Caffeic acid enhanced levels of the antioxidant enzyme catalase, glutathione (GSH), and glutathione S transferase (GST).[59] In PC12 cells, caffeic acid demonstrated neuroprotective effects against Abeta(25-35)-induced toxicity and inhibited self-induced aggregation of Abeta(1-42).[60]

Chrysophanol is found in *chuan xiong, da huang* 大黄 (*Rheum palmatum* L.), and other plants and fungi. In BV2 murine microglia treated with LPS, treatment with chrysophanol reduced the release of pro-inflammatory mediators, including iNOS, prostaglandin E2 (PGE2), and TNF-α, and reduced cell damage from intracellular ROS and oxidation of DNA.[61]

Beta-sitosterol is found in many plants and is well-known for its cholesterol-lowering effects. In human blood, β-sitosterol inhibited release of Abeta from platelets induced by high cholesterol, probably via maintenance of membrane cholesterol homeostasis.[62]

Experimental Studies on *dang gui* 当归

Angelica sinensis (Oliv.) Diels is the official source of *dang gui* 当归. Its chemical constituents predominantly consist of ferulic acid, Z-ligustilide, E-ligustilide, butylidenephthalide, senkyunolide I, senkyunolide H, and coniferyl ferulate.[34,63,64]

An alcohol extract of *Angelica sinensis* root showed a dose-dependent neuroprotective effect in Neuro 2A neuroblastoma cells treated with Abeta(25-35) and reduced production of ROS.[65] In a common carotid artery occlusion rat model of neurodegenerative disease, *A. sinensis* extract improved cognitive decline, enhanced hippocampal neurogenesis, and restored expression of BDNF.[66]

Ferulic Acid

Ferulic acid is an antioxidant that is found in many herbs and foods and has been shown to inhibit aggregation of Abeta.[67] Ferulic acid attenuated cognitive deficits induced by mecamylamine (MECA), scopolamine (scop), and Abeta(1-40) in rats. It also reversed deterioration in the activity of SOD and AChE.[68] In rats with cerebral ischemia induced by occlusion of the right middle cerebral artery followed by reperfusion, daily treatment with ferulic acid reduced neurological deficits, attenuated nerve injury in the hippocampus, and increased erythropoietin (EPO) in both the hippocampus and peripheral blood.[69] Pre-treatment of PC12 cells with ferulic acid improved cell viability in response to damage from Abeta(25-35), increased the activity level of SOD, and attenuated release of TNF-α and IL-1β. In response to LPS, pre-incubation with ferulic acid protected PC12 cell from LPS toxicity, inhibited reduction of cyclic adenosine monophosphate (cAMP), and attenuated the increase in calcium ions (Ca^{2+}) in response to LPS.[70] In rats with cadmium-induced brain damage, co-administration of ferulic acid reduced the cadmium-induced increases in monoamine oxidase (MAO), AChE, butyrylcholinesterase (BChE), and sodium-potassium adenosine triphosphatase (Na^+/K^+-ATPase), indicating neuroprotective effects against cadmium injury.[71]

Ligustilide

Ligustilide has shown neuroprotective activity in a number of models of brain injury. In rats with experimentally-induced chronic cerebral hypoperfusion, oral administration of Z-ligustilide for 40 days post-surgery ameliorated cognitive dysfunction and improved performance in a Morris water maze. In the brains of Z-ligustilide-treated rats, there were increased antioxidant effects and improved cholinergic activity.[72] In a similar model, rats given oral Z-ligustilide (in soybean oil) for seven days showed improved spatial learning in a Morris water maze. Post-mortem tests showed that there was a reduction in neuronal loss and dendrite damage in the parietal cortex and hippocampus, along with reduced astrocyte activation and proliferation.[73]

In a rat model of subarachnoid haemorrhage, injection of ligustilide reduced post-operative mortality, brain oedema, blood-brain barrier permeability, and cerebral vasospasm. Neurobehavioral deficits were attenuated and the histological appearance of vascular endothelial cells within the basilar artery was improved. Ligustilide decreased expression of p53 and cleaved caspase-3, suggesting that it was protective against apoptosis.[74] In rats with experimental AD induced by intra-cerebroventricular injections of Abeta(25-35), oral administration of ligustilide improved Morris water maze performance, reduced the neurotoxic effects of Abeta, and modulated the TNF-α-activated NF-κB signalling pathway.[75] In a mouse model of thromboembolic stroke treated with adipose-derived stem cells (ADSC) transplanted into mouse brains, pre-treatment of the ADSCs with ligustilide resulted in greater therapeutic efficacy and improved behaviour and locomotor performance.[76]

Senkyunolide I

In a cerebral ischemia-reperfusion model in rats, intravenous senkyunolide I reduced the severity of neurological deficits and reduced infarct volume, brain oedema, and injury in the cortex and hippocampus. Oxidative stress due to reduced cerebral blood flow and subsequent reperfusion was attenuated, as indicated by the decreased

MDA formation and elevated SOD activity in the treated group. Senkyunolide I also inhibited the expression of cleaved caspase-3 and caspase-9 and improvement in the ratio of Bcl/Bax, suggesting that cells were protected against apoptosis.[77]

For butylidenephthalide, see *chuan xiong* 川芎.

Experimental Studies on *he shou wu* 何首乌

The official botanical source of *he shou wu* 何首乌 is *Polygonum multiflorum* Thunb. Its major constituents are stilbenes (including resveratrol and 2,3,5,4′-tetrahydroxystilbene-2-O-beta-D-glucoside), quinones and anthraquinones (including emodins, chrysophanol, physcion, and rhein), and flavonoids (including rutin and quercetin). Other compounds include gallic acid and N-trans-feruloyltyramine, and around 100 different compounds have been reported.[34,78,79] Extracts of *Polygonum multiflorum* have been investigated in numerous animal and cell-line studies relevant to dementia and ageing.

Extracts

In gerbils with cerebral ischemia induced by middle cerebral artery occlusion, treatment with a dried 50% ethanol extract of *Polygonum multiflorum* for two weeks pre-surgery significantly reduced infarct size, but there were no significant differences between groups on locomotor tests.[80] Senescence-accelerated (SAMP8) mice fed an ethanol extract of *he shou wu* that had been dried and mixed with protein, sugar, and vitamins performed better in an active (shuttle) avoidance test. Their brains showed less spongy degeneration and had lower MDA concentrations and lipofuscin accumulation, suggesting an anti-oxidant mechanism.[81,82]

Mice fed an experimental diet that included a freeze-dried water extract of *P. multiflorum* for four weeks and were administered an single intra-cerebroventricular injection of Abeta(25-35) performed better than controls on passive avoidance and Morris water maze tasks. Furthermore, Abeta-induced increases in AChE activity were attenuated.[83] In a screen of ethanol extracts of 15 herbs using mouse neuroblastoma cells expressing Swedish amyloid precursor protein (N2a-SweAPP), *P. multiflorum* extract showed inhibition of Abeta production via modulation of amyloid precursor protein (APP), up-regulation of secreted APP-alpha (sAPPα), and down-regulation of secreted APP-beta (sAPPβ).[84]

Membrane fluidity is understood to play an important role in AD development.[85] Rats injected with Abeta(1-40) into the hippocampus and treated with intra-gastric *P. multiflorum* extract showed attenuation of Abeta-induced deficits in learning and memory. There was reduced viscosity in the mitochondria membrane of the hippocampus and enhanced COX activity.[86]

In human U373-MG astrocytoma cells, an ethanol extract of *P. multiflorum* protected cells from H_2O_2 injury. This effect was related to the antioxidant activity of the phenolic fraction, but this did not account for the total effect.[87] In a rat-derived primary cortical neuronal cell culture, pre-treatment with a hexane extract of *P. multiflorum* inhibited glutamate-induced apoptosis by decreasing glutamate-induced death receptor (DR)4 expression and enhancing the expression of anti-apoptotic proteins Bcl-2 and the X-linked inhibitor of apoptosis protein (XIAP).[88]

A formulation known as PMC-12, which has *P. multiflorum* as its main constituent plus *Polygala tenuifolia, Rehmannia glutinosa* and *Acorus gramineus* root, was orally administered to normal young C57BL/6 mice for two weeks. Performance was improved in Morris water maze tests compared to controls. Newly generated cells in the dentate gyrus were significantly increased in treated mice. They showed increased survival and differentiation of new neurons in the hippocampus, which also had increased levels of BDNF, cAMP response element-binding protein (p-CREB), and SYP.[89]

2,3,5,4′-tetrahydroxystilbene-2-*O*-beta-D-glucoside

The polyphenolic compound 2,3,5,4′-tetrahydroxystilbene-2-O-beta-D-glucoside (TSG) has received considerable research attention. It has shown important antioxidant properties and can inhibit the formation of advanced glycation end products (AGEs).[90] In rats with middle cerebral artery occlusion, TSG significantly reduced brain infarct volume. In primary-cultured cortical neurons from neonatal rats subjected to ischemia by oxygen-glucose deprivation followed by reperfusion, TSG protected neurons against damage from ROS, inhibited iNOS gene expression, and reduced apoptosis.[91]

In coronary arterial smooth cells, TSG reduced lipoprotein oxidation and NO content, suggesting it may facilitate the prevention of atherosclerosis.[92] In the nematode *Caenorhabditis elegans*, TSG exerted greater antioxidative activity than resveratrol, was protective against heat stress, alleviated the accumulation of lipofuscin, and prolonged the mean life span of the nematode by 23.5%.[93] To investigate the effects of TSG on rats at different ages, five groups aged one to 24 months were tested in a Morris water maze. The older rats showed improved spatial learning as well as increases in the number of synaptic vesicles and elevated expression of SYP in the hippocampus.[94] In aged mice, intra-gastric administration of TSG for three months improved performance on passive avoidance and rotarod tasks. In rat brains, there was protection of the synaptic ultrastructure and increased synaptic connections in the hippocampal CA1 region and striatum.[94]

In addition, TSG inhibited overexpression and aggregation of alpha-synuclein in the hippocampus, striatum, and cerebral cortex.[95] If left to aggregate, alpha-synuclein causes toxic damage to surrounding cells and has been linked to neurodegenerative disorders including PD.[96] In rat PC12 cells treated with 1-methyl-4-phenylpyridinium (MPP+) to produce a model of PD, pre-incubation with TSG improved cell viability and attenuated apoptosis. These effects were probably induced via inhibition of ROS generation and modulation of c-Jun N-terminal Kinase (JNK) activation.[97,98] A similar result was found in human dopaminergic neuroblastoma SH-SY5Y cells.[99]

In APP transgenic mice used as models of AD, administration of TSG reduced learning and memory deficits in both younger and older mice.[100] In rats injected with Abeta(1-42) intra-cerebroventricularly, intra-gastric treatment with TSG improved performance in a Morris water maze test and up-regulated expression of Proto-oncogene tyrosine-protein kinase Src and the ionotropic glutamate receptor subunit (NR2B).[101]

Resveratrol

Resveratrol has also received considerable research attention for its antioxidant effects and potential for cardiovascular diseases associated with ageing.[102] In healthy adults who have been administered single doses of trans-resveratrol, cerebral blood flow was dose-dependently increased during task performance measured by near-infrared spectroscopy compared to placebo.[103] Longer term administration (28 days) showed similar effects on cerebral blood flow but only small beneficial effects on cognition.[104] In adults with type 2 diabetes who are known to have endothelial dysfunction, trans-resveratrol improved cerebral vasodilator responsiveness in the middle and posterior cerebral arteries as measured by Transcranial Doppler ultrasound, and this effect was most evident at the lowest dosage (75 mg, once a week for 4 weeks).[105] Following traumatic brain injury, rats administered resveratrol showed reduced oedema, reduced neurological impairment, and improved spatial cognitive function.[106]

Other Compounds

Other compounds found in *he shou wu* have shown activities of relevance to VaD, including N-trans-feruloyltyramine, emodin, and beta-sitosterol (for beta-sitosterol, see the section on *chuan xiong* 川芎). In primary cortical cultures of neurons derived from rat embryos treated with Abeta(25-35), pre-treatment with emodin reduced Abeta(25-35)-induced cell death and reduced release of lactate dehydrogenase (LDH), indicating a neuroprotective effect.[107] In murine hippocampal HT22 cells treated with glutamate to induce cell death, pre-treatment with emodin reduced cytotoxicity, LDH levels, and DNA fragmentation. In male C57BL/6 mice with surgically induced cortical ischemia, intra-cortical injection of emodin prior to ischemia reduced infarct volume and improved neurological function via reduction of Bax and active caspase-3.[108] In rat primary cortical cell cultures, pre-treatment with n-trans-feruloyltyramine (25-250 M) attenuated the cytotoxicity of Abeta(1-42) in a dose-dependent manner, reduced levels of caspase-3 and Bax, and prevented increase in intracellular ROS.[109]

Experimental Studies on *huang qi* 黄芪

The official botanical sources of *huang qi* 黄芪 are the roots of *Astragalus membranaceus* (Fisch.) Bge. or *A. membranaceus* (Fisch.) Bge. var. *mongholicus* (Bge.) Hsiao, which contain astragalosides (ASTs) including ATS I-IV and the isoflavones calycosin, calycosin-7-O-β-d-glucoside (CG), and formononetin.[34,110,111]

Astragalosides

Mice administered D-galactose for 10 weeks to accelerate ageing and middle-aged mice (aged 17 months) that received oral ASTs daily for 10 weeks performed better on rotarod and passive avoidance tests than control mice, indicating improvements in memory and motor function.[112]

In rats with induced transient focal cerebral ischemia, injection of AST IV immediately post-surgery showed attenuation of increased blood-brain barrier permeability due to ischemia/reperfusion injury.[113] In a focal ischemia/reperfusion model in rats, i.p. injections of AST IV immediately as well as 12 hours after onset of reperfusion attenuated neurological deficits, reduced brain oedema, and reduced permeability of the blood-brain barrier via inhibition of the up-regulation of matrix metallopeptidase 9 (MMP-9) and aquaporin 4 (AQP4).[114]

In experimentally-induced subarachnoid haemorrhage in rats, intra-peritoneal injection of AST IV did not affect lesion severity but reduced neurological deficits and attenuated brain oedema and neural death at the cortex. At 24 hours post-surgery, activities of antioxidant enzymes were up-regulated and expression of cleaved caspase-3 was down-regulated.[115]

In APP/PS1 double-transgenic mice as a model of AD that were administered AST IV intra-gastrically for three months, there was a significant reduction in plaque count and Abeta burden. This effect was reduced via blockade of peroxisome proliferator-activated receptor gamma (PPARγ) signalling. In cultured SH-SY5Y cells, AST IV increased activity of PPARγ, and inhibited beta-site APP cleaving enzyme 1 (BACE1) expression.[116]

Extracts and Other Compounds

In a rat model of embolic cerebral ischemia, intra-peritoneal injection of a combination of *A. membranaceus* extract and ligustrazine (from *chuan xiong*) and separate administration of these compounds showed reduced infarct volumes and cerebral haemorrhage in all three treatment groups without significant differences between groups and improved blood-brain barrier protection for the combination group.[117]

In a cerebral artery occlusion plus reperfusion model in rats, intra-peritoneal injection of calycosin-7-O-β-D-glucoside reduced infarct volume and histological damage while enhancing the integrity of the blood-brain barrier. It scavenged NO, inhibited MMP activity, and secured expression of caveolin-1 and tight-junction proteins.[118]

A combination of extracts of *A. membranaceus* and *Salvia miltiorrhiza* known as 'Myelophil' was orally administered to ten-week-old male C57BL/6N mice for seven days prior to injection with scopolamine to induce memory impairment. The treated mice performed better in a Morris water maze and showed attenuated increases in AChE activity in the brain, levels of ROS in serum and the brain, and MDA levels.[119]

Experimental studies on *dan shen* 丹参

Salvia miltiorrhiza Bge. is the official source for *dan shen* 丹参. Its main constituents consist of danshensu (salvianic acid A), protocatechuic aldehyde, rosmarinic acid (an ester of caffeic acid), 3,4-dihydroxyphenyllactic acid,[34] and salvianolic acids A and B, along with lipophilic compounds including cryptotanshinone, dihydrotanshinone I, and tanshinones I and IIA.[120,121]

The majority of studies investigated compounds from *dan shen* were in models of ischemia and neurological damage.

Danshensu

In rats with ischemia induced by middle cerebral artery occlusion, injection of the sodium salt of danshensu at the onset of reperfusion for five days attenuated neurological deficits, reduced infarct volume and histological damage, decreased the number of apoptotic cells, and increased the ratio of Bcl-2 to Bax.[122] In a similar model, danshensu derivatives decreased the overall infarct volume whilst increasing cell viability, reducing lactate dehydrogenase leakage, increasing SOD activity, and decreasing ROS levels.[123]

Salvianolic Acids

In a cerebral ischemia-reperfusion injury in mice, salvianolic acid A (3 and 10 mg/kg injection) improved memory function, reduced MDA in the brain (cortex, hippocampus, and corpus striatum), inhibited lipid peroxidation, and scavenged free hydroxyl radicals.[124] In rats with middle cerebral artery occlusion, post-surgical injection of salvianolic acid A diminished neurological deficits and inhibited soluble epoxide hydrolase (sEH) to increase levels of epoxyeicosatrienoic acids (EETs).[125]

In myocardial ischemia/reperfusion (I/R) injury in rats, treatment with salvianolic acid B and ginsenoside Rg1 (10 mg/kg) reduced myocardial infarct size, improved maintenance of myocardium structure, improved cardiac function and decreased secretion of the cytokines TNF-α, IL-1β, regulated on activation, normal T cell expressed and secreted (RANTES), and soluble vascular cell adhesion molecule-1 (sVCAM-1), which suggests that the combination of salvianolic acid B and ginsenoside Rg1 protected endothelial barrier function and regulated inflammatory cytokines.[126]

Salvianolic acid B inhibited Abeta(1-40) fibril formation and disaggregated preformed fibrils of Abeta(1-42) in an enzyme-linked immunosorbent assay (ELISA) and protected human neuroblastoma SH-SY5Y cells and PC-12 cells against Abeta(1-42)-induced cytotoxicity. In a comparison with ferulic acid and curcumin, salvianolic acid B showed greater inhibition of Abeta aggregation than ferulic acid but less than that of curcumin.[127] In order to overcome the relative impermeability of the blood-brain barrier to salvianolic acid B, nanoparticles loaded with salvianolic acid B were administered to rats and mice. When administered systemically, the particles passed through the blood-brain barrier and showed prolonged release of salvianolic acid B in the brain without apparent toxicity, suggesting a promising strategy for enhancing salvianolic acid B's neuroprotective potential.[128]

A study of the effects of fractions and compounds from *S. miltiorrhiza* on Abeta(25-35)-induced toxicity and inhibition of AChE examined total polyphenols and the compounds salvianolic acid B, danshensu and protocatechuic aldehyde, total tanshinones, and the compounds tanshinone I, tanshinone IIA, and cryptotanshinone in a rat pheochromocytoma PC-12 cell line. Cytoprotective activity was more evident in the polyphenol fraction with danshensu and salvianolic acid B, blocking the cytotoxic effects of Abeta(25-35), inhibiting LDH release, and reducing pathological changes in the cells. In rat brains, the tanshinone fraction blocked AChE activity with the main activity being due to tanshinone I and dihydrotanshinone I.[129]

Rosmarinic Acid

Botanical extracts containing high levels of rosmarinic acid have been reported to improve recognition[130] and attention in humans with dementia.[131] In PC-12 cells treated with Abeta(42), incubation with rosmarinic acid reduced the cytotoxic effects of Abeta, concentration-dependently reduced ROS formation, reduced lipid peroxidation (MDA level), reduced Abeta-induced tau hyperphosphorylation, and reduced DNA fragmentation and caspase-3 activation.[132]

In mice injected with Abeta(25-35) into the brain, post-treatment with rosmarinic acid for nine days improved memory and performance in a Y maze and enhanced the scavenging of peroxynitrites in the hippocampus.[133] In a model of AD using ovariectomised female rats injected with D-galactose and intra-gastric rosmarinic acid for 60 days showed restoration of locomotor activity and short-term spatial memory, normalisation of cell structure, and reduced Abeta deposits. Inhibition of lipid peroxidation and COX-2 expression in the hippocampus were proposed as a possible mechanism of action.[134]

In N2A mouse neuroblastoma cells with oxidative damage induced by H_2O_2, pre-treatment with rosmarinic acid reduced cytotoxicity and genotoxicity, attenuated LDH leakage, reduced ROS production, and reduced loss of mitochondrial membrane potential, indicating neuroprotective effects.[135]

In mice with permanent middle cerebral artery occlusion, pre-treatment with rosmarinic acid which continued for five days attenuated ischemia-induced deficits in working, spatial, and recognition memory, reduced infarct size and neurological impairments, suppressed inflammatory response and astroglial activation, prevented decrease in synaptophysin in the striatum, and increased levels of BDNF in the hippocampus. Together, this suggests protective effects against neurodegenerative changes resulting from cerebral ischemia.[136]

In diabetic rats with cerebral ischemia induced by middle cerebral artery occlusion, injection of rosmarinic acid following reperfusion decreased neurological deficit scores, infarct volume, and brain oedema. Rosmarinic acid inhibited inflammatory response by reducing myeloperoxidase (MPO) activity, blocking NF-κB activation, and reducing the expression of high-mobility group box1 (HMGB1) in rat brains.[137]

Protocatechuic Aldehyde

The effect of protocatechuic aldehyde has been investigated in human neuroblastoma SH-SY5Y cells and DJ-1-knockdown SH-SY5Y cells treated with H_2O_2 to induce oxidative injury. Pre-treatment with protocatechuic aldehyde attenuated cell death dose-dependently and inhibited ROS production in SH-SY5Y cells but not in DJ-1-knockdown SH-SY5Y cells, suggesting activity via the protein deglycase (DJ-1) gene. This gene has a role in transcriptional regulation of mitochondrial function and anti-oxidative stress via the RAC-α serine/threonine-protein kinase (AKT1)-signalling pathway.[138] Increased DJ-1 activity may protect dopaminergic neurons from oxidative stress in PD. In cell and animal models of PD, protocatechuic aldehyde showed protection against neurotoxicity induced by oxidopamine (6-OHDA).[139]

Cryptotanshinone

In a primary culture of rat cortical neurons, pre-treatment with cryptotanshinone reversed neuronal toxicity induced by glutamate, reduced LDH release, and protected cells against apoptosis via activation of the PI3K/AKT-signalling pathway.[140] In an AD model using rat cortical neurons overexpressing Swedish mutant human APP695, cryptotanshinone decreased intra- and extra-cellular levels of Abeta(42), increased alpha-secretase activity, and increased sAPPα release.[141] In human neuroblastoma SH-SY5Y cells treated with Abeta(42), cryptotanshinone inhibited Abeta aggregation and fibril formation, reduced cytotoxicity, and protected against apoptosis.[142]

In apolipoprotein E-deficient mice fed a high cholesterol diet as a model of atherosclerotic cardiovascular disease, cryptotanshinone by daily oral gavage reduced formation of atherosclerotic plaques in the aorta, enhanced plaque stability, and inhibited ROS generation and NF-κB activation, suggesting a potential for treatment in cardiovascular diseases.[143]

Tanshinones I and IIA

In primary cultured cortical neurons treated with Abeta(1-42), pre-treatment with tanshinone IIA increased survival, protected cells from morphological damage,[144] and decreased expression of phosphorylated Tau.[145] Tanshinones I and IIA both inhibited Abeta(1-42) fibril aggregation assessed by atomic force microscopy (AFM) and thioflavin-T fluorescence (ThT). In human neuroblastoma SY5Y cells, low doses of both tanshinones inhibited Abeta-induced toxicity.[146]

In mice with streptozotocin (STZ)-induced memory deficits, treatment with tanshinone IIA improved performance in a Morris water maze. Subsequent examination of rat brains found that tanshinone IIA protected against the following adverse effects of STZ: damage to hippocampal neurons, elevated acetylcholinesterase activity and MDA levels, and reduced SOD and GSH peroxidase (GSH-Px) activities.[147] In rats with cerebral ischemia followed by reperfusion induced by cerebral artery occlusion, injection of tanshinone IIA dose-dependently reduced infarct size and reduced expression of caspase-3 and caspase-8.[148]

In immortalized C17.2 neuronal stem cells, rat embryonic cortical NSCs, and rat PC-12 pheochromocytoma cells, tanshinone IIA promoted neuronal differentiation and up-regulated expression of BDNF and nerve growth factor (NGF).[149]

Experimental Studies on *yuan zhi* 远志

Polygala tenuifolia Willd. is the official source of *yuan zhi* 远志. Major constituents are tenuifolin, saponins, polygalaxanthone III, 3, 6′-disinapoly sucrose,[34, 150] and oligosaccharides (such as tenuifoliside B).[151]

Extracts and Fractions

An ethanol extract of *P. tenuifolia* root, called BT11, reduced cytotoxicity induced by glutamate and Abeta in a rat primary neuron culture. In rats with scopolamine-induced memory and cognitive impairment, intra-peritoneal BT11 improved performance in passive avoidance and water maze tasks and reduced AChE activity in rat brains.[152] In an eight-arm radial maze, rats orally administered a glycoside-rich extract of *P. tenuifolia* root showed reduced scopolamine-induced memory impairment and improved spatial cognition.[153] A water extract of *P. tenuifolia* root attenuated Abeta

(25-35)-induced cell damage in rat primary cortical neurons. Axon length was increased, but there was no effect on dendrite damage or on reconstruction of synapses.[154]

In mice with anoxia induced by potassium cyanide (KCN), an acylated oligosaccharide fraction shortened coma time, indicating a protective effect against cerebral injury. In mice and rats with scopolamine-induced memory impairment, oral tenuifoliside B reduced impaired performance in passive avoidance tasks.[151] In rat embryo astrocytes, a saponin fraction and the compounds onjisaponin A, B, E, F, and G prepared from *P. tenuifolia* root increased the level of NGF.[155] A fractionated extract from *P. tenuifolia* containing oligosaccharide esters fed to Senescence Accelerated Mouse-Prone 8 (SAMP8) mice significantly enhanced serum and liver SOD and GSH-Px activity, indicating *in vivo* antioxidant activity.[156]

Tenuigenin

In neuroblastoma cells transfected with the C-terminal 99 amino acid residues of APP plus the signal peptide (SH-SY5Y SPA4CT) as a model of Abeta secretion in AD (i.e., SH-SY5Y APP695 cells), incubation with tenuigenin (aka senegenin) extracted from *P. tenuifolia* inhibited the secretion of Abeta via beta-secretase 1 (BACE1) inhibition.[157]

Tenuifolin

In COS-7 fibroblast-like cells transfected with either APP695 cDNA (COS 695 WT), Swedish mutation (COS 695 Swe), or C-terminal 99 amino acid residues plus the signal peptide (COS SPA4CT) to form three cell-line models of Abeta secretion, treatment with tenuifolin did not produce cytotoxicity in any cell-line, ELISA indicated lowered secretion of Abeta(1-40) and Abeta(1-42), and the BACE inhibition assay indicated a dose-dependent increase.[158]

In aged mice and young mice with memory deficits induced by scopolamine, sodium nitrite, and ethanol (4 groups), oral administration of tenuifolin for 15 days improved performance in passive avoidance and Y maze tests at the higher dose of 0.08 g/kg per day. In the brains of aged mice, cortical AChE activity was decreased dose-dependently and there were increases in hippocampal norepinephrine (NE) and dopamine (DA).[159] In PC-12 cells treated with Abeta(25-35), pre-treatment with tenuifolin demonstrated dose-dependent neuroprotective effects. In mice that were administered hippocampal injections of Abeta(25-35), oral administration of tenuifolin (3 and 9 mg/kg) or galantamine (2 mg/kg) 24 hours post-injection resulted in no effect in an open-field test, but tenuifolin and galantamine reduced spatial learning deficits in the Morris water maze and passive-avoidance tasks, indicating similar degrees of memory enhancement.[160]

Experimental Studies on *shui zhi* 水蛭

Shui zhi 水蛭 typically refers to leeches of the species *Hirudo nipponica* Whitman and *Whitemania pigra* Whitman. Its anticoagulant effects have been linked to its most abundant constituent compound, hirudin.[161] Hirudin inhibits blood coagulation by forming a tight complex with thrombin[162] and is considered the most potent natural thrombin inhibitor.[163]

Hirudin

In an RCT of patients with acute myocardial ischemia, hirudin (medium dose) was superior to heparin in preventing ischemic events.[164] In rats with induced myocardial ischemia and reperfusion, r-hirudin attenuated post-ischemic endothelial leukocyte adhesion and inhibited emigration of adherent leukocytes, thus attenuating the post-ischemic inflammatory response.[165] In pigs that were administered a normothermic cardiopulmonary bypass operation, r-hirudin improved cardiac recovery and reduced cardiomyocyte apoptosis and anti-inflammatory effects.[166]

In rats with cerebral ischemia induced by middle cerebral artery occlusion, brain thrombin activity was elevated and administration of thrombin exacerbated brain oedema while intra-cerebral injection of hirudin reduced neurological deficits due to ischemic injury.[167] In hippocampal slice cultures from immature rats subjected to oxygen and glucose deprivation as a model of ischemic injury, addition of hirudin reduced cell death. This suggested that thrombin was a mediator of ischemic cell death while hirudin protected neurons following ischemic injury.[168]

Tongxinluo

The Chinese formula *Tongxinluo* 通心络, which includes *H. nipponica* as one of its 12 ingredients, was administered to rats for three days prior to middle cerebral artery occlusion. It reduced neurological deficit scores, ischemic area, brain oedema, and post-ischemic inflammation.[169]

Experimental Studies on *di huang* 地黄

Rehmannia glutinosa Libosch is the botanical source for *di huang* 地黄 and contains iridoids and iridoid glycosides (such as catalpol), saccharides (such as mannotriose), amino acids, and other constituents. Polysaccharides and oligosaccharides are the most abundant compounds.[34,170]

Catalpol

Most studies investigated catalpol in animal and cell models. In gerbils with transient global cerebral ischemia induced by bilateral occlusion of the common carotid arteries, injection of catalpol immediately following reperfusion improved performance in a Y maze and there was significant rescue of neurons in the hippocampus. The neuroprotective effect extended to 35 days after ischemic damage.[171] In the same model, there was a dose-dependent reduction in errors in the Y maze and an increase in the survival of hippocampal neurons at doses of up to 10 mg/kg. The effects of catalpol (5 mg/kg) were evident when administered three hours post-reperfusion, but were not significant when administered at six hours.[172] In a similar model, injection of catalpol three days prior to common carotid artery occlusion reduced stroke index, increased SOD activity, and decreased MDA content in the brain and endothelin-1 plasma levels.[173]

In primary cultured astrocytes exposed to oxygen-glucose deprivation followed by reperfusion as a model of ischemia, treatment with catalpol increased survival, decreased mitochondrial membrane potential, suppressed free radical production, and elevated antioxidant capacity.[174] A recent review of catalpol concluded that its therapeutic potential for the treatment of ischemic injury was via enhancement of antioxidant, anti-inflammatory, and anti-apoptotic activity.[175]

Oxidative stress has been implicated as a key factor in age-related neurodegenerative disease development. In cultured mesencephalic neurons treated with 1-methyl-4-phenylpyridinium to induce oxidative stress, catalpol increased cell viability in a dose-dependent manner, reduced lipid peroxidation, and increased the activity of GSH-Px and SOD.[176] In astrocytes from neonatal mice with oxidant stress induced by H_2O_2, treatment with catalpol increased cell viability in a dose-dependent manner, reduced ROS formation, and increased activity of GSH-Px and GSH reductase.[177] In neuron-glia cultures prepared from ventral mesencephalic tissues of embryonic mice activated with LPS to induce inflammation-mediated neurodegeneration, catalpol protected neurones by inhibiting microglial activation and reduced release of ROS, NO, and TNF-α.[178]

To induce a model of age-related cognitive dysfunction, mice were injected with D-galactose for six weeks. From week five, daily injection of catalpol reversed learning and memory deficits in a passive-avoidance test, improved neuronal densities in the hippocampus, and increased the activities of GSH S-transferase (GSH-ST), glutamine synthetase (GS), and creatine kinase (CK) in the cortex and hippocampus.[178] In the same model, catalpol elevated the decreased activities of SOD, LDH, GS, and other endogenous antioxidants in the Liver and Spleen, suggesting potential as an anti-ageing agent.[179] In a similar study, catalpol reversed increases in AChE activity in the cerebral cortex and hippocampus and decreases in choline acetyltransferase (ChAT) activity whilst reducing elevations in TNF-α,

IL-1β, and advanced glycation endproducts (AGEs).[180] In aged rats showing age-related neuronal decline, catalpol attenuated the decline by modulating presynaptic protein expression and increasing protein kinase C (PKC) and BDNF in the hippocampus.[181]

In a primary cortical neuron culture treated with Abeta(1-42), pre-treatment with catalpol attenuated neuronal apoptosis by reversing increases in intracellular ROS accumulation and collapse of mitochondrial membrane potential and reducing cleavage of caspase-3 and 9.[182]

In mice injected with Abeta(25-35) plus ibotenic acid, gastric administration of catalpol reduced memory deficits in a Y maze but did not inhibit AChE activity. It elevated the decline in ChAT and BDNF levels, indicating that its action was different from that of donepezil.[183] In the same model, catalpol improved learning ability and memory in Y maze tests after administration for two to three months. It rescued declines in brain muscarinic acetylcholine receptor (M receptor) density and ChAT activity, whereas donepezil showed much smaller effects. This study also indicated that the actions of catalpol were via a different mechanism from that of donepezil.[184] Intra-cerebroventricular injection of Abeta(25-35) in rats and treatment of PC-12 cells with Abeta(25-35) produced both decreased expression and activity of ChAT. In both models, catalpol increased ChAT dose-dependently, but there was no corresponding effect on muscarinic cholinergic receptors (M receptor) indicating a likely mode of action for catalpol.[185]

Other Compounds

Mannotriose, which is a *R. glutinosa*-derived trisaccharide, protected cultured rat hippocampal neurons against injury induced by high concentrations of corticosterone. Western blot analysis showed increased expression of glucocorticoid receptors (GCR), serum and glucocorticoid-regulated protein kinase (SGK), and BDNF.[186] In a similar model, treatment with 5-hydroxymethylfurfural derived from *R. glutinosa* improved survival rates and reversed increases in beta-galactosidase activity.[187]

Experimental Studies on *gou qi zi* 枸杞子

Lycium barbarum L. fruit is the official source of *gou qi zi* 枸杞子. Its bioactive isolates include a diversity of polysaccharides, carotenoids (beta-carotene, zeaxanthin, and zeaxanthin dipalmitate), vitamins (riboflavin, thiamine, and ascorbic acid), flavonoids (myricetin, quercetin, kaempferol, and rutin), amino acids (betaine, taurine and GABA), fatty acids (hexadecanoic acid, linoleic acid, beta-elemene, myristic acid, and ethylhexadecanoate), and phenolic acids (chlorogenic acid, caffeoylquinic acid, caffeic acid, and p-coumaric acid).[34,188–193]

Extracts and Fractions

L. barbarum fruits have been noted for their antioxidant properties.[193,194] Oral administration of *L. barbarum* polysaccharides to aged mice counteracted increases in endogenous lipid peroxidation and decreases in antioxidant activities associated with ageing[195] and reduced abnormal oxidative indices in rats that have been administered streptozotocin.[196]

Mice with cerebral ischemia induced by middle cerebral artery occlusion that were fed *L. barbarum* extract showed reduced neurological deficits, decreased infarct size and hemispheric swelling, and reduced blood-brain barrier disruption, suggesting prophylactic effects.[197] In similar models, treatment with *L. barbarum* polysaccharides attenuated brain damage, decreased MDA activity, increased activity of endogenous antioxidants,[198] and attenuated neuronal apoptosis.[199] In neonatal rat primary cultured hippocampal neurons with ischemia-reperfusion injury induced by oxygen-glucose deprivation, treatment with *L. barbarum* polysaccharides inhibited LDH release, attenuated neuronal damage, enhanced SOD activity, inhibited elevation of intracellular Ca^{2+}, and stabilised mitochondrial membrane potential.[200]

Rats with induced hypoxia as a model of sleep apnoea that were fed *L. barbarum* polysaccharides prior to hypoxic episodes showed normal performance in a Morris water maze, no histological evidence of hippocampal apoptosis, lowered levels of pro-apoptotic proteins, and attenuation of oxidative stress, indicating neuroprotective activities against hypoxia injury.[201] In rat hearts with induced ischemia/reperfusion injury, pre-feeding of rats with *L. barbarum* polysaccharides increased myocardium Na(+)-K(+)-ATPase and Ca(2+)-ATPase activity and reduced the level of apoptosis.[202]

In primary rat cortical neurons treated with Abeta(1-42) and Abeta(25-35) as a model of neurotoxicity in AD, pre-treatment with *L. barbarum* extract produced cytoprotective effects, reduced LDH release, and attenuated caspase-3 activation.[203] In primary cultures of rat cortical neurons exposed to glutamate excitotoxicity, pre-treatment with *L. barbarum* polysaccharides abrogated cell death induced by glutamate and inhibited caspase-3 activation[204] and showed a similar protective effect against homocysteine as well as reduced homocysteine-induced Tau phosphorylation.[205] In rats with scopolamine-induced memory impairment, gastric perfusion of *L. barbarum* polysaccharides for two weeks prior to injury improved performance in a Morris water maze, decreased scopolamine-induced oxidative stress in the hippocampus, and reduced apoptosis, but did not alter AChE levels.[206]

In rats administered electrical trauma, pre-administration of *L. barbarum* polysaccharides for three days prior to shocks showed a reduction in stress behaviours and improved maze test results. Stress-induced morphological changes in the hippocampus were reduced and there was recovery of the regeneration/apoptosis imbalance.[207] A review of *L. barbarum*'s neuroprotective effects found its main activities to be alleviation of oxidative stress, inflammation, and apoptosis.[208]

Summary of Evidence From *in Vivo* and *in Vitro* Studies

Experimental evidence shows that the extracts and/or constituent compounds from each of the ten herbs most frequently included in formulae tested in the RCTs in Chapter 5 have potential therapeutic benefits for VaD. In animal models of learning, memory, and ischemic injury, a number of herbs have shown benefits and *in vitro* studies have identified herbal constituents with neuroprotective, neurogenic, anti-oxidant, anti-apoptotic, anti-amyloid, or anti-inflammatory actions.

Notably, asarones from *shi chang pu* 石菖蒲 crossed the blood-brain barrier and had neuroprotective effects. From *chuan xiong*, TMP promoted neurogenesis and L-NBP showed protective effects in ischemic and AD models. Similarly, ferulic acid and ligustilide from *dang gui* 当归 reduced the effects of reperfusion injury and Abeta toxicity, whereas TSG from *he shou wu* 何首乌 showed significant antioxidant and neuroprotective effects as well as benefits in the prevention of atherosclerosis. From *huang qi* 黄芪, AST IV was neuroprotective and acted on the blood-brain barrier to modulate its permeability. Salvianolic acid from *dan shen* 丹参 inhibited Abeta-(1-40) toxicity and fibril formation. Tenuifolin from *yuan zhi* 远志 improved memory and protected neurons from Abeta toxicity. The inhibitory effects of hirudin from *shui zhi* 水蛭 on thrombin activity protected the brain against ischemic injury and oedema. Catalpol from *di huang* 地黄 reduced oxidative stress and inflammation and protected cells from apoptosis. Polysaccharides from *gou qi zi* 枸杞子 showed neuroprotective, anti-inflammatory, and antioxidant activities. The evidence indicates that these Chinese herbs and their constituent compounds warrant further research as potential therapies for cognitive impairment and VaD.

References

1. Zhang F, Qi P, Xue R, *et al.* (2015) Qualitative and quantitative analysis of the major constituents in Acorus tatarinowii schott by HPLC/ESI-QTOF-MS/MS. *Biomed Chromatogr* **29**(6):890–901.
2. Lu Y, Xue Y, Chen S, *et al.* (2016) Antioxidant lignans and neolignans from acorus tatarinowii. *Sci Rep* **6**:22909.
3. Ni G, Shi GR, Zhang D, *et al.* (2016) Cytotoxic lignans and sesquiterpenoids from the rhizomes of Acorus tatarinowii. *Planta Med* **82**(7):632–638.
4. Liu SJ, Yang C, Zhang Y, *et al.* (2016) Neuroprotective effect of beta-asarone against Alzheimer's disease: Regulation of synaptic plasticity by increased expression of SYP and GLUR1. *Drug Des Dev Ther* **10**:1461–1469.

5. An HM, Li GW, Lin C, *et al.* (2014) Acorus tatarinowii schott extract protects PC12 cells from amyloid-beta induced neurotoxicity. *Pharmazie* **69**(5):391–395.
6. Zhu M, Zhu H, Tan N, *et al.* (2014) The effects of Acorus tatarinowii schott on 5-HT concentrations, TPH2 and 5-HT1b expression in the dorsal raphe of exercised rats. *J Ethnopharmacol* **158 (P + A)**: 431–436.
7. Fang YQ, Shi C, Liu L, Fang RM. (2012) Pharmacokinetics of beta-asarone in rabbit blood, hippocampus, cortex, brain stem, thalamus and cerebellum. *Pharmazie* **67**(2):120–123.
8. Lu J, Fu T, Qian Y, *et al.* (2014) Distribution of alpha-asarone in brain following three different routes of administration in rats. *Eur J Pharm Sci* **63**:63–70.
9. Liu J, Li C, Xing G, *et al.* (2010) Beta-asarone attenuates neuronal apoptosis induced by beta amyloid in rat hippocampus. *Yakugaku Zasshi* **130**(5):737–746.
10. Li Z, Zhao G, Qian S, *et al.* (2012) Cerebrovascular protection of beta-asarone in Alzheimer's disease rats: A behavioral, cerebral blood flow, biochemical and genic study. *J Ethnopharmacol* **144**(2):305–312.
11. Zhang S, Gui XH, Huang LP, *et al.* (2016) Neuroprotective effects of beta-asarone against 6-hydroxy dopamine-induced parkinsonism via jnk/bcl-2/beclin-1 pathway. *Mol Neurobiol* **53**(1):83–94.
12. Ning B, Deng M, Zhang Q, Wang N, *et al.* (2016) Beta-asarone inhibits IRE1/XBP1 endoplasmic reticulum stress pathway in 6-OHDA-induced parkinsonian rats. *Neurochem Res* **41**(8):2097–2101.
13. Huang L, Deng M, He Y, Lu S, *et al.* (2016) Beta-asarone and levodopa co-administration increase striatal dopamine level in 6-hydroxydopamine induced rats by modulating p-glycoprotein and tight junction proteins at the blood-brain barrier and promoting levodopa into the brain. *Clin Exp Pharmacol Physiol* **43**(6):634–643.
14. Kumar H, Kim BW, Song SY, *et al.* (2012) Cognitive enhancing effects of alpha asarone in amnesic mice by influencing cholinergic and antioxidant defense mechanisms. *Biosci Biotechnol Biochem* **76**(8):1518–1522.
15. Sundaramahalingam M, Ramasundaram S, Rathinasamy SD, Natarajan RP, *et al.* (2013) Role of Acorus calamus and alpha-asarone on hippocampal dependent memory in noise stress exposed rats. *Pak J Biol Sci* **16**(16):770–778.

16. Limon ID, Mendieta L, Diaz A, *et al.* (2009) Neuroprotective effect of alpha-asarone on spatial memory and nitric oxide levels in rats injected with amyloid-beta(25–35). *Neurosci Lett* **453**(2):98–103.
17. Kim BW, Koppula S, Kumar H, *et al.* (2015) Alpha-asarone attenuates microglia-mediated neuroinflammation by inhibiting NF Kappa b activation and mitigates MPTP-induced behavioral deficits in a mouse model of Parkinson's disease. *Neuropharmacology* **97**:46–57.
18. Rodriguez-Paez L, Juarez-Sanchez M, Antunez-Solis J, Baeza I, *et al.* (2003) Alpha-asarone inhibits HMG-COa reductase, lowers serum LDL-cholesterol levels and reduces biliary CSI in hypercholesterolemic rats. *Phytomedicine* **10**(5):397–404.
19. Qiu G, Chen S, Guo J, Wu J, *et al.* (2016) Alpha-asarone improves striatal cholinergic function and locomotor hyperactivity in *fmr1* knockout mice. *Behav Brain Res* **312**:212–218.
20. Chellian R, Pandy V, Mohamed Z. (2016) Biphasic effects of alpha-asarone on immobility in the tail suspension test: Evidence for the involvement of the noradrenergic and serotonergic systems in its antidepressant-like activity. *Front Pharmacol* **7**:72.
21. Mendez M, Lim G. (2003) Seizures in elderly patients with dementia: Epidemiology and management. *Drugs Aging* **20**(11):791–803.
22. Huang C, Li WG, Zhang XB, *et al.* (2013) Alpha-asarone from Acorus gramineus alleviates epilepsy by modulating a-type gaba receptors. *Neuropharmacology* **65**:1–11.
23. Wang ZJ, Levinson SR, Sun L, Heinbockel T. (2014) Identification of both GABAa receptors and voltage-activated Na(+) channels as molecular targets of anticonvulsant alpha-asarone. *Front Pharmacol* **5**:40.
24. Lee B, Sur B, Yeom M, Shim I, *et al.* (2014) Alpha-asarone, a major component of Acorus gramineus, attenuates corticosterone-induced anxiety-like behaviours via modulating TRKB signaling process. *Korean J Physiol Pharmacol* **18**(3):191–200.
25. Wiseman RW, Miller EC, Miller JA, Liem A. (1987) Structure-activity studies of the hepatocarcinogenicities of alkenylbenzene derivatives related to estragole and safrole on administration to preweanling male C57BL/6J x C3H/HeJ F1 mice. *Cancer Res* **47**(9):2275–2283.
26. European Commission (2002) Opinion of the scientific committee on food on the presence of beta-asarone in flavourings and other food ingredients with flavouring properties. European Commission, Brussels, Belgium.

27. U.S. Food and Drug Administration (2005) Title 21-Food and drugs: Chapter 1 — Food and drug administration. U.S. Food and Drug Administration, Silver Spring, Maryland.
28. Cartus AT, Stegmuller S, Simson N, *et al.* (2015) Hepatic metabolism of carcinogenic beta-asarone. *Chem Res Toxicol* **28**(9):1760–1773.
29. Cho JY, Yoo ES, Baik KU, Park MH. (1999) Eudesmin inhibits tumor necrosis factor-alpha production and T cell proliferation. *Arch Pharm Res* **22**(4):348–353.
30. Raimundo JM, Trindade AP, Velozo LS, Kaplan MA, *et al.* (2009) The lignan eudesmin extracted from Piper truncatum induced vascular relaxation via activation of endothelial histamine H1 receptors. *Eur J Pharmacol* **606**(1–3):150–154.
31. Liu H, Song Z, Liao DG, *et al.* (2015) Anticonvulsant and sedative effects of eudesmin isolated from Acorus tatarinowii on mice and rats. *Phytother Res* **29**(7):996–1003.
32. Liu JL, Zheng SL, Fan QJ, Yuan JC, *et al.* (2014) Optimization of high-pressure ultrasonic-assisted simultaneous extraction of six major constituents from Ligusticum chuan xiong rhizome using response surface methodology. *Molecules* **19**(2):1887–1911.
33. Zhao YX, Ding MY, Liu DL. (2005) Phenolic acids analysis in Ligusticum chuan xiong using HPLC. *J Chromatogr Sci* **43**(8):389–393.
34. Bensky D, Clavey S, Stoger E. (2004) Eastland Press, Inc, Seattle, US.
35. Li SL, Chan SS, Lin G, *et al.* (2003) Simultaneous analysis of seventeen chemical ingredients of Ligusticum chuan xiong by on-line high performance liquid chromatography-diode array detector-mass spectrometry. *Planta Med* **69**(5):445–451.
36. Yan R, Li SL, Chung HS, Tam YK, *et al.* (2005) Simultaneous quantification of 12 bioactive components of Ligusticum chuan xiong Hort. By high-performance liquid chromatography. *J Pharm Biomed Anal* **37**(1):87–95.
37. Ran X, Ma L, Peng C, Zhang H, *et al.* (2011) Ligusticum chuan xiong Hort: A review of chemistry and pharmacology. *Pharm Biol* **49**(11):1180–1189.
38. Wang Q, Li S, Liu P, *et al.* (2012) HPLC evaluation on 3-n-butylphthalide distribution. *J Appl Pharm Sci* **2**(10):16–20.
39. Zhang C, Liu RQ, He J, Ma ZQ, *et al.* (2016) Chemical compositions of Ligusticum chuan xiong oil and lemongrass oil and their joint action against Aphis citricola Van Der Goot (hemiptera: Aphididae). *Molecules* **21**(10).

40. Liu SY, Sylvester DM. (1994) Antiplatelet activity of tetramethylpyrazine. *Thromb Res* **75**(1):51–62.
41. Sheu JR, Kan YC, Hung WC, Ko WC, *et al.* (1997) Mechanisms involved in the antiplatelet activity of tetramethylpyrazine in human platelets. *Thromb Res* **88**(3):259–70.
42. Sheu JR, Hsiao G, Lee YM, Yen MH. (2001) Antithrombotic effects of tetramethylpyrazine in *in vivo* experiments. *Int J Hematol* **73**(3): 393–398.
43. Li M, Handa S, Ikeda Y, Goto S. (2001) Specific inhibiting characteristics of tetramethylpyrazine, one of the active ingredients of the Chinese herbal medicine 'chuan xiong,' on platelet thrombus formation under high shear rates. *Thromb Res* **104**(1):15–28.
44. Liao SL, Kao TK, Chen WY, *et al.* (2004) Tetramethylpyrazine reduces ischemic brain injury in rats. *Neurosci Lett* **372**(1–2):40–45.
45. Kao TK, Chang CY, Ou YC, *et al.* (2013) Tetramethylpyrazine reduces cellular inflammatory response following permanent focal cerebral ischemia in rats. *Exp Neurol* **247**:188–201.
46. Ding Y, Hou X, Chen L, *et al.* (2013) Protective action of tetramethylpyrazine on the medulla oblongata in rats with chronic hypoxia. *Auton Neurosci* **173**(1–2):45–52.
47. Chang CY, Kao TK, Chen WY, *et al.* (2015) Tetramethylpyrazine inhibits neutrophil activation following permanent cerebral ischemia in rats. *Biochem Biophys Res Commun* **463**(3):421–427.
48. Xiao X, Liu Y, Qi C, *et al.* (2010) Neuroprotection and enhanced neurogenesis by tetramethylpyrazine in adult rat brain after focal ischemia. *Neurol Res* **32**(5):547–555.
49. Yan Y, Zhao J, Cao C, *et al.* (2014) Tetramethylpyrazine promotes SH-SY5Y cell differentiation into neurons through epigenetic regulation of topoisomerase IIbeta. *Neuroscience* **278**:179–193.
50. Zhang M, Gao F, Teng F, Zhang C. (2014) Tetramethylpyrazine promotes the proliferation and migration of brain endothelial cells. *Mol Med Rep* **10**(1):29–32.
51. Kong X, Zhong M, Su X, *et al.* (2015) Tetramethylpyrazine promotes migration of neural precursor cells via activating the phosphatidylinositol 3-kinase pathway. *Mol Neurobiol* **53**(9):6526–6539.
52. Xiang J, Pan J, Chen F, *et al.* (2014) L-3-n-butylphthalide improves cognitive impairment of APP/PS1 mice by BDNF/TRKB/PI3K/AKT pathway. *Int J Clin Exp Med* **7**(7):1706–1713.

53. Peng Y, Xu S, Chen G, Wang L, *et al.* (2007) L-3-n-butylphthalide improves cognitive impairment induced by chronic cerebral hypoperfusion in rats. *J Pharmacol Exp Ther* **321**(3):902–910.
54. Peng Y, Xing C, Lemere CA, *et al.* (2008) L-3-n-butylphthalide ameliorates beta-amyloid-induced neuronal toxicity in cultured neuronal cells. *Neurosci Lett* **434**(2):224–229.
55. Peng Y, Xing C, Xu S, *et al.* (2009) L-3-n-butylphthalide improves cognitive impairment induced by intracerebroventricular infusion of amyloid-beta peptide in rats. *Eur J Pharmacol* **621**(1–3):38–45.
56. Peng Y, Hu Y, Feng N, Wang L, *et al.* (2011) L-3-n-butyl-phthalide alleviates hydrogen peroxide-induced apoptosis by PKC pathway in human neuroblastoma SK-N-SH cells. *Naunyn Schmiedebergs Arch Pharmacol* **383**(1):91–99.
57. Teng CM, Chen WY, Ko WC, Ouyang CH. (1987) Antiplatelet effect of butylidenephthalide. *Biochim Biophys Acta* **924**(3):375–382.
58. Nam KN, Kim KP, Cho KH, *et al.* (2013) Prevention of inflammation-mediated neurotoxicity by butylidenephthalide and its role in microglial activation. *Cell Biochem Funct* **31**(8):707–712.
59. Khan KA, Kumar N, Nayak PG, *et al.* (2013) Impact of caffeic acid on aluminium chloride-induced dementia in rats. *J Pharm Pharmacol* **65**(12):1745–1752.
60. Wei M, Chen L, Liu J, Zhao J, *et al.* (2016) Protective effects of a chotosan fraction and its active components on beta-amyloid-induced neurotoxicity. *Neurosci Lett* **617**:143–149.
61. Lin F, Zhang C, Chen X, *et al.* (2015) Chrysophanol affords neuroprotection against microglial activation and free radical-mediated oxidative damage in BV2 murine microglia. *Int J Clin Exp Med* **8**(3):3447–3455.
62. Shi C, Liu J, Wu F, Zhu X, *et al.* (2011) Beta-sitosterol inhibits high cholesterol-induced platelet beta-amyloid release. *J Bioenerg Biomembr* **43**(6):691–697.
63. Chao WW, Lin BF. (2011) Bioactivities of major constituents isolated from Angelica sinensis (danggui). *Chin Med* **6**:29.
64. Ying L, Si-Wang W, Hong-Hai T, Wei C. (2013) Simultaneous quantification of six main active constituents in Chinese angelica by high-performance liquid chromatography with photodiode array detector. *Pharmacogn Mag* **9**(34):114–119.
65. Huang SH, Lin CM, Chiang BH. (2008) Protective effects of Angelica sinensis extract on amyloid beta-peptide-induced neurotoxicity. *Phytomedicine* **15**(9):710–721.

66. Xin J, Zhang J, Yang Y, Deng M, *et al.* (2013) Radix angelica sinensis that contains the component Z-ligustilide promotes adult neurogenesis to mediate recovery from cognitive impairment. *Curr Neurovasc Res* **10**(4):304–315.
67. Sgarbossa A, Giacomazza D, Di Carlo M. (2015) Ferulic acid: A hope for Alzheimer's disease therapy from plants. *Nutrients* **7**(7):5764–5782.
68. Tsai FS, Wu LY, Yang SE, *et al.* (2015) Ferulic acid reverses the cognitive dysfunction caused by amyloid beta peptide 1–40 through anti-oxidant activity and cholinergic activation in rats. *Am J Chin Med* **43**(2):319–335.
69. Zhang L, Wang H, Wang T, *et al.* (2015) Ferulic acid ameliorates nerve injury induced by cerebral ischemia in rats. *Exp Ther Med* **9**(3):972–976.
70. Huang H, Ma ZC, Wang YG, *et al.* (2015) Ferulic acid alleviates abeta (25–35) and lipopolysaccharide-induced PC12 cellular damage: A potential role in Alzheimer's disease by PDE inhibition. *Int J Clin Pharmacol Ther* **53**(10):828–837.
71. Adefegha SA, Omojokun OS, Oboh G, Fasakin O, *et al.* (2015) Modulatory effects of ferulic acid on cadmium-induced brain damage. *J Evid Based Complement Altern Med* **21**(4):NP56–NP61.
72. Kuang X, Du JR, Liu YX, Zhang GY, *et al.* (2008) Postischemic administration of Z-ligustilide ameliorates cognitive dysfunction and brain damage induced by permanent forebrain ischemia in rats. *Pharmacol Biochem Behav* **88**(3):213–221.
73. Feng Z, Lu Y, Wu X, *et al.* (2012) Ligustilide alleviates brain damage and improves cognitive function in rats of chronic cerebral hypoperfusion. *J Ethnopharmacol* **144**(2):313–321.
74. Chen D, Tang J, Khatibi NH, *et al.* (2011) Treatment with z-ligustilide, a component of Angelica sinensis, reduces brain injury after a subarachnoid hemorrhage in rats. *J Pharmacol Exp Ther* **337**(3):663–672.
75. Kuang X, Du JR, Chen YS, Wang J, *et al.* (2009) Protective effect of z-ligustilide against amyloid beta-induced neurotoxicity is associated with decreased pro-inflammatory markers in rat brains. *Pharmacol Biochem Behav* **92**(4):635–641.
76. Chi K, Fu RH, Huang YC, *et al.* (2016) Therapeutic effect of ligustilide-stimulated adipose-derived stem cells in a mouse thromboembolic stroke model. *Cell Transplant* **25**(5):899–912.
77. Hu Y, Duan M, Liang S, Wang Y, *et al.* (2015) Senkyunolide I protects rat brain against focal cerebral ischemia-reperfusion injury by up-regulating p-ERK1/2, NRF2/HO-1 and inhibiting caspase-3. *Brain Res* **1605**:39–48.

78. Lin L, Ni B, Lin H, *et al.* (2015) Traditional usages, botany, phytochemistry, pharmacology and toxicology of Polygonum multiflorum thunb.: A review. *J Ethnopharmacol* **159**:158–183.
79. Yao S, Li Y, Kong L. (2006) Preparative isolation and purification of chemical constituents from the root of Polygonum multiflorum by high-speed counter-current chromatography. *J Chromatogr A* **1115**(1–2): 64–71.
80. Chan YC, Wang MF, Chen YC, Yang DY, *et al.* (2003) Long-term administration of Polygonum multiflorum thunb. Reduces cerebral ischemia-induced infarct volume in gerbils. *Am J Chin Med* **31**(1): 71–77.
81. Chan YC, Cheng FC, Wang MF. (2002) Beneficial effects of different Polygonum multiflorum thunb. Extracts on memory and hippocampus morphology. *J Nutr Sci Vitaminol (Tokyo)* **48**(6):491–497.
82. Chan YC, Wang MF, Chang HC. (2003) Polygonum multiflorum extracts improve cognitive performance in senescence accelerated mice. *Am J Chin Med* **31**(2):171–179.
83. Um MY, Choi WH, Aan JY, Kim SR, *et al.* (2006) Protective effect of Polygonum multiflorum thunb on amyloid beta-peptide 25-35 induced cognitive deficits in mice. *J Ethnopharmacol* **104**(1–2):144–148.
84. Liu LF, Durairajan SS, Lu JH, Koo I, *et al.* (2012) In vitro screening on amyloid precursor protein modulation of plants used in Ayurvedic and traditional Chinese medicine for memory improvement. *J Ethnopharmacol* **141**(2):754–760.
85. Zhu D, Bungart BL, Yang X, Zhumadilov Z, *et al.* (2015) Role of membrane biophysics in Alzheimer's-related cell pathways. *Front Neurosci* **9**:186.
86. Hou DR, Wang Y, Xue L, *et al.* (2008) Effect of Polygonum multiflorum on the fluidity of the mitochondria membrane and activity of COX in the hippocampus of rats with abeta (1-40)-induced Alzheimer's disease. *Zhong Nan Da Xue Xue Bao Yi Xue Ban* **33**(11):987–992.
87. Steele ML, Truong J, Govindaraghavan S, Ooi L, *et al.* (2013) Cytoprotective properties of traditional Chinese medicinal herbal extracts in hydrogen peroxide challenged human U373 astroglia cells. *Neurochem Int* **62**(5):522–529.
88. Jang JY, Kim HN, Kim YR, *et al.* (2013) Hexane extract from polygonum multiflorum attenuates glutamate-induced apoptosis in primary cultured cortical neurons. *J Ethnopharmacol* **145**(1):261–268.

89. Park HR, Kim JY, Lee Y, *et al.* (2016) PMC-12, a traditional herbal medicine, enhances learning memory and hippocampal neurogenesis in mice. *Neurosci Lett* **617**:254–263.
90. Lv L, Shao X, Wang L, Huang D, *et al.* (2010) Stilbene glucoside from Polygonum multiflorum thunb.: A novel natural inhibitor of advanced glycation end product formation by trapping of methylglyoxal. *J Agric Food Chem* **58**(4):2239–2245.
91. Wang T, Gu J, Wu PF, *et al.* (2009) Protection by tetrahydroxystilbene glucoside against cerebral ischemia: Involvement of JNK, SIRT1, and NF-κB pathways and inhibition of intracellular ROS/RNS generation. *Free Radic Biol Med* **47**(3):229–240.
92. Liu QL, Xiao JH, Ma R, Ban Y, *et al.* (2007) Effect of 2,3,5,4′-tetrahydroxystilbene-2-o-beta-d-glucoside on lipoprotein oxidation and proliferation of coronary arterial smooth cells. *J Asian Nat Prod Res* **9**(6–8):689–697.
93. Buchter C, Zhao L, Havermann S, *et al.* (2015) TSG (2,3,5,4′-tetrahydroxystilbene-2-o-beta-d-glucoside) from the Chinese herb Polygonum multiflorum increases life span and stress resistance of Caenorhabditis elegans. *Oxid Med Cell Longev* **2015**:124357.
94. Wang R, Tang Y, Feng B, *et al.* (2007) Changes in hippocampal synapses and learning-memory abilities in age-increasing rats and effects of tetrahydroxystilbene glucoside in aged rats. *Neuroscience* **149**(4): 739–746.
95. Shen C, Sun FL, Zhang RY, *et al.* (2015) Tetrahydroxystilbene glucoside ameliorates memory and movement functions, protects synapses and inhibits alpha-synuclein aggregation in hippocampus and striatum in aged mice. *Restor Neurol Neurosci* **33**(4):531–541.
96. Stefanis L. (2012) Alpha-synuclein in Parkinson's disease. *Cold Spring Harb Perspect Med* **2**(2):a009399.
97. Li X, Li Y, Chen J, *et al.* (2010) Tetrahydroxystilbene glucoside attenuates MPP+-induced apoptosis in PC12 cells by inhibiting ROS generation and modulating JNK activation. *Neurosci Lett* **483**(1):1–5.
98. Qin R, Li X, Li G, *et al.* (2011) Protection by tetrahydroxystilbene glucoside against neurotoxicity induced by MPP+: The involvement of PI3K/AKT pathway activation. *Toxicol Lett* **202**(1):1–7.
99. Sun FL, Zhang L, Zhang RY, Li L. (2011) Tetrahydroxystilbene glucoside protects human neuroblastoma SH-SY5Y cells against MPP+-induced cytotoxicity. *Eur J Pharmacol* **660**(2–3):283–290.

100. Zhang L, Xing Y, Ye CF, Ai HX, *et al.* (2006) Learning-memory deficit with aging in APP transgenic mice of Alzheimer's disease and intervention by using tetrahydroxystilbene glucoside. *Behav Brain Res* **173**(2):246–254.
101. Zhou L, Hou Y, Yang Q, *et al.* (2012) Tetrahydroxystilbene glucoside improves the learning and memory of amyloid-beta(1)(-)(4)(2)-injected rats and may be connected to synaptic changes in the hippocampus. *Can J Physiol Pharmacol* **90**(11):1446–1455.
102. Diaz M, Degens H, Vanhees L, Austin C, *et al.* (2016) The effects of resveratrol on aging vessels. *Exp Gerontol* **85**:41–47.
103. Kennedy DO, Wightman EL, Reay JL, *et al.* (2010) Effects of resveratrol on cerebral blood flow variables and cognitive performance in humans: A double-blind, placebo-controlled, crossover investigation. *Am J Clin Nutr* **91**(6):1590–1597.
104. Wightman EL, Haskell-Ramsay CF, Reay JL, *et al.* (2015) The effects of chronic trans-resveratrol supplementation on aspects of cognitive function, mood, sleep, health and cerebral blood flow in healthy, young humans. *Br J Nutr* **114**(9):1427–1437.
105. Wong RH, Nealon RS, Scholey A, Howe PR. (2016) Low dose resveratrol improves cerebrovascular function in type 2 diabetes mellitus. *Nutr Metab Cardiovasc Dis* **26**(5):393–399.
106. Feng Y, Cui Y, Gao JL, *et al.* (2016) Neuroprotective effects of resveratrol against traumatic brain injury in rats: Involvement of synaptic proteins and neuronal autophagy. *Mol Med Rep* **13**(6):5248–5254.
107. Liu J, Hu XG, Yang Q, *et al.* (2010) Comparison of the immunoregulatory function of different constituents in Radix astragali and Radix hedysari. *J Biomed Biotechnol* **2010**:479426.
108. Ahn SM, Kim HN, Kim YR, *et al.* (2016) Emodin from Polygonum multiflorum ameliorates oxidative toxicity in HT22 cells and deficits in photothrombotic ischemia. *J Ethnopharmacol* **188**:13–20.
109. Thangnipon W, Suwanna N, Kitiyanant N, *et al.* (2012) Protective role of n-trans-feruloyltyramine against beta-amyloid peptide-induced neurotoxicity in rat cultured cortical neurons. *Neurosci Lett* **513**(2):229–232.
110. Park YJ, Thwe AA, Li X, *et al.* (2015) Triterpene and flavonoid biosynthesis and metabolic profiling of hairy roots, adventitious roots, and seedling roots of Astragalus membranaceus. *J Agric Food Chem* **63**(40):8862–8869.

111. Zhang X, Xiao HB, Xue XY, Sun YG, *et al.* (2007) Simultaneous characterization of isoflavonoids and astragalosides in two Astragalus species by high-performance liquid chromatography coupled with atmospheric pressure chemical ionization tandem mass spectrometry. *J Sep Sci* **30**(13):2059–2069.
112. Lei H, Wang B, Li WP, Yang Y, *et al.* (2003) Anti-aging effect of astragalosides and its mechanism of action. *Acta Pharmacol Sin* **24**(3):230–234.
113. Qu YZ, Li M, Zhao YL, *et al.* (2009) Astragaloside IV attenuates cerebral ischemia-reperfusion-induced increase in permeability of the blood-brain barrier in rats. *Eur J Pharmacol* **606**(1–3):137–141.
114. Li M, Ma RN, Li LH, Qu YZ, *et al.* (2013) Astragaloside IV reduces cerebral edema post-ischemia/reperfusion correlating the suppression of MMP-9 and AQP4. *Eur J Pharmacol* **715**(1–3):189–195.
115. Shao A, Guo S, Tu S, *et al.* (2014) Astragaloside IV alleviates early brain injury following experimental subarachnoid hemorrhage in rats. *Int J Med Sci* **11**(10):1073–1081.
116. Wang X, Wang Y, Hu JP, *et al.* (2016) Astragaloside IV, a natural PPARgamma agonist, reduces abeta production in Alzheimer's disease through inhibition of BACE1. Mol *Neurobiol* **54**(4):2939–2949.
117. Cai J, Pan R, Jia X, *et al.* (2014) The combination of Astragalus membranaceus and ligustrazine ameliorates micro-haemorrhage by maintaining blood-brain barrier integrity in cerebrally ischaemic rats. *J Ethnopharmacol* **158**(Pt A):301–309.
118. Fu S, Gu Y, Jiang JQ, *et al.* (2014) Calycosin-7-o-beta-d-glucoside regulates nitric oxide/caveolin-1/matrix metalloproteinases pathway and protects blood-brain barrier integrity in experimental cerebral ischemia-reperfusion injury. *J Ethnopharmacol* **155**(1):692–701.
119. Lee JS, Kim HG, Han JM, *et al.* (2014) Ethanol extract of Astragali radix and salviae miltiorrhizae radix, myelophil, exerts anti-amnesic effect in a mouse model of scopolamine-induced memory deficits. *J Ethnopharmacol* **153**(3):782–792.
120. Petersen M, Simmonds MS. (2003) Rosmarinic acid. *Phytochemistry* **62**(2):121–125.
121. Luo H, Kong W, Hu Y, *et al.* (2015) Quality evaluation of Salvia miltiorrhiza bge. By ultrahigh performance liquid chromatography with photodiode array detection and chemical finger printing coupled with chemometric analysis. *J Sep Sci* **38**(9):1544–1551.

122. Guo C, Yin Y, Duan J, *et al.* (2015) Neuroprotective effect and underlying mechanism of sodium dan shen su [3-(3,4-dihydroxyphenyl) lactic acid from radix and Rhizoma salviae miltiorrhizae = dan shen] against cerebral ischemia and reperfusion injury in rats. *Phytomedicine* **22**(2):283–289.
123. Seetapun S, Yaoling J, Wang Y, Zhu YZ. (2013) Neuroprotective effect of dan shen su derivatives as anti-ischaemia agents on SH-SY5Y cells and rat brain. *Biosci Rep* **33**(4): e00062.
124. Du G, Zhang J. (1997) Protective effects of salvianolic acid a against impairment of memory induced by cerebral ischemia-reperfusion in mice. *Chin Med J (Engl)* **110**(1):65–68.
125. Wang SB, Pang XB, Zhao Y, *et al.* (2012) Protection of salvianolic acid a on rat brain from ischemic damage via soluble epoxide hydrolase inhibition. *J Asian Nat Prod Res* **14**(11):1084–1092.
126. Deng Y, Yang M, Xu F, *et al.* (2015) Combined salvianolic acid b and ginsenoside RG1 exerts cardioprotection against ischemia/reperfusion injury in rats. *PLoS One* **10**(8):e0135435.
127. Durairajan SS, Yuan Q, Xie L, *et al.* (2008) Salvianolic acid b inhibits abeta fibril formation and disaggregates preformed fibrils and protects against abeta-induced cytotoxicty. *Neurochem Int* **52**(4–5):741–750.
128. Grossi C, Guccione C, Isacchi B, *et al.* (2016) Development of blood-brain barrier permeable nanoparticles as potential carriers for salvianolic acid b to CNS. *Planta Med* **83**(5):382–391.
129. Zhou YQ, Li WX, Xu L, Chen LY. (2011) In Salvia miltiorrhiza, phenolic acids possess protective properties against amyloid beta-induced cytotoxicity, and tanshinones act as acetylcholinesterase inhibitors. *Environ Toxicol Pharmacol* **31**(3):443–452.
130. Akhondzadeh S, Noroozian M, Mohammadi M, Ohadinia S, *et al.* (2003) Salvia officinalis extract in the treatment of patients with mild to moderate Alzheimer's disease: A double blind, randomized and placebo-controlled trial. *J Clin Pharm Ther* **28**(1):53–59.
131. Perry NS, Bollen C, Perry EK, Ballard C. (2003) Salvia for dementia therapy: Review of pharmacological activity and pilot tolerability clinical trial. *Pharmacol Biochem Behav* **75**(3):651–659.
132. Iuvone T, De Filippis D, Esposito G, D'Amico A, *et al.* (2006) The spice sage and its active ingredient rosmarinic acid protect PC12 cells from amyloid-beta peptide-induced neurotoxicity. *J Pharmacol Exp Ther* **317**(3):1143–1149.

133. Alkam T, Nitta A, Mizoguchi H, Itoh A, *et al.* (2007) A natural scavenger of peroxynitrites, rosmarinic acid, protects against impairment of memory induced by abeta(25–35). *Behav Brain Res* **180**(2):139–145.
134. Kantar G D̀, Ozturk N, Er H, *et al.* (2015) Effects of rosmarinic acid on cognitive and biochemical alterations in ovariectomized rats treated with d-galactose. *Folia Histochem Cytobiol* **53**(4): 283–293.
135. Ghaffari H, Venkataramana M, Jalali GB, *et al.* (2014) Rosmarinic acid mediated neuroprotective effects against H_2O_2-induced neuronal cell damage in n2a cells. *Life Sci* **113**(1–2):7–13.
136. Fonteles AA, De Souza CM, De Sousa Neves JC, *et al.* (2016) Rosmarinic acid prevents against memory deficits in ischemic mice. *Behav Brain Res* **297**:91–103.
137. Luan H, Kan Z, Xu Y, Lv C, *et al.* (2013) Rosmarinic acid protects against experimental diabetes with cerebral ischemia: Relation to inflammation response. *J Neuroinflamm* **10**:28.
138. Gao JW, Yamane T, Maita H, *et al.* (2011) DJ-1-mediated protective effect of protocatechuic aldehyde against oxidative stress in SH-SY5Y cells. *J Pharmacol Sci* **115**(1):36–44.
139. Zhao X, Zhai S, An MS, *et al.* (2013) Neuroprotective effects of protocatechuic aldehyde against neurotoxin-induced cellular and animal models of Parkinson's disease. *PLoS One* **8**(10):e78220.
140. Zhang F, Zheng W, Pi R, *et al.* (2009) Cryptotanshinone protects primary rat cortical neurons from glutamate-induced neurotoxicity via the activation of the phosphatidylinositol 3-kinase/AKT signaling pathway. *Exp Brain Res* **193**(1):109–118.
141. Mei Z, Situ B, Tan X, *et al.* (2010) Cryptotanshinione upregulates alpha-secretase by activation PI3k pathway in cortical neurons. *Brain Res* **1348**:165–173.
142. Mei Z, Yan P, Situ B, Mou Y, *et al.* (2012) Cryptotanshinione inhibits beta-amyloid aggregation and protects damage from beta-amyloid in SH-SY5Y cells. *Neurochem Res* **37**(3):622–628.
143. Liu Z, Xu S, Huang X, *et al.* (2015) Cryptotanshinone, an orally bioactive herbal compound from danshen, attenuates atherosclerosis in apolipoprotein e-deficient mice: Role of lectin-like oxidized LDL receptor-1 (Lox-1). *Br J Pharmacol* **172**(23):5661–5675.
144. Qian YH, Xiao Q, Xu J. (2012) The protective effects of tanshinone IIa on beta-amyloid protein (1–42)-induced cytotoxicity via activation of the Bcl-xl pathway in neuron. *Brain Res Bull* **88**(4):354–358.

145. Shi LL, Yang WN, Chen XL, *et al.* (2012) The protective effects of tanshinone IIA on neurotoxicity induced by beta-amyloid protein through calpain and the p35/Cdk5 pathway in primary cortical neurons. *Neurochem Int* **61**(2):227–235.
146. Wang QM, Yu X, Patal K, *et al.* (2013) Tanshinones inhibit amyloid aggregation by amyloid-beta peptide, disaggregate amyloid fibrils, and protect cultured cells. *ACS Chem Neurosci* **4**(6):1004–1015.
147. Liu C, Wu Y, Zha S, *et al.* (2016) Treatment effects of tanshinone IIa against intracerebroventricular streptozotocin induced memory deficits in mice. *Brain Res* **1631**:137–146.
148. Zhou L, Bondy SC, Jian L, *et al.* (2015) Tanshinone IIa attenuates the cerebral ischemic injury-induced increase in levels of GFAP and of caspases-3 and -8. *Neuroscience* **288**:105–111.
149. Zhao Y, Xu P, Hu S, *et al.* (2015) Tanshinone IIa, a multiple target neuroprotectant, promotes caveolae-dependent neuronal differentiation. *Eur J Pharmacol* **765**:437–446.
150. Zhang YH, Bai L, Li ZY, Zhang FS, *et al.* (2015) [HPLC fingerprint and active components determination of Polygala tenuifolia root bark and root]. *Zhong Yao Cai* **38**(7):1408–1412.
151. Ikeya Y, Takeda S, Tunakawa M, *et al.* (2004) Cognitive improving and cerebral protective effects of acylated oligosaccharides in Polygala tenuifolia. *Biol Pharm Bull* **27**(7):1081–1085.
152. Park CH, Choi SH, Koo JW, *et al.* (2002) Novel cognitive improving and neuroprotective activities of Polygala tenuifolia willdenow extract, BT-11. *J Neurosci Res* **70**(3):484–492.
153. Sun XL, Ito H, Masuoka T, Kamei C, *et al.* (2007) Effect of Polygala tenuifolia root extract on scopolamine-induced impairment of rat spatial cognition in an eight-arm radial maze task. *Biol Pharm Bull* **30**(9):1727–1731.
154. Naito R, Tohda C. (2006) Characterization of anti-neurodegenerative effects of Polygala tenuifolia in a beta(25-35)-treated cortical neurons. *Biol Pharm Bull* **29**(9):1892–1896.
155. Yabe T, Tuchida H, Kiyohara H, Takeda T, *et al.* (2003) Induction of NGF synthesis in astrocytes by onjisaponins of Polygala tenuifolia, constituents of kampo (Japanese herbal) medicine, ninjin-yoei-to. *Phytomedicine* **10**(2–3):106–114.
156. Liu P, Hu Y, Guo DH, *et al.* (2010) Antioxidant activity of oligosaccharide ester extracted from Polygala tenuifolia roots in senescence-accelerated mice. *Pharm Biol* **48**(7):828–833.

157. Jia H, Jiang Y, Ruan Y, *et al.* (2004) Tenuigenin treatment decreases secretion of the Alzheimer's disease amyloid beta-protein in cultured cells. *Neurosci Lett* **367**(1):123–128.
158. Lv J, Jia H, Jiang Y, *et al.* (2009) Tenuifolin, an extract derived from tenuigenin, inhibits amyloid-beta secretion *in vitro. Acta Physiol (Oxford)* **196**(4):419–425.
159. Zhang H, Han T, Zhang L, *et al.* (2008) Effects of tenuifolin extracted from radix polygalae on learning and memory: A behavioral and biochemical study on aged and amnesic mice. *Phytomedicine* **15**(8): 587–594.
160. Liu YM, Li ZY, Hu H, *et al.* (2015) Tenuifolin, a secondary saponin from hydrolysates of polygalasaponins, counteracts the neurotoxicity induced by abeta (25-35) peptides *in vitro* and *in vivo. Pharmacol Biochem Behav* **128**:14–22.
161. Walsmann P. (1991) Isolation and characterization of hirudin from Hirudo medicinalis. *Semin Thromb Hemost* **17**(2):83–87.
162. Mao SJ, Yates MT, Blankenship DT, *et al.* (1987) Rapid purification and revised amino-terminal sequence of hirudin: A specific thrombin inhibitor of the bloodsucking leech. *Anal Biochem* **161**(2):514–518.
163. Markwardt F. (2002) Hirudin as alternative anticoagulant — A historical review. *Semin Thromb Hemost* **28**(5):405–414.
164. Berger P. (1998) Medium-dose hirudin was superior to heparin in preventing ischemic events in patients with acute myocardial ischemia. *Evid Based Cardiovasc Med* **1**(1):12.
165. Habazettl H, Lindert J, Baeter S, *et al.* (2004) Effects of unfractionated heparin, low molecular weight heparin and r-hirudin on leukocyte adhesion in ischemia/reperfusion. *Blood Coagul Fibrinol* **15**(5): 375–381.
166. Jormalainen M, Vento AE, Lukkarinen H, *et al.* (2007) Inhibition of thrombin during reperfusion improves immediate postischemic myocardial function and modulates apoptosis in a porcine model of cardiopulmonary bypass. *J Cardiothorac Vasc Anesth* **21**(2):224–231.
167. Hua Y, Wu J, Keep RF, Hoff JT, *et al.* (2003) Thrombin exacerbates brain edema in focal cerebral ischemia. *Acta Neurochir Suppl* **86**:163–166.
168. De Castro R M, Badaut J, Price M, *et al.* (2006) Thrombin in ischemic neuronal death. *Exp Neurol* **198**(1):199–203.
169. Cai M, Yu Z, Wang L, *et al.* (2016) Tong xin luo reduces brain edema and inhibits post-ischemic inflammation after middle cerebral artery occlusion in rats. *J Ethnopharmacol* **181**:136–145.

170. Zhang RX, Li MX, Jia ZP. (2008) Rehmannia glutinosa: Review of botany, chemistry and pharmacology. *J Ethnopharmacol* **117**(2):199–214.
171. Li DQ, Bao YM, Zhao JJ, Liu CP, *et al.* (2004) Neuroprotective properties of catalpol in transient global cerebral ischemia in gerbils: Dose-response, therapeutic time-window and long-term efficacy. *Brain Res* **1029**(2):179–185.
172. Li DQ, Li Y, Liu Y, Bao YM, *et al.* (2005) Catalpol prevents the loss of CA1 hippocampal neurons and reduces working errors in gerbils after ischemia-reperfusion injury. *Toxicon.* **46**(8):845–851.
173. Liu YR, Li PW, Suo JJ, *et al.* (2014) Catalpol provides protective effects against cerebral ischaemia/reperfusion injury in gerbils. *J Pharm Pharmacol* **66**(9):1265–1270.
174. Li Y, Bao Y, Jiang B, *et al.* (2008) Catalpol protects primary cultured astrocytes from *in vitro* ischemia-induced damage. *Int J Dev Neurosci* **26**(3–4):309–317.
175. Jiang B, Shen RF, Bi J, Tian XS, *et al.* (2015) Catalpol: A potential therapeutic for neurodegenerative diseases. *Curr Med Chem* **22**(10):1278–1291.
176. Tian YY, Jiang B, An LJ, Bao YM. (2007) Neuroprotective effect of catalpol against MPP(+)-induced oxidative stress in mesencephalic neurons. *Eur J Pharmacol* **568**(1–3):142–148.
177. Bi J, Jiang B, Liu JH, Lei C, *et al.* (2008) Protective effects of catalpol against H_2O_2-induced oxidative stress in astrocytes primary cultures. *Neurosci Lett* **442**(3):224–227.
178. Tian YY, An LJ, Jiang L, Duan YL, *et al.* (2006) Catalpol protects dopaminergic neurons from LPS-induced neurotoxicity in mesencephalic neuron-glia cultures. *Life Sci* **80**(3):193–199.
179. Zhang XL, Zhang AH, Jiang B, Bao YM, *et al.* (2008) Further pharmacological evidence of the neuroprotective effect of catalpol from Rehmannia glutinosa. *Phytomedicine* **15**(6–7):484–490.
180. Zhang X, Jin C, Li Y, Guan S, *et al.* (2013) Catalpol improves cholinergic function and reduces inflammatory cytokines in the senescent mice induced by d-galactose. *Food Chem Toxicol* **58**:50–55.
181. Liu J, He QJ, Zou W, *et al.* (2006) Catalpol increases hippocampal neuroplasticity and up-regulates PKC and BDNF in the aged rats. *Brain Res* **1123**(1):68–79.
182. Liang JH, Du J, Xu LD, *et al.* (2009) Catalpol protects primary cultured cortical neurons induced by abeta(1-42) through a mitochondrial-dependent caspase pathway. *Neurochem Int* **55**(8):741–746.

183. Wang Z, Liu Q, Zhang R, Liu S, *et al.* (2009) Catalpol ameliorates beta amyloid-induced degeneration of cholinergic neurons by elevating brain-derived neurotrophic factors. *Neuroscience* **163**(4):1363–1372.
184. Xia Z, Zhang R, Wu P, Xia Z, *et al.* (2012) Memory defect induced by beta-amyloid plus glutamate receptor agonist is alleviated by catalpol and donepezil through different mechanisms. *Brain Res* **1441**:27–37.
185. Wang JH, Xie H, Zhao TK, Kang B. (2015) Catalpol regulates cholinergic nerve system function through effect on choline acetyl-transferase not m receptor affinity. *Biomed Pharmacother* **69**:291–296.
186. Zhang L, Dai W, Zhang X, Gong Z, *et al.* (2013) Mannotriose regulates learning and memory signal transduction in the hippocampus. *Neural Regen Res* **8**(32):3020–3026.
187. Zhang LN, Jin GQ, Zhang XL, Gong ZB, *et al.* (2014) Effects of 5-hydroxymethylfurfural extracted from Rehmannia glutinosa libosch on the expression of signaling molecules relevant to learning and memory among hippocampal neurons exposed to high concentration of corticosterone. *Chin J Integr Med* **20**(11):844–849.
188. Lu W, Jiang Q, Shi H, Niu Y, Gao B, *et al.* (2014) Partial least-squares-discriminant analysis differentiating Chinese wolfberries by UPLC-MS and flow injection mass spectrometric (FIMS) fingerprints. *J Agric Food Chem* **62**(37):9073–9080.
189. Peng Y, Ma C, Li Y, Leung KS, *et al.* (2005) Quantification of zeaxanthin dipalmitate and total carotenoids in Lycium fruits (Fructus lycii). *Plant Foods Hum Nutr* **60**(4):161–164.
190. Potterat O. (2010) Goji (and L. Chinense): Phytochemistry, pharmacology and safety in the perspective of traditional uses and recent popularity. *Planta Med* **76**(1):7–19.
191. Inbaraj BS, Lu H, Hung CF, Wu WB, *et al.* (2008) Determination of carotenoids and their esters in fruits of Lycium barbarum linnaeus by HPLC-DAD-APCI-MS. *J Pharm Biomed Anal* **47**(4–5):812–818.
192. Inbaraj BS, Lu H, Kao TH, Chen BH. (2010) Simultaneous determination of phenolic acids and flavonoids in Lycium barbarum linnaeus by HPLC-DAD-ESI-MS. *J Pharm Biomed Anal* **51**(3):549–556.
193. Wang CC, Chang SC, Inbaraj BS, Chen BH. (2010) Isolation of carotenoids, flavonoids and polysaccharides from Lycium barbarum l. And evaluation of antioxidant activity. *Food Chem* **120**(1):184–192.

194. Le K, Chiu F, Ng K. (2007) Identification and quantification of antioxidants in Fructus lycii. *Food Chem* **105**(1):353–363.
195. Li Y, Xie DM, ed. (2007) Gu jin zhong yi nao bing bian zhi jing yao 'Essentials of the treatment of brain disorders in ancient and modern Chinese medicine'. Ren min jun yi chu ban she, Beijing.
196. Li XM. (2007) Protective effect of Lycium barbarum polysaccharides on streptozotocin-induced oxidative stress in rats. *Int J Biol Macromol* **40**(5):461–465.
197. Yang D, Li SY, Yeung CM, *et al.* (2012) Lycium barbarum extracts protect the brain from blood-brain barrier disruption and cerebral edema in experimental stroke. *PLoS One* **7**(3):e33596.
198. Wang HB, Li YX, Hao YJ, *et al.* (2013) Neuroprotective effects of LBP on brain ischemic reperfusion neurodegeneration. *Eur Rev Med Pharmacol Sci* **17**(20):2760–2765.
199. Wang T, Li Y, Wang Y, *et al.* (2014) Lycium barbarum polysaccharide prevents focal cerebral ischemic injury by inhibiting neuronal apoptosis in mice. *PLoS One* **9**(3):e90780.
200. Rui C, Yuxiang L, Yinju H, *et al.* (2012) Protective effects of Lycium barbarum polysaccharide on neonatal rat primary cultured hippocampal neurons injured by oxygen-glucose deprivation and reperfusion. *J Mol Histol* **43**(5):535–542.
201. Lam CS, Tipoe GL, So KF, Fung ML. (2015) Neuroprotective mechanism of Lycium barbarum polysaccharides against hippocampal-dependent spatial memory deficits in a rat model of obstructive sleep apnea. *PLoS One* **10**(2):e0117990.
202. Lu SP, Zhao PT. (2010) Chemical characterization of Lycium barbarum polysaccharides and their reducing myocardial injury in ischemia/reperfusion of rat heart. *Int J Biol Macromol* **47**(5):681–684.
203. Yu MS, Leung SK, Lai SW, *et al.* (2005) Neuroprotective effects of anti-aging oriental medicine Lycium barbarum against beta-amyloid peptide neurotoxicity. *Exp Gerontol* **40**(8–9):716–727.
204. Ho YS, Yu MS, Yik SY, So KF, *et al.* (2009) Polysaccharides from wolfberry antagonizes glutamate excitotoxicity in rat cortical neurons. *Cell Mol Neurobiol* **29**(8):1233–1244.
205. Ho YS, Yu MS, Yang XF, So KF, *et al.* (2010) Neuroprotective effects of polysaccharides from wolfberry, the fruits of Lycium barbarum, against homocysteine-induced toxicity in rat cortical neurons. *J Alzheimers Dis* **19**(3):813–827.

206. Chen W, Cheng X, Chen J, *et al.* (2014) Lycium barbarum polysaccharides prevent memory and neurogenesis impairments in scopolamine-treated rats. *PLoS One* **9**(2):e88076.
207. Gao J, Chen C, Liu Y, *et al.* (2015) Lycium barbarum polysaccharide improves traumatic cognition via reversing imbalance of apoptosis/regeneration in hippocampal neurons after stress. *Life Sci* **121**:124–134.
208. Xing X, Liu F, Xiao J, So KF. (2016) Neuro-protective mechanisms of Lycium barbarum. *Neuromol Med* **18**(3):253–263.

7

Clinical Evidence for Acupuncture and Related Therapies

OVERVIEW

Seventy studies of acupuncture, electro-acupuncture, scalp acupuncture, moxibustion, and ear acupressure for vascular dementia were identified. These included 47 randomised controlled trials, two controlled clinical trials, and 21 non-controlled studies. Meta-analyses of outcome data were conducted to evaluate the efficacy and safety of acupuncture therapies for vascular dementia. Both controlled and non-controlled studies were examined to identify the interventions used and to explore the safety profiles. The results suggest that certain acupuncture therapies appear to improve outcomes in vascular dementia. However, the studies tended to be small, of short duration, and of variable methodological quality.

Introduction

Acupuncture is part of a family of techniques that stimulate acupoints to correct imbalances of energy and restore health to the body. Methods of stimulating acupoints include:

- Manual acupuncture: Insertion of an acupuncture needle into acupoints.
- Electro-acupuncture: Application of electrical stimulation to acupoints.
- Scalp acupuncture: Oblique insertion of acupuncture needles into the scalp along specified scalp zones.

- Moxibustion: Burning of a herb (usually *ai ye* 艾叶 *Artemesia vulgaris* L.) close to or on the skin to induce a warming sensation.
- Ear acupuncture: Insertion of small needles into points or zones located on the ear.
- Acupressure: Application of pressure to acupoints on the body or the ear.

Whilst many of these therapies have ancient roots, several have emerged as new techniques in the last century including scalp acupuncture, electro-acupuncture, and ear acupuncture.

Previous Systematic Reviews

One Cochrane review identified 95 clinical studies of acupuncture for vascular dementia (VaD). Of these, 17 were classified as randomised controlled trials (RCTs), but none employed a comparison with placebo or no treatment. Since this was the criteria for inclusion, the review did not report meta-analysis results for any of the studies.[1] Other systematic reviews and meta-analyses of acupuncture[2,3] have reported benefits compared to controls, as have meta-analyses that focused on electro-acupuncture[4] and head and scalp acupuncture.[5] A systematic review of acupuncture for cognitive impairment after stroke, which included 21 RCTs, reported a statistically significant improvement in outcomes from the Mini-Mental State Examination (MMSE) based on 4 studies and other measures when acupuncture or electro-acupuncture was added to conventional treatment.[6]

In addition to these systematic reviews of outcomes, a study of 185 controlled and 53 non-controlled studies aimed to identify the acupoints used in studies for which a benefit for using acupuncture was reported. In controlled studies, this was defined as an improvement in the acupuncture group while in non-controlled studies, this was defined as an improvement after treatment. The outcome measures used and statistical tests were not specified. The frequently used points included GV20 *Baihui* 百会, EX-HN1 *Sishencong* 四神聪, GB20 *Fengchi* 风池, GV24 *Shenting* 神庭, GV26 *Shuigou* 水沟, and ST36 *Zusanli* 足三里.[7]

Identification of Clinical Studies

Seventy clinical trials of acupuncture and related therapies that reported results for the effects of acupuncture on VaD were located. These included 47 RCTs, two controlled clinical trials (CCTs), and 21 non-controlled studies (see Figure 7.1). The interventions tested in the studies include:

- Acupuncture, with or without electro-stimulation or moxibustion, on traditional points (40 RCTs, 2 CCTs, 20 non-controlled studies).
- Scalp acupuncture using modern scalp zones (4 RCTs, 1 non-controlled study).
- Moxibustion alone (2 RCTs).
- Ear acupressure alone (2 RCTs).

The results of studies are presented separately for acupuncture, scalp acupuncture, moxibustion, and ear acupressure.

Risk of Bias

All 47 RCTs of acupuncture and related therapies were described as using randomisation, but only 19 reported adequate details and were judged as 'low' risk for sequence generation (SG). Seven used an inappropriate method for SG and were judged as 'high' risk for SG. Four studies adequately described the method of allocation concealment and were judged as 'low' risk (Table 7.1). Those that did not report details pertaining to these domains were assessed as having 'unclear' risk of bias. One study used a sham acupuncture intervention but did not adequately describe the procedure for blinding participants, so it was judged as having 'unclear' risk. Blinding of study personnel or outcome assessors was not described in any study. This is difficult to achieve in acupuncture studies, so all studies were judged as having 'high' risk of bias. All studies that indicated having no dropouts were assessed as 'low' risk of bias for incomplete outcome data. Two studies were judged as 'high' risk since there was a marked imbalance between groups and intent-to-treat analysis was not used. No protocols could be located, so all studies were assessed

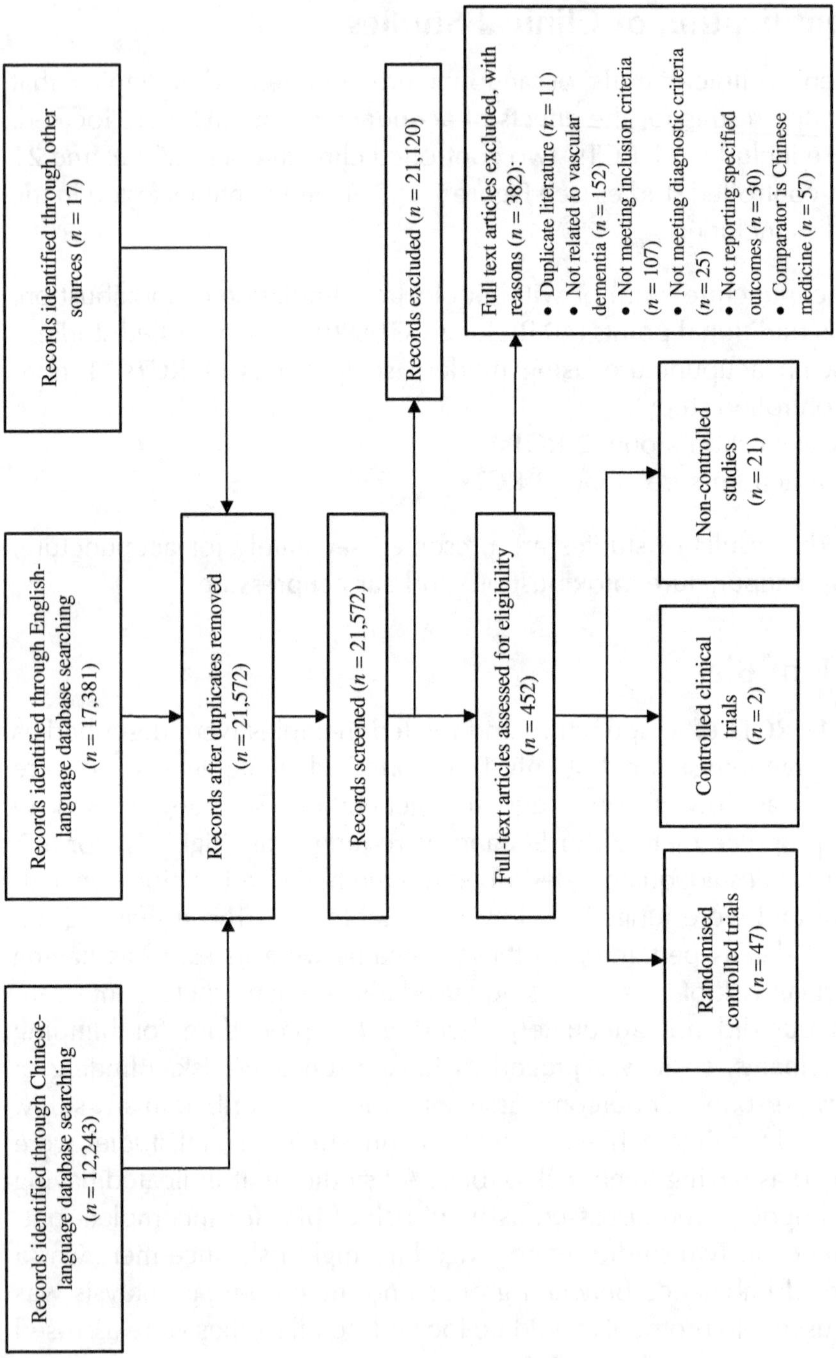

Figure 7.1 Flow Chart of Study Selection Process: Acupuncture and Related Therapies

Table 7.1 Risk of Bias of Randomised Controlled Trials

Risk of Bias Domain	Low Risk *n* (%)	Unclear Risk *n* (%)	High Risk *n* (%)
Sequence generation	19 (40.4)	21 (44.7)	7 (14.9)
Allocation concealment	4 (8.5)	43 (91.5)	0 (0)
Blinding of participants	0 (0)	1 (2.1)	46 (97.9)
Blinding of personnel*	0 (0)	0 (0)	47 (100)
Blinding of outcome assessors	0 (0)	0 (0)	47 (100)
Incomplete outcome data	44 (93.6)	1 (2.1)	2 (4.3)
Selective outcome reporting	0 (0)	47 (100)	0 (0)

*Blinding of personnel (acupuncturists) is challenging in manual therapies.

as having 'unclear' risk of bias for selective outcome reporting. Overall, judgements of the methodological quality of the included studies were limited by lack of detail in the published reports.

Studies of Acupuncture

In the studies of acupuncture using needling of traditional points (manual only or with electrical stimulation), there were 40 RCTs (A1–A40), two CCTs (A41, A42), and 20 non-controlled studies (A43–A62). None of the RCTs or CCTs combined acupuncture with moxibustion, but this was done in two of the non-controlled studies. Data from RCTs, CCTs, and non-controlled studies are presented separately below. All studies were conducted in China.

Randomised Controlled Trials of Acupuncture

In total, 3,131 participants diagnosed with VaD were enrolled in the 40 RCTs of acupuncture or electro-acupuncture (A1-A40). Based on the reported mean ages, the majority of participants were between 60 and 70 years old. The overall age range was between 45 to 79 years, but age range was not reported in most studies. Duration of treatment ranged from two to 24 weeks.

Test interventions were traditional acupuncture using needles, with 13 RCTs also using electro-acupuncture. Nine studies included more than two intervention groups, so data were included in the relevant comparisons, which included sham acupuncture (1 study; A1), no treatment (1 study; A2), and a range of pharmacotherapies (38 studies). Pharmacotherapies included donepezil, huperzine A, nimodipine, co-dergocrine mesylate, dihydroergotamine, nicergoline, piracetam, aniractam, citicoline injection, neurokinin injection, cerebroprotein hydrolysate injection, and sodium monosialotetrahexosylganglioside injection. Of these, nimodipine was the most frequent control intervention. Studies that employed almitrine-raubasine as a comparator were excluded. Seventeen studies included an integrative medicine approach that employed acupuncture therapy in conjunction with pharmacotherapy. In three studies, inconsistencies in the data made them unsuitable for inclusion in certain meta-analysis pools (A8, A12, A40).

Outcome data suitable for analysis include the Mini-Mental State Examination (MMSE), Alzheimer's Disease Assessment Scale ADAS — cognitive subscale (ADAS-cog), Hasegawa's Dementia Scale (HDS/HDS-R), activities of daily living (ADL) scales, Functional Activities Questionnaire (FAQ), Memory Quotient (MQ), and Wechsler Adult Intelligence Scale — Revised by China (WAIS-RC).

Syndromes

Ten studies reported the use of Chinese medicine (CM) syndrome differentiation. Eight used acupuncture (A2, A3, A9, A12, A13, A25, A34, A39) and two included electro-stimulation (A24, A26).

The most frequently mentioned syndromes were:

- Turbid phlegm obstructing the Orifices 痰浊阻窍/痰浊蒙窍 (9 studies).
- *Qi* stagnation and Blood stasis 气滞血瘀 (6 studies).
- Spleen and Kidney dual deficiency 脾肾两虚 (5 studies).
- Deficiency of 'Sea of Marrow' 髓海不足 (5 studies).
- Heart and Liver fire 心肝火盛 (5 studies).
- Liver and Kidney insufficiency 肝肾不足/肝肾亏虚 (5 studies).
- Deficiency of Kidney and Essence 肾精亏虚/肾精亏损 (3 studies).
- Liver *yang* ascendant hyperactivity 肝阳上亢/肝阳暴亢 (3 studies).

Frequently Used Points in Randomised Controlled Trials of Acupuncture

The points that were most frequently included in the 40 RCTs were GV20 *Baihui* 百会, EX-HN1 *Sishencong* 四神聪, GV24 *Shenting* 神庭, and GB20 *Fengchi* 风池 (Table 7.2). All points were stimulated

Table 7.2 Frequently Used Acupuncture Points in the Randomised Controlled Trials

Point Name	Frequency of Use
GV20 *Baihui* 百会	27
EX-HN1 *Sishencong* 四神聪	26
GV24 *Shenting* 神庭	16
GB20 *Fengchi* 风池	14
GV26 *Shiugou* 水沟	12
ST36 *Zusanli* 足三里	11
PC6 *Neiguan* 内关	10
GB13 *Benshen* 本神	8
SP6 *Sanyinjiao* 三阴交	7
SP10 *Xuehai* 血海	7
CV6 *Qihai* 气海	5
CV12 *Zhongwan* 中脘	5
CV17 *Tanzhong* 膻中	5
HT7 *Shenmen* 神门	4
TE5 *Waiguan* 外关	4
KI3 *Taixi* 太溪	4
LR3 *Taichong* 太冲	4
GV14 *Dazhui* 大椎	4
GV16 *Fengfu* 风府	4
GB8 *Shuaigu* 率谷	4

Notes: (1) Analysis is based on the main points and does not include extra points added for certain symptoms or syndromes; (2) point names have been standardised and (3) the list includes 40 studies and 41 groups; one 3-armed study (A35) used different points in each group, so both groups were counted. In the other 3-group studies, the points were the same or similar, so these were not double counted.

using needles (with or without electro-stimulation). None received additional moxibustion.

Acupuncture vs. Sham Acupuncture

A single study involving 10 participants (A1) compared real acupuncture at CV17 *Danzhong* 膻中, CV12 *Zhongwan* 中脘, CV6 *Qihai* 气海, SP10 *Xuehai* 血海, TE5 *Waiguan* 外关, and ST36 *Zusanli* 足三里 with sham acupuncture, which involved needling at locations 0.5 cm lateral to the real points. For MMSE scores, after eight weeks of treatment, the real acupuncture group fared better than the sham group (mean difference (MD): 5.20 [2.55, 7.85]). The study also reported that imaging with positron emission tomography (PET) revealed changes in glucose metabolism in both the affected and unaffected brain hemispheres. Adverse events (AEs) were not mentioned.

Acupuncture vs. No Treatment

One study ($n = 60$ participants) compared a group that received acupuncture with a group that received no acupuncture (A2). Both groups received usual supportive care. The acupuncture method was described as 'replenish *qi*, regulate Blood, reinforce the Root, and build up the source *qi*' (*yi qi tiao xue fu ben pei yuan* 益气调血扶本培元) and used the points CV17 *Danzhong* 膻中, CV12 *Zhongwan* 中脘, CV6 *Qihai* 气海, SP10 *Xuehai* 血海, and ST36 *Zusanli* 足三里. After six weeks of treatment, the authors reported improvements in the MMSE and HDS scores in the acupuncture groups, but the random effects analysis found no significant differences between groups for the MMSE (MD: 2.56 [–1.15, 6.27]), HDS (MD: 2.25 [–2.36, 6.86]) or 'lower is better' ADL scores (MD: –0.09 [–0.60, 0.42]). The study did not report on AEs.

Acupuncture vs. Pharmacotherapy

Twenty-four studies included a comparison between acupuncture or electro-acupuncture and a pharmacotherapy. The meta-analysis results are reported according to the outcome measures: MMSE, ADAS-cog, HDS, ADL, FAQ, BBS, and WAIS-RC.

Mini-Mental State Examination

Thirteen RCTs (A3-A15) compared acupuncture (without electro-stimulation) with a pharmacotherapy (donepezil, nicergoline, nimodipine, piracetam, aniracetam, or co-dergocrine mesylate) for VaD using the MMSE as an outcome. Three studies employed two different acupuncture interventions (A4, A9, A13), so there were 16 intervention groups in total. To avoid double counting of participants in the meta-analysis, the control group numbers were halved here and in subsequent meta-analyses.

The pooled results showed no significant difference for acupuncture compared to donepezil or aniracetam, while the acupuncture groups showed significant increases in outcomes on the MMSE for the comparisons with other pharmacotherapies. The pooled result (13 studies, 16 groups) showed a significant difference compared to pharmacotherapies in favour of acupuncture (MD: 2.11 [1.33, 2.88], $I^2 = 84\%$); however, heterogeneity was considerable (Table 7.3).

In the six studies that used electro-acupuncture (A16-A21), there were significant differences when compared to co-dergocrine mesylate and nimodipine but no significant difference when compared to piracetam (Table 7.3). The total pool for electro-acupuncture revealed that electro-acupuncture was beneficial compared to pharmacotherapies (MD: 2.35 [1.32, 3.37], $I^2 = 23\%$), without significant heterogeneity. For the pooled result of 19 studies (22 groups) of acupuncture and electro-acupuncture with durations ranging from three to 12 weeks, there was a significant improvement in MMSE scores compared to the pharmacotherapy groups (MD 2.17 [1.52, 2.83], $I^2 = 80\%$), albeit with considerable heterogeneity in the pooled results (Table 7.3).

Nine studies that investigated acupuncture or electro-acupuncture over durations of four to 12 weeks were judged as 'low' risk for SG (A3, A4, A8, A10, A15, A17–A20). The pooled result showed a significant benefit in the acupuncture groups compared to pharmacotherapy

Table 7.3 Acupuncture vs. Pharmacotherapy: Mini-Mental State Examination

Comparator	No. of Studies (Participants), Duration	Effect Size (MD [95% CI], I^2)	Included Studies
Acupuncture			
Donepezil	1 (38), 12 wks	2.26 [−0.45, 4.97]	A3
Nimodipine	3 RCTs, 4 gps (447), 4 wks	1.69 [0.38, 3.00]*, 81%	A7–A9
Nicergoline	2 RCTs, 3 gps (120), 8–12 wks	1.48 [0.12, 2.84]*, 0%	A4, A5
Piracetam	2 (186), 4 wks	2.98 [0.30, 5.66]*, 54%	A10, A11
Aniracetam	2 RCTs, 3 gps (204), 3–6 wks	1.70 [−0.61, 4.00], 95%	A12, A13
Co-dergocrine mesylate	3 (166), 6–12 wks	3.28 [1.40, 5.17]*, 66%	A6, A14, A15
Pharmacotherapy	13 RCTs, 16 gps (1,161), 3–12 wks	2.11 [1.33, 2.88]*, 84%	All above
Electro-acupuncture			
Nimodipine	2 (212), 6 wks	3.48 [2.16, 4.81]*, 0%	A17, A18
co-dergocrine mesylate	1 (68), 4 wks	2.43 [0.15, 4.71]*	A16
Nimodipine plus co-dergocrine mesylate	1 (64), 12 wks	1.33 [0.19, 2.47]*	A19
Piracetam	2 (128), 4–12 wks	1.70 [−0.94, 4.34], 22%	A20, A21
Pharmacotherapy	6 (472), 4–12 wks	2.35 [1.32, 3.37]*, 32%	A16–A21
Total pool (acupuncture/electro-acupuncture)			
Pharmacotherapy	19 RCTs, 22 gps (1,633), 4–12 wks	2.17 [1.52, 2.83]*, 80%	All above

*Statistically significant. Abbreviations: CI, confidence interval; gps, groups; MD, mean difference; RCTs, randomised controlled trials; wks, weeks.

controls with reduced heterogeneity (MD: 2.33 [1.59, 3.07], $I^2 = 51\%$, $n = 870$ participants).

Alzheimer's Disease Assessment Scale — Cognitive Subscale

One study provided data for the ADAS-cog in addition to MMSE (A3). This was a three-armed 12-week study with a sixth-month follow-up that compared acupuncture against donepezil as well as the combination of acupuncture and Chinese herbal medicine (CHM). This study is reported in greater detail below as well as in Chapter 9. For acupuncture vs. donepezil, there was no significant difference between groups at the end of treatment (MD: –2.42 [–5.02, 0.18], $n = 38$ participants) or at the sixth-month follow-up (MD: –2.79 [–5.61, 0.03], $n = 38$ participants).

Hasegawa Dementia Scale

Seven studies of acupuncture (A4, A7–11, A22) and five studies of electro-acupuncture (A20, A21, A23–A25) reported data for the HDS. The comparators in the acupuncture studies were nimodipine, nicergoline, piracetam, and sodium monosialotetrahexosylganglioside injection. The pooled result showed a greater improvement in HDS scores for the acupuncture groups compared to the pharmacotherapies (MD: 1.56 [0.53, 2.60], $I^2 = 74\%$); however, there was considerable heterogeneity. Of the subgroups, only the comparison with piracetam showed a significant difference between groups (Table 7.4).

The electro-acupuncture interventions were compared with nimodipine, co-dergocrine mesylate, dihydroergotamine, or piracetam. These subgroups showed significant differences in favour of electro-acupuncture except for the comparison with nimodipine. The pool of five studies found a significant increase in HDS scores in the electro-acupuncture groups compared to the pharmacotherapy controls (MD: 3.96 [1.94, 5.97], $I^2 = 46\%$). In the total pool of 12 studies, the acupuncture or electro-acupuncture interventions were significantly

Table 7.4 Acupuncture vs. Pharmacotherapy: Hasegawa Dementia Scale

Comparator	No. of Studies (Participants), Duration	Effect Size (MD [95% CI], I^2)	Included Studies
Acupuncture			
Nimodipine	3 RCTs, 4 gps (447), 4 wks	1.61 [–0.09, 3.31], 89%	A7–A9
Nicergoline	1 RCTs, 2 gps (60), 8 wks	1.85 [–1.27, 4.98], 0%	A4
Piracetam	2 (186), 4 wks	1.60 [0.51, 2.68]*, 0%	A10, A11
Sodium monosialotetrahexosy-lganglioside injection	1 (63), 4 wks	1.45 [–0.63, 3.53]	A22
Pharmacotherapy	7 RCTs, 9 gps (756), 4–8 wks	1.56 [0.53, 2.60]*, 74%	All above
Electro-acupuncture			
Nimodipine	1 (46), 4 wks	1.91 [–0.41, 4.23]	A25
Co-dergocrine mesylate	1 (66), 6 wks	5.10 [1.47, 8.73]*	A23
Dihydroergotamine	1 (60), 6 wks	6.73 [3.54, 9.92]*	A24
Piracetam	2 (128), 4–12 wks	3.12 [0.40, 5.84]*, 0%	A20, A21
Pharmacotherapy	5 (300), 4–12 wks	3.96 [1.94, 5.97]*, 46%	A20, A21, A23–A25
Total pool (acupuncture/electro-acupuncture)			
Pharmacotherapy	12 RCTs, 14 gps (1,011), 4–12 wks	2.22 [1.20, 3.23]*, 74%	All above

*Statistically significant. Abbreviations: CI, confidence interval; gps, groups; MD, mean difference; RCTs, randomised controlled trials; wks, weeks.

different from the pharmacotherapy controls (MD: 2.22 [1.20, 3.23], $I^2 = 74\%$); however, the heterogeneity was substantial (Table 7.4).

In the five studies (4–8 weeks duration) of acupuncture or electro-acupuncture that were judged as 'low' risk of bias for SG (A4, A8, A10, A20, A22), there was a significant increase in HDS scores in the acupuncture groups (MD: 2.45 [1.29, 3.61], $I^2 = 36\%$, $n = 559$ participants), with reduced heterogeneity.

Activities of Daily Living

Thirteen studies compared acupuncture or electro-acupuncture with a pharmacotherapy and reported ADL outcomes. Eight studies (A3, A5, A10, A13, A14, A17, A18, A21) used ADL scales whereby lower scores indicated improvement ('lower is better') and five studies (A19, A20, A24, A25) used ADL scales whereby higher scores indicated improvement ('higher is better'). These were pooled separately using the standardised mean difference (SMD).

For 'lower is better' ADL, the acupuncture interventions were significantly better in the comparisons with piracetam and aniracetam, but there were no significant differences when compared to other pharmacotherapies (Table 7.5). The pool of five studies found that acupuncture interventions showed significant improvements in ADL outcomes compared to pharmacotherapies (SMD: –0.66 [–0.98, –0.34], $I^2 = 58\%$), with moderate heterogeneity. Electro-acupuncture was significantly better than piracetam but not significantly different when compared to nimodipine, and there was no significant difference between groups in the pool of three studies (SMD: –0.36 [–0.75, 0.04], $I^2 = 55\%$). In the total pool of eight studies, there was a significant benefit for the acupuncture and electro-acupuncture groups (SMD: –0.56 [–0.81, –0.30], $I^2 = 50\%$).

In the two studies of acupuncture (4–8 weeks duration) judged as 'low' risk of bias for SG (A3, A10) the result for acupuncture was similar to that of the total acupuncture pool, but without heterogeneity (SMD: –0.60 [–0.91, –0.29] $I^2 = 0\%$, $n = 166$ participants). For electro-acupuncture, the two studies judged as 'low' risk of bias for SG were in the nimodipine subgroup, and these showed a similar outcome to the electro-acupuncture pool, but without heterogeneity (SMD: –0.22 [–0.49, 0.05], $I^2 = 0\%$, $n = 212$ participants). In the total pool, there were four studies judged as 'low' risk for SG (A3, A10, A17, A18). The pool for these studies (SMD: –0.38 [–0.63, –0.13], $I^2 = 26\%$ $n = 378$ participants) showed a similar result to that for all studies, without substantial heterogeneity.

Five studies (one with two acupuncture groups and four with electro-acupuncture) reported results using ADL scales whereby

Table 7.5 Acupuncture vs. Pharmacotherapy: 'Lower is Better' Activities of Daily Living

Comparator	No. of Studies (Participants), Duration	Effect Size (SMD [95% CI], I²)	Included Studies
Acupuncture			
Donepezil	1 (38), 12 wks	–0.59 [–1.24, 0.06]	A3
Nicergoline	1 (60), 12 wks	–0.39 [–0.90, 0.12]	A5
Piracetam	1 (128), 4 wks	–0.60 [–0.96, –0.25]*	A10
Aniracetam	1 RCT, 2 gps (150), 6 wks	–1.04 [–1.90, –0.19]*, 82%	A13
Co-dergocrine mesylate	1 (60), 6 wks	–0.32 [–0.83, 0.19]	A14
Pharmacotherapy	5 RCTs, 6 gps (436), 4–12 wks	–0.66 [–0.97, –0.35]*, 58%	All above
Electro-acupuncture			
Nimodipine	2 (212), 6 wks	–0.22 [–0.49, 0.05], 0%	A17, A18
Piracetam	1 (60), 12 wks	–0.82 [–1.38, -0.27]*	A21
Pharmacotherapy	3 (272), 6–12 wks	–0.36 [–0.75, 0.04], 55%	A17, A18, A21
Total pool (acupuncture/electro-acupuncture)			
Pharmacotherapy	8 RCTs, 9 gps (708), 4–12 wks	–0.56 [–0.81, –0.30]*, 60%	All above

*Statistically significant. Abbreviations: CI, confidence interval; gps, groups; SMD, standardised mean difference; RCTs, randomised controlled trials; wks, weeks.

higher scores indicated better results (Table 7.6). In the acupuncture group, one study included two different acupuncture interventions that were compared with nimodipine (A9). A data error appeared in another study that compared acupuncture with aniracetam (A12), so this study was not included in the meta-analysis. For electro-acupuncture, each study used a different comparator. The pooled data showed a significant increase in the electro-acupuncture groups for ADL scores compared to the pharmacotherapy groups (SMD: 0.57 [0.19, 0.96], I^2 = 54%). The total pool of five studies of acupuncture or electro-acupuncture

Table 7.6 Acupuncture vs. Pharmacotherapy: 'Higher is Better' Activities of Daily Living

Comparator	No. of Studies (Participants), Duration	Effect Size (SMD [95% CI], I^2)	Included Studies
Acupuncture			
Nimodipine	1 RCT, 2 gps (147), 4 wks	1.24 [0.15, 2.34]*, 88%	A9
Electro-acupuncture			
Nimodipine	1 (46), 4 wks	0.49 [–0.10, 1.08]	A25
Nimodipine plus co-dergocrine mesylate	1 (64), 12 wks	0.47 [–0.03, 0.97]	A19
Piracetam	1 (68), 4 wks	1.11 [0.60, 1.62]*	A20
Dihydroergotamine	1 (60), 6 wks	0.21 [–0.30, 0.71]	A24
Pharmacotherapy	4 (238), 4–12 wks	0.57 [0.19, 0.96]*, 54%	A19, A20, A24, A25
Total pool (acupuncture/electro-acupuncture)			
Pharmacotherapy	5 RCTs, 6 gps (385), 4–12 wks	0.79 [0.34, 1.24]*, 77%	All above

*Statistically significant. Abbreviations: CI, confidence interval; gps, groups; RCTs, randomised controlled trials; SMD, standardised mean difference; wks, weeks.

showed a significant benefit based on 'higher is better' ADL, but with considerable heterogeneity (SMD: 0.79 [0.34, 1.24], $I^2 = 77\%$, $n = 385$ participants) (Table 7.6).

Three studies of electro-acupuncture (A19, A20, A25) and no studies of acupuncture were judged as 'low' risk of bias for SG. The pooled result showed a significant increase in ADL scores (SMD: 0.70 [0.28, 1.12], $I^2 = 47\%$, $n = 178$ participants), with reduced heterogeneity.

Functional Activities Questionnaire

Two RCTs that compared acupuncture with piracetam (A11) or nicergoline (A4) used the FAQ as an outcome measure. The pooled result

Table 7.7 Acupuncture vs. Pharmacotherapy: Functional Activities Questionnaire

Comparator	No. of Studies (Participants), Duration	Effect Size (MD [95% CI], I^2)	Included Studies
Acupuncture			
Piracetam	1 (58), 8 wks	–0.65 [–3.80, 2.50]	A11
Nicergoline	1 RCT, 2 gps (60), 8 wks	–1.60 [–4.49, 1.29], 0%	A4
Pharmacotherapy	2 RCTs, 3 gps (118), 8 wks	–1.17 [–3.30, 0.96], 0%	A4, A11
Electro-acupuncture			
Piracetam	1 (60), 12 wks	–4.74 [–7.32, –2.16]*	A21
Co-dergocrine mesylate	1 (66), 6 wks	–2.12 [–5.11, 0.87]	A23
Dihydroergotamine	1 (60), 6 wks	–0.55 [–3.36, 2.26]	A24
Pharmacotherapy	3 (186) 6–12 wks	–2.53 [–5.02, –0.04]*, 58%	A21, A23, A24
Total pool (acupuncture/electro-acupuncture)			
Pharmacotherapy	5 RCTs, 6 gps (304), 6–12 wks	–2.05 [–3.48, –0.61]*, 18%	All above

*Statistically significant. Abbreviations: CI, confidence interval; gps, groups; MD, mean difference; RCTs, randomised controlled trials; wks, weeks.

found no significant difference between groups after eight weeks (MD: –1.17 [–3.30, 0.96], I^2 = 0%) (Table 7.7). The three studies of electro-acupuncture each used different comparators. The pooled data found a significant decrease (i.e., improvement) in FAQ scores compared to the pharmacotherapies (MD: –2.53 [–5.02, –0.04], I^2 = 58%). In the total pool of five studies, there was significant improvement in FAQ scores (MD: –2.05 [–3.48, –0.61], I^2 = 18%), without substantial heterogeneity.

One three-armed study that compared acupuncture to nicergoline (A4) was judged as 'low' risk of bias for SG. Both groups used the same three points: GV21 *Qianding* 前顶, GV24 *Shenting* 神庭, and BL6 *Chengguang* 承光, but one group (n = 20 participants) used a 30-minutes retention time, as is usual in practice, while the other group ($n = 20$ participants) used an extended retention time. The results were very similar in both groups. After eight weeks, the pooled result for the two acupuncture groups was not significantly different from nicergoline (MD: –1.60 [–4.49, 1.29], $I^2 = 0\%$, $n = 60$ participants).

Blessed Behaviour Scale

One study of acupuncture (A15) and one study of electro-acupuncture (A16) reported BBS scores whereby lower scores indicate improvement. In both studies, comparisons were made with co-dergocrine mesylate. The acupuncture study was judged as 'low' risk of bias for SG. The points that were used include CV17 *Danzhong* 膻中, CV12 *Zhongwan* 中脘, CV6 *Qihai* 气海, SP10 *Xuehai* 血海, ST36 *Zusanli* 足三里, and TE5 *Waiguan* 外关 (30-minutes retention), and a significant difference between groups (MD: –1.67 [–2.77, –0.57], $n = 60$ participants) was documented in favour of acupuncture after 12 weeks. The electro-acupuncture study, which used GV20 *Baihui* 百会, BL23 *Shenshu* 肾俞, and BL17 *Geshu* 膈俞 for 20 minutes, also showed a significant reduction in BBS scores (MD: –3.08 [–5.96, –0.20], $n = 68$) after 30 days. The pooled result of the two studies (MD: –1.85 [–2.88, –0.82], $I^2 = 0\%$, $n = 128$ participants) showed a significant improvement in the acupuncture groups.

Wechsler Adult Intelligence Scale — Revised by China

One six-week study (A26) of electro-acupuncture at EX-HN1 *Sishencong* 四神聪, GB13 *Benshen* 本神, GV20 *Baihui* 百会, and GB20 *Fengchi* 风池 compared to nimodipine found that the scores on the WAIS-RC were significantly higher in the electro-acupuncture group (MD: 26.33 [21.89, 30.77], $n = 46$). This study was judged as 'unclear' risk for SG.

Integrative Acupuncture vs. Pharmacotherapy

Seventeen RCTs included a comparison between the combination of acupuncture or electro-acupuncture and a pharmacotherapy vs. the same pharmacotherapy alone. Four of these studies used electro-acupuncture. Outcome data were available for the MMSE, HDS, ADL, and FAQ.

Mini-Mental State Examination

Nine RCTs of acupuncture (A27-A35) reported data on MMSE scores. Two of these studies used two acupuncture intervention groups (A32, A35). In the pool of nine studies of acupuncture, there was a significant increase in MMSE scores in the integrative therapy group (MD: 1.91 [1.38, 2.45], $I^2 = 0\%$) (Table 7.8). For four studies of electro-acupuncture (A17, A18, A21, A36), there was a significant increase in MMSE scores in the comparison with nimodipine (2 studies) as well as in the pool of four studies that compared acupuncture with pharmacotherapy (MD: 2.23 [1.65, 2.81], $I^2 = 0\%$). In the total pool for acupuncture and electro-acupuncture, there was a significant improvement in MMSE scores in the acupuncture/electro-acupuncture plus pharmacotherapy groups vs. the various pharmacotherapies (MD: 2.23 [1.65, 2.81], $I^2 = 21\%$), without substantial heterogeneity.

In the acupuncture groups, three studies (A28, A31, A34) were judged as 'low' risk of bias for SG and the pooled result was significant in favour of integrative acupuncture (MD: 2.01 [0.38, 3.65], 0%, $n = 179$). For electro-acupuncture, only the two studies in the nimodipine subgroup were judged as 'low' risk for SG. These studies showed a significant difference in favour of the integrative group. In the total pool of five studies judged as 'low' risk for SG, there was a significant difference between groups with reduced heterogeneity (MD: 3.05 [1.96, 4.13], $I^2 = 5\%$, $n = 392$ participants).

Hasegawa Dementia Scale

Six studies of integrative acupuncture (A31, A34, A35, A37–A39) and one of integrative electro-acupuncture (A21) reported HDS scores for comparisons with five different pharmacotherapies (Table 7.9). Significant differences were found for the citicoline injection and cerebroprotein hydrolysate injection subgroups as

Table 7.8 Integrative Acupuncture vs. Pharmacotherapy: Mini-Mental State Examination

Comparator	No. of Studies (Participants), Duration	Effect Size (MD [95% CI], I^2)	Included Studies
Acupuncture			
Nimodipine	1 (48), 13 wks	3.23 [0.18, 6.28]*	A28
Nicergoline	1 (48), 4 wks	1.53 [0.29, 2.77]*	A27
Huperzine A	1 (85), 24 wks	2.12 [1.05, 3.19]	A29
Piracetam plus citicoline injection	1 (62), 8 wks	2.00 [0.18, 3.82]*	A30
Oxiracetam	2 RCTs, 3 gps (160), 4 wks	1.61 [0.63, 2.58], 0%	A31, A32
Co-dergocrine mesylate	1 (123), 8 wks	1.52 [−1.13, 4.17]	A33
Co-dergocrine mesylate plus pyritinol	1 (61), 8 wks	1.93 [−0.26, 4.12]	A34
Neurokinin injection	1 RCT, 2 gps (98), 2 wks	3.44 [−1.85, 8.74], 80%	A35
Pharmacotherapy	9 RCTs, 11 gps (685), 2–24 wks	1.91 [1.38, 2.45]*, 0%	A27–A35
Electro-acupuncture			
Nimodipine	2 (213), 6 wks	3.79 [2.44, 5.14]*, 0%	A17, A18
Co-dergocrine mesylate	1 (63), 8 wks	0.35 [−2.15, 2.85]	A36
Piracetam	1 (50), 12 wks	0.10 [−3.73, 3.93]	A21
Pharmacotherapy	4 (326), 6–12 wks	3.49 [2.33, 4.65]*, 0%	A17, A18, A21, A36
Total pool (acupuncture/electro-acupuncture)			
Pharmacotherapy	13 RCTs, 15 gps (1,011), 2–24 wks	2.23 [1.65, 2.81]*, 21%	All above

*Statistically significant. Abbreviations: CI, confidence interval; gps, groups; MD, mean difference; RCTs, randomised controlled trials; wks, weeks.

well as for the pool of six integrative acupuncture studies (MD: 2.00 [1.05, 2.96], $I^2 = 0\%$). The single integrative electro-acupuncture study (A21) found no significant difference between groups. In the total pool of seven studies, there was a significant increase in HDS scores in favour of acupuncture or electro-acupuncture plus pharmacotherapy compared to pharmacotherapy without any acupuncture (MD: 2.02 [1.10, 2.94], $I^2 = 0\%$).

Table 7.9 Integrative Acupuncture vs. Pharmacotherapy: Hasegawa Dementia Scale

Comparator	No. of Studies (Participants), Duration	Effect Size (MD [95% CI], I^2)	Included Studies
Acupuncture			
Oxiracetam	1 (70), 4 wks	1.00 [–1.81, 3.81]	A31
Co-dergocrine mesylate plus pyritinol	1 (61), 8 wks	2.01 [–0.83, 4.85]	A34
Citicoline injection	1 (62), 3 wks	4.30 [1.91, 6.69]*	A37
Cerebroprotein hydrolysate injection	2 (102), 2 wks	1.62 [0.06, 3.17]*, 0%	A38, A39
Neurokinin injection	1 RCT, 2 gps (98), 2 wks	1.56 [–0.41, 3.53], 0%	A35
Pharmacotherapy	6 RCTs, 7 gps (393), 2–8 wks	2.00 [1.05, 2.96]*, 0%	All above
Electro-acupuncture			
Piracetam	1 (50), 12 wks	2.29 [–1.22, 5.80]	A21
Total pool (acupuncture/electro-acupuncture)			
Pharmacotherapy	7 RCTs, 8 gps (443), 2–12 wks	2.02 [1.10, 2.94]*, 0%	All above

*Statistically significant. Abbreviations: CI, confidence interval; gps, groups; MD, mean difference; RCTs, randomised controlled trials; wks, weeks.

In the seven studies, two of the acupuncture studies were judged as 'low' risk of bias for SG (A31, A34). When pooled, there was no significant difference between groups (MD: 1.50 [–0.50, 3.50], I^2 = 0%, $n = 131$ participants).

Activities of Daily Living

Six studies used ADL scales on which lower values indicate improvement and five studies used 'higher is better' ADL scales. These were pooled separately using SMD. On the 'lower is better' ADL scales (Table 7.10), the pool of three studies of acupuncture plus

Table 7.10 Integrative Acupuncture vs. Pharmacotherapy: 'Lower is Better' Activities of Daily Living

Comparator	No. of Studies (Participants), Duration	Effect Size (SMD [95% CI], I^2)	Included Studies
Acupuncture			
Nicergoline	1 (48), 4 wks	–0.63 [–1.21, –0.05]*	A27
Oxiracetam	1 (70), 4 wks	–0.13 [–0.60, 0.34]	A31
Citicoline injection	1 (62), 8 wks	–0.55 [–1.06, –0.04]*	A30
Pharmacotherapy	3 (180), 4–8 wks	–0.41 [–0.72, –0.10]*, 9%	All above
Electro-acupuncture			
Nimodipine	2 (213), 6 wks	–0.27 [–0.54, 0.00], 0%	A17, A18
Piracetam	1 (50), 12 wks	–0.73 [–1.32, –0.15]*	A21
Pharmacotherapy	3 (263), 6–12 wks	–0.35 [–0.60, –0.10]*, 4%	A17, A18, A21
Total pool (acupuncture/electro-acupuncture)			
Pharmacotherapy	6 (443), 4–12 wks	–0.37 [–0.56, –0.18]*, 0%	All above

*Statistically significant. Abbreviations: CI, confidence interval; SMD, standardized mean difference; wks, weeks.

pharmacotherapy vs. the same pharmacotherapy (A27, A30, A31) showed a significant benefit for integrative acupuncture vs. pharmacotherapy without acupuncture (SMD: –0.41 [–0.72, –0.10], I^2 = 9%). There was a similar result for the three studies (A17, A18, A21) of integrative electro-acupuncture vs. pharmacotherapy (SMD: –0.35 [–0.60, –0.10], $I^2 = 4\%$) and the total pool of six studies (SMD: –0.37 [–0.56, –0.18], $I^2 = 0\%$).

Of the acupuncture studies, one was judged as 'low' risk for SG (A31). The two studies of electro-acupuncture in the nimodipine subgroup were also judged to have 'low' risk (A17, A18). In the pool of three studies, the result was marginally significant (SMD: –0.23 [–0.47, 0.00], $I^2 = 0\%$, $n = 283$ participants).

Five studies of acupuncture plus pharmacotherapy (A28, A29, A32, A34, A38) reported ADL using 'higher is better' scales (Table 7.11). Each of the five studies used a different comparator.

Table 7.11 Integrative Acupuncture vs. Pharmacotherapy: 'Higher is Better' Activities of Daily Living

Comparator	No. of Studies (Participants), Duration	Effect Size (SMD [95% CI], I^2)	Included Studies
Nimodipine	1 (48), 13 wks	0.60 [0.02, 1.18]*	A28
Oxiracetam	1 RCT, 2 gps (90), 4 wks	0.12 [–0.32, 0.56], 0%	A32
Huperzine A	1 (85), 24 wks	0.56 [0.13, 1.00]*	A29
Co-dergocrine mesylate plus pyritinol	1 (61), 8 wks	0.78 [0.25, 1.30]*	A34
Cerebroprotein hydrolysate injection	1 (60), 2 wks	0.78 [0.25, 1.30]*	A38
Pharmacotherapy	5 RCTs, 6 gps (344), 2–24 wks	0.53 [0.31, 0.75]*, 2%	All above

*Statistically significant. Abbreviations: CI, confidence interval; gps, groups; RCTs, randomised controlled trial; SMD, standardised mean difference; wks, weeks.

One study used two different acupuncture groups in comparison with oxiracetam (A32). Both groups used the points GV20 *Baihui* 百会, EX-HN1 *Sishencong* 四神聪, EX-HN5 *Taiyang* 太阳, and GB20 *Fengchi* 风池, with one group using manipulation to stimulate the points and the other group not receiving any manipulation. There was little difference between the two acupuncture groups, so they were combined in the analysis. The total pool of five studies revealed a significant difference between groups in favour of acupuncture plus pharmacotherapy vs. the same pharmacotherapy without acupuncture (SMD: 0.53 [0.31, 0.75], $I^2 = 2\%$).

Two studies were judged as 'low' risk of bias for SG (A28, A34). The pooled result showed a significant benefit for integrative acupuncture (SMD: 0.70 [0.31, 1.09], $I^2 = 0\%$, $n = 109$) without heterogeneity.

Functional Activities Questionnaire

One 12-week study of electro-acupuncture plus piracetam reported FAQ scores (A21). This study compared electro-acupuncture at

GV20 *Baihui* 百会, GV24 *Shenting* 神庭, and EX-HN1 *Sishencong* 四神聪 plus piracetam with piracetam alone and reported a significant benefit for the integrative approach (MD: –4.64 [–7.57, –1.71], *n* = 50).

Frequently Reported Acupuncture Points in Meta-analyses

This section examines the points frequently used in the studies included in the meta-analysis pools for which there was a significant difference between groups. Outcomes are divided into cognitive outcomes as measured by the MMSE, ADAS-cog, and/or HDS and daily living activities as measured by 'lower is better' ADL, 'higher is better' ADL, or the FAQ. Results are presented separately for studies of acupuncture or electro-acupuncture vs. pharmacotherapy (Table 7.12) and studies of integrative acupuncture or electro-acupuncture vs. pharmacotherapy (Table 7.13).

In the 23 studies that included a comparison between acupuncture or electro-acupuncture and a pharmacotherapy that reported cognitive outcome measures, the points most frequently used in the RCTs were EX-HN1 *Sishencong* 四神聪, GV20 *Baihui* 百会, GV24 *Shenting* 神庭, and GB20 *Fengchi* 风池 (Table 7.12). A very similar group of points was used in the 17 studies that reported outcomes for ADL. There is considerable overlap in the studies included in these two groups since many studies reported on both types of outcome measures.

In the integrative medicine comparisons, the most frequently used points in the 16 studies that reported cognitive outcomes were GV20 *Baihui* 百会, EX-HN1 *Sishencong* 四神聪, PC6 *Neiguan* 内关, GV24 *Shenting* 神庭, and GB20 *Fengchi* 风池 (Table 7.13). In the 11 studies that reported on ADL, the most frequent points were GV20 *Baihui* 百会, EX-HN1 *Sishencong* 四神聪, GB20 *Fengchi* 风池, and GV24 *Shenting* 神庭. Again, the integrative acupuncture studies that reported cognitive outcomes tended to also report ADL scores, so there was considerable overlap between studies.

Table 7.12 Frequently Used Acupuncture Points in the Randomised Controlled Trials that Compared Acupuncture or Electro-acupuncture with a Pharmacotherapy

Outcome	Point Name	Frequency of Use
Cognitive: MMSE, HDS. 23 studies[1]	EX-HN1 *Sishencong* 四神聪	16
	GV20 *Baihui* 百会	15
	GV24 *Shenting* 神庭	11
	GB20 *Fengchi* 风池	9
	GV26 *Shuigou* 水沟	7
	GB13 *Benshen* 本神	5
	ST36 *Zusanli* 足三里	4
	GB8 *Shuaigu* 率谷	4
	SP10 *Xuehai* 血海	4
	PC6 *Neiguan* 内关	4
Activities of daily living: 'lower is better' ADL, 'higher is better' ADL, FAQ. 17 studies[2]	EX-HN1 *Sishencong* 四神聪	13
	GV20 *Baihui* 百会	11
	GV24 *Shenting* 神庭	10
	GB20 *Fengchi* 风池	8
	GB13 *Benshen* 本神	5
	GV26 *Shuigou* 水沟	5
	ST36 *Zusanli* 足三里	3
	GV16 *Fengfu* 风府	3

Notes: (1) For references to studies reporting MMSE and HDS, see Tables 7.3 and 7.4 and (2) for references to studies reporting ADL and FAQ, see Tables 7.5, 7.6 and 7.7.

Abbreviations: ADL, activities of daily living; FAQ, Functional Activities Questionnaire; HDS, Hasegawa Dementia Scale; MMSE, Mini-Mental State Examination.

Assessment of Acupuncture Using GRADE

The evidence for the most clinically relevant comparisons was assessed using the Grading of Recommendations Assessment, Development, and Evaluation (GRADE). Interventions, comparators, and outcomes to be included were selected based on the consensus process described in Chapter 4. The outcome measures — MMSE, HDS, ADAS-cog, MoCA, 'lower is better' ADL, 'higher is better' ADL, and FAQ — were selected

Table 7.13 Frequently Used Acupuncture Points in the Randomised Controlled Trials that Compared Integrative Acupuncture or Electro-acupuncture with a Pharmacotherapy

Outcome	Point Name	Frequency of Use
Cognitive: MMSE, HDS. 16 studies[1]	GV20 *Baihui* 百会	13
	EX-HN1 *Sishencong* 四神聪	10
	PC6 *Neiguan* 内关	6
	GV24 *Shenting* 神庭	6
	GB20 *Fengchi* 风池	6
	GV26 *Shuigou* 水沟	5
	SP6 *Sanyinjiao* 三阴交	5
	ST36 *Zusanli* 足三里	4
	HT7 *Shenmen* 神门	4
	KI3 *Taixi* 太溪	3
Activities of daily living: 'lower is better' ADL, 'higher is better' ADL, FAQ. 11 studies[2]	GV20 *Baihui* 百会	10
	EX-HN1 *Sishencong* 四神聪	8
	GB20 *Fengchi* 风池	5
	GV24 *Shenting* 神庭	5

Notes: (1) For references to studies reporting MMSE and HDS, see Tables 7.8 and 7.9 and (2) for references to studies reporting ADL studies, see Tables 7.10 and 7.11.

Abbreviations: Abbreviations: ADL, activities of daily living; FAQ, Functional Activities Questionnaire; HDS, Hasegawa Dementia Scale; MMSE, Mini-Mental State Examination.

if available. The comparison was acupuncture vs. donepezil. One GRADE table is presented below (Table 7.14).

Acupuncture vs. Donepezil

One study (A3) compared acupuncture to donepezil (5 mg/day) in a three-armed study that included an acupuncture arm (n = 19 participants), an acupuncture plus CHM arm (n = 19 participants), and a donepezil arm (n = 19 participants). The comparison between acupuncture plus CHM and donepezil is reported in Chapter 9. Placebos were used for the CHM and donepezil groups, so participants were

Table 7.14 GRADE: Acupuncture Therapy Compared to Donepezil

Outcomes (Treatment Duration)	No of Participants (Studies)	Certainty of Evidence (GRADE)	Anticipated Absolute Effects	
			Risk with Donepezil	Risk Difference with Acupuncture[3]
MMSE (12 weeks)	38 (1 RCT)	⊕⊕◯◯ LOW[1,2]	Mean MMSE in control group = **19.37**	MD **2.26 higher** (0.45 lower to 4.97 higher)
ADAS-cog (12 weeks)	38 (1 RCT)	⊕⊕◯◯ LOW[1,2]	Mean ADAS-cog in control group = **21.16**	MD **2.42 lower** (5.02 lower to 0.18 higher)
'Lower is better' ADL (12 weeks)	38 (1 RCT)	⊕⊕◯◯ LOW[1,2]	Mean 'lower is better' ADL in control group = **44.31**	SMD **0.59 SD lower** (1.24 lower to 0.06 higher)

Notes: (1) Lack of blinding; (2) small sample size limits certainty of results and (3) the risk in the intervention group (and its 95% confidence interval) is based on the assumed risk in the comparison group and the relative effect of the intervention (and its 95% CI).

Abbreviations: ADAS-cog, Alzheimer's Disease Assessment Scale — cognitive subscale; ADL, activities of daily living; FAQ, Functional Activities Questionnaire; HDS, Hasegawa Dementia Scale; MD, mean difference; MMSE, Mini-Mental State Examination; SD, standard deviation; SMD, standardised mean difference; RCT, randomised controlled trial.

Adverse events: In the acupuncture group, there were two dropouts because they felt cold and could not tolerate the pain of acupuncture. In the donepezil group, there were three dropouts, all of whom died, but the reasons for death were not specified.

Study Reference: A3.

blind to whether they received acupuncture alone or acupuncture plus CHM, but the other comparisons were not blinded. Central randomisation was used but there was no description of allocation concealment. The treatment period was 12 weeks and there was a follow-up at six months.

Syndrome differentiation was used as an inclusion criterion. All participants were required to have dual deficiency of *qi* and Blood 气血亏虚. Additional syndromes were allowed and treatment was modified accordingly. The main acupuncture points were CV17

Tanzhong 膻中, CV12 *Zhongwan* 中脘, CV6 *Qihai* 气海, SP10 *Xuehai* 血海, ST36 *Zusanli* 足三里, TE5 *Waiguan* 外关, EX-HN1 *Sishencong* 四神聪, and GV20 *Baihui* 百会. Additional points were added according to additional syndromes as follows: GB39 *Juegu* 绝骨 (*Xuanzhong* 悬钟) was added for deficiency of Kidney and Essence 肾精亏虚, ST40 *Fenglong* 丰隆 was added for turbid phlegm obstructing the Orifices 痰浊阻窍, BL17 *Geshu* 膈俞 was added for Blood stasis obstructing the collaterals 瘀血阻络, LR3 *Taichong* 太冲 was added for Liver *yang* ascendant hyperactivity 肝阳上亢, ST44 *Neiting* 内庭 was added for fire and heat exuberant internally 火热内盛, and ST25 *Tianshu* 天枢 was added for Bowel stagnation turbidity retention *fu zhi zhuo liu* 腑滞浊留. Treatment was done in three 30-minute sessions per week. The author reported that both the donepezil and acupuncture groups improved over the 12 weeks of treatment, with greater improvements in the acupuncture group in outcomes for ADAS-cog, MMSE, and 'lower is better' ADL. However, the meta-analyses of these outcome measures did not detect significant differences between groups (Tables 7.3 and 7.5). At the six-month follow-up, there was no significant difference between groups for the MMSE (MD: 1.89 [–0.26, 4.04]), ADAS cog (MD: –2.79 [–5.61, 0.03]), or 'lower is better' ADL (SMD: –0.77 [–1.43, –0.11]).

In the acupuncture group, there were two dropouts because they felt cold and could not tolerate the pain of acupuncture. In the donepezil group, there were three dropouts, all of whom died but the reasons for death were not specified. The report also did not indicate when, during the course of the study, the dropouts occurred. In addition, the treatment of the dropouts in the data analysis was not specified. The data tables include 19 participants per group, so it appears that an intent-to-treat approach was used but no details were given so this cannot be confirmed. A sensitivity analysis with participant numbers adjusted for dropouts found no substantive difference in the outcomes.

Overall, the evidence for acupuncture vs. donepezil for VaD was of 'low' certainty (Table 7.14). The acupuncture treatments were neither inferior nor superior to donepezil based on the outcomes for the MMSE,

ADAS cog, or 'lower is better' ADL at the end of treatment. Other outcome measures were not reported. No integrative medicine studies that provided a comparison with donepezil were identified.

Clinical Evidence from Non-randomised Controlled Trials of Acupuncture

No non-randomised CCTs of acupuncture for VaD were identified in the searches. However, there were two non-randomised CCTs of electro-acupuncture for VaD. Neither study mentioned syndrome differentiation.

One study (A41) compared electro-acupuncture at EX-HN3 *Yintang* 印堂, GV20 *Baihui* 百会, GV16 *Fengfu* 风府, GB20 *Fengchi* 风池, EX-HN5 *Taiyang* 太阳, LI4 *Hegu* 合谷, and LR3 *Taichong* 太冲 with dihydroergotoxine methanesulfonate-sustained release tablets. After four weeks of treatment there was no significant difference between groups based on MMSE scores (MD: 1.14 [–1.36, 3.64], $n = 60$ participants) or 'lower is better' ADL scores (SMD: –0.32 [–0.83, 0.19]).

The other study (A42) applied electro-acupuncture at PC6 *Neiguan* 内关 and HT7 *Shenmen* 神门 as the main points, with ST36 *Zusanli* 足三里, GB34 *Yanglingquan* 阳陵泉, SI3 *Houxi* 后溪, BL60 *Kunlun* 昆仑, and GB39 *Xuanzhong* 悬钟 as additional points. Both groups received conventional routine therapy including medications for thrombolysis, anticoagulation, brain protection, blood circulation, and cerebral circulation, as well as the Bobath technique-based rehabilitation (also referred to as 'neurodevelopmental treatment', NDT). After six weeks, there was a significant increase in MMSE scores in the electro-acupuncture plus conventional routine therapy group (MD: 2.37 [0.69, 4.05]). Neither study reported on AEs.

Clinical Evidence from Non-controlled Studies of Acupuncture/Moxibustion

Acupuncture, with or without moxibustion, was assessed for VaD in 20 non-controlled studies (A43–A62). One of these studies used electro-acupuncture (A43) and two studies combined acupuncture and moxibustion (A44, A45). One study combined acupuncture with huperzine A (A46) and one study combined acupuncture with hyperbaric oxygen therapy (A47). All studies were conducted in China. The total number of participants enrolled in the studies was 864.

Two studies reported CM syndromes. In one study (A48), participants were divided into two groups according to syndrome: (1) Heat and turbidity obstructing the Orifices 热浊阻窍, which is an excess syndrome (*shi zheng* 实证), and (2) *yin* and Essence insufficiency 阴精亏损 which is a deficient syndrome (*xu zheng* 虚证). The acupuncture treatment was different for each group: (1) PC4 *Ximen* 郄门, HT5 *Tongli* 通里, GV26 *Shuigou* 水沟, ST40 *Fenglong* 丰隆, LR2 *Xingjian* 行间, and ST44 *Neiting* 内庭; and (2) GV23 *Shangxing* 上星, EX-HN3 *Yintang* 印堂, PC6 *Neiguan* 内关, HT7 *Shenmen* 神门, CV23 *Lianquan* 廉泉, KI7 *Fuliu* 复溜, and ST36 *Zusanli* 足三里.

The other study (A49) required all 30 participants to have the syndromes of Liver and Kidney insufficiency 肝肾亏损 and *qi* stagnation and Blood stasis 气滞血瘀. In addition, 14 participants had phlegm heat with excess in the hollow organs 痰热腑实, while 10 participants had Liver *yang* hyperactivity 肝阳亢盛. The main points and their actions were as follows: KI3 *Taixi* 太溪, BL23 *Shenshu* 肾俞, SP6 *Sanyinjiao* 三阴交, and CV6 *Qihai* 气海 were used to tonify Kidney and replenish Essence; ST36 *Zusanli* 足三里, SP10 *Xuehai* 血海, PC6 *Neiguan* 内关, and LI4 *Hegu* 合谷 were used to move Blood and resolve stasis 活血化瘀; and GV20 *Baihui* 百会, GB20 *Fengchi* 风池, GV24 *Shenting* 神庭, and GB8 *Shuaigu* 率谷 were used to awaken the Brain and open the Orifices 醒脑开窍. Additional points were added for specific syndromes.

The most frequently used acupuncture points in the 21 non-controlled studies were GV20 *Baihui* 百会, KI3 *Taixi* 太溪, ST36 *Zusanli* 足三里, GB20 *Fengchi* 风池, EX-HN1 *Sishencong* 四神聪, and GV26 *Shuigou* 水沟, all of which were used in eight or more studies (Table 7.15).

Two studies combined acupuncture with moxibustion. In one of the studies (A45), the acupuncture was applied to EX-HN1 *Sishencong* 四神聪, GB13 *Benshen* 本神, GV26 *Shuigou* 水沟, ST40

Table 7.15 Frequently Used Acupuncture Points in the Non-controlled Studies

Acupuncture Point	Frequency of Use
GV20 *Baihui* 百会	14
KI3 *Taixi* 太溪	9
ST36 *Zusanli* 足三里	9
GB20 *Fengchi* 风池	8
EX-HN1 *Sishencong* 四神聪	8
GV26 *Shuigou* 水沟	8
SP6 *Sanyinjiao* 三阴交	7
LR3 *Taichong* 太冲	7
GB13 *Benshen* 本神	6
GV24 *Shenting* 神庭	6
BL23 *Shenshu* 肾俞	6
PC6 *Neiguan* 内关	5
HT7 *Shenmen* 神门	5
ST40 *Fenglong* 丰隆	4
LI4 *Hegu* 合谷	4
GV14 *Dazhui* 大椎	3
LI11 *Quchi* 曲池	3
GV16 *Fengfu* 风府	2
GV4 *Mingmen* 命门	2
GB39 *Xuanzhong* 悬钟	2
SP10 *Xuehai* 血海	2
EX-HN3 *Yintang* 印堂	2

Note: Analysis is based on the main points and does not include extra points added for certain symptoms or syndromes.

Fenglong 丰隆, SP6 *Sanyinjiao* 三阴交, KI3 *Taixi* 太溪, BL23 *Shenshu* 肾俞, and a moxa-stick was applied to GV20 *Baihui* 百会 and ST36 *Zusanli* 足三里 (A45). In the other study (A44), acupuncture and a moxa-stick were used as alternating therapies on two groups of points: (1) GV26 *Shuigou* 水沟, EX-HN1 *Sishencong* 四神聪, GV24 *Shenting* 神庭, GB13 *Benshen* 本神, ST36 *Zusanli* 足三里, KI3 *Taixi* 太溪, and GB39 *Xuanzhong* 悬钟; and (2) GV20 *Baihui*

百会, GV14 *Dazhui* 大椎, GV4 *Mingmen* 命门, BL18 *Ganshu* 肝俞, and BL23 *Shenshu* 肾俞.

Safety of Acupuncture and Electro-acupuncture

Most RCTs did not mention AEs, one study stated that there were no AEs (A27), and one three-armed study provided a more detailed report on AEs and dropouts (A18). In the electro-acupuncture group, one person had dizziness and nausea which resolved after needles were removed. Another had fever, but this was unlikely to have been associated with the acupuncture. This study also reported numbers of dropouts due to other reasons including returning to hometown, not attending due to cold weather, or not having family members available to help them. However, it was not specified which group these dropouts were in. Another three-armed study reported that two people withdrew from the acupuncture group due to feeling cold and the pain of acupuncture, and the donepezil control group lost three individuals who died due to unspecified causes (A3). Neither of the two CCTs mentioned AEs, while AEs were mentioned in only one of the non-controlled studies, which specified that there were no AEs (A54).

Studies of Scalp Acupuncture

Four RCTs employed scalp acupuncture using the modern scalp zones. No CCTs and one non-controlled study of scalp acupuncture for VaD were identified. One RCT (A63) involved four groups (n = 180 participants) and the other three RCTs involved two groups and tested comparisons with pharmacotherapies. The most commonly used scalp zones in the RCTs were:

- MS1 *Ezhongxian* 额中线: 2 studies (A63, A64).
- MS5 *Dingzhongxian* 顶中线: 2 studies (A63, A64).
- MS6 *Dingnieqianxiexian* 顶颞前斜线: 2 studies (A64, A65).

None of the scalp acupuncture RCTs reported syndrome differentiation. The available outcome measures that provided suitable data for meta-analyses were the MMSE, HDS, ADL, and MQ.

Scalp Acupuncture vs. No Treatment

The four-armed RCT (n = 180 participants) reported on scalp acupuncture with electro-stimulation vs. no treatment and scalp electro-acupuncture with the addition of nimodipine vs. no treatment (i.e., two treatment groups, each of eight weeks). Conventional supportive treatment was provided in all groups (A63). The zones used in this study were MS5 *Dingzhongxian* 顶中线, MS1–MS3 *Epang1-3xian* 额旁1～3线, MS10 *Nieqianxian* 颞前线, and MS11 *Niehouxian* 颞后线.

For the MMSE, there was a significant increase in outcomes in the scalp electro-acupuncture group and a greater increase in the scalp electro-acupuncture plus nimodipine group at eight weeks. For 'lower score is better' ADL, there were significant reductions in both groups. Similarly, MQ scores improved in both groups (Table 7.16).

Scalp Acupuncture vs. Pharmacotherapy

Four RCTs included comparisons with nimodipine, piracetam, or citicoline.

Table 7.16 Scalp Electro-acupuncture vs. No Treatment

Outcome	Intervention	No. of Participants[1]	Effect Size (MD or SMD [95% CI])
MMSE	Scalp electro-acupuncture	90	MD: 2.68 [0.97, 4.39]*
	Scalp electro-acupuncture plus nimodipine	60	MD: 3.07 [1.13, 5.01]*
'Lower is better' ADL	Scalp electro-acupuncture	90	SMD: –0.60 [–1.05, –0.15]*
	Scalp electro-acupuncture plus nimodipine	60	SMD: –0.85 [–1.38, –0.32]*
MQ	Scalp electro-acupuncture	90	MD: 10.97 [7.49, 14.45]*
	Scalp electro-acupuncture plus nimodipine	60	MD: 12.50 [7.23, 17.77]*

*Statistically significant. *Note*: (1) Data from one RCT (A63). Abbreviations: ADL, activities of daily living; CI, confidence interval; MD, mean difference; MMSE, Mini-Mental State Examination; MQ, memory quotient; SMD, standardised mean difference.

Mini-Mental State Examination

Three studies of scalp acupuncture (A64–A66) and one of scalp electro-acupuncture (A63) tested comparisons with pharmacotherapies and reported data for the MMSE (Table 7.17). There was a small but significant difference between groups for the comparison with piracetam, but there was no difference between groups for the other comparisons. The pooled result for the four studies found a small but significant benefit at the end of treatment for scalp acupuncture or electro-acupuncture interventions compared to pharmacotherapies (MD: 0.81 [0.21, 1.41], $I^2 = 0\%$).

The only study that was judged as 'low' risk for SG compared scalp acupuncture with nimodipine and found no difference between groups (A65).

Hasegawa Dementia Scale

Only one four-week study (A65) of scalp acupuncture at MS6 *Dingnieqianxiexian* 顶颞前斜线 and MS7 *Dingniehouxiexian*

Table 7.17 Scalp Acupuncture *vs.* Pharmacotherapy: Mini-Mental State Examination

Comparator	No. of Studies (Participants), Duration	Effect Size (MD [95% CI], I^2)	Included Studies
Scalp acupuncture			
Nimodipine	1 (92), 4 wks	–0.29 [–1.96, 1.38]	A65
Piracetam	1 (60), 6 wks	0.92 [0.11, 1.73]*	A66
Citicoline	1 (77), 5 wks	1.80 [–0.12, 3.72]	A64
Scalp electro-acupuncture			
Nimodipine	1 (120), 8 wks	0.73 [–0.55, 2.01]	A63
Total pool (scalp acupuncture/scalp electro-acupuncture)			
Pharmacotherapy	4 (349), 4–8 wks	0.81 [0.21, 1.41]*, 0%	All above

*Statistically significant. Abbreviations: CI, confidence interval; MD, mean difference; wks, weeks.

顶颞后斜线 reported data on the HDS. In comparison with nimodipine, there was no difference between groups at the end of treatment (MD: –0.11 [–2.48, 2.26], $n = 92$ participants). This study was judged to be 'low' risk for SG.

Activities of Daily Living

One study of scalp acupuncture (A65) and one of scalp electro-acupuncture (A63) reported 'lower is better' ADL scores (Table 7.18). Nimodipine was the comparator in both studies and there was no significant difference between groups in either study or in the pool of two studies (SMD: 0.15 [–0.23, 0.52], $I^2 = 47\%$).

Two studies reported 'higher is better' ADL data (A64, A66) and revealed a significant difference in the comparison with piracetam but not the comparison with citicoline. The pool of the two studies showed a small but significant benefit for scalp acupuncture (SMD: 0.40 [0.06, 0.74], $I^2 = 0\%$) (Table 7.19). Neither study was judged to have 'low' risk of bias for SG.

Memory Quotient

One study that lasted eight weeks (A63) compared scalp electro-acupuncture with nimodipine and measured MQ. There were

Table 7.18 Scalp Acupuncture vs. Pharmacotherapy: 'Lower is Better' Activities of Daily Living

Comparator	No. of Studies (Participants), Duration	Effect Size (SMD [95% CI], I^2)	Included Studies
Scalp acupuncture			
Nimodipine	1 (120), 4 wks	–0.06 [–0.46, 0.35]	A65
Scalp electro-acupuncture			
Nimodipine	1 (120), 8 wks	0.33 [–0.03, 0.69]	A63
Total pool (scalp acupuncture/scalp electro-acupuncture)			
Nimodipine	2 (240), 4–8 wks	0.15 [–0.23, 0.52], 47%	All above

Abbreviations: CI, confidence interval; SMD, standardised mean difference, wks, weeks.

Table 7.19 Scalp Acupuncture vs. Pharmacotherapy: 'Higher is Better' Activities of Daily Living

Comparator	No. of Studies (Participants), Duration	Effect Size (SMD [95% CI], I^2)	Included Studies
Piracetam	1 (60), 6 wks	0.59 [0.08, 1.11]*	A66
Citicoline	1 (77), 5 wks	0.25 [–0.20, 0.70]	A64
Pharmacotherapy	2 (137), 5–6 wks	0.40 [0.06, 0.74]*, 0%	All above

*Statistically significant. Abbreviations: CI, confidence interval; SMD, standardised mean difference, wks, weeks.

Table 7.20 Integrative Scalp acupuncture vs. Nimodipine

Outcome	Intervention	No. of Participants[1]	Effect size (MD or SMD [95% CI])
MMSE	Scalp electro-acupuncture	90	MD: 1.12 [–0.45, 2.69]
'Lower is better' ADL	Scalp electro-acupuncture	90	SMD: –0.15 [–0.59, 0.29]
MQ	Scalp electro-acupuncture	90	MD: 1.12 [–4.28, 6.52]

Note: (1) All in one RCT (A63). Abbreviations: ADL, activities of daily living; CI, confidence interval; MD, mean difference; MMSE, Mini-Mental State Examination; MQ, memory quotient; SMD, standardised mean difference.

no differences between groups (MD: –0.41 [–4.09, 3.27], $n = 120$ participants).

Integrative Scalp Acupuncture

Only one study (A63) compared scalp electro-acupuncture plus nimodipine with nimodipine alone for eight weeks and reported results for the MMSE, 'lower is better' ADL, and MQ (Table 7.20). There were no significant differences between groups for any of these outcomes.

Non-controlled Studies of Scalp Acupuncture

One study reported on the use of scalp acupuncture in 32 people with VaD who were treated for 56 days (A67). The scalp zones used were the vertex zone *Ding qu* 顶区, anterior vertex zone *Ding qian qu* 顶前区, and frontal zone *E qu* 额区. The authors reported that the treatment was effective based on effective rate but did not report other outcome measures.

Safety of Scalp Acupuncture

Only one of the RCTs reported on AEs (A64). There were two dropouts in the scalp acupuncture group. In one case, the family withdrew the patient after the patient fainted, and in the other case, the person completed less than half of the treatment course and was excluded. There was one dropout in the citicoline injection group due to a red rash at the injection site, which may have been due to an allergic reaction. There was no mention of AEs in the single non-controlled study.

Frequently Reported Scalp Acupuncture Zones in Meta-analyses

The meta-analysis pool for MMSE (Table 7.17) showed a significant result in favour of scalp acupuncture vs. pharmacotherapy. It included four studies. Three scalp zones were used in two studies each, namely MS1 *Ezhongxian* 额中线 (A63, A64), MS5 *Dingzhongxian* 顶中线 (A63, A64), and MS6 *Dingnieqianxiexian* 顶颞前斜线 (A64, A65).

Moxibustion

Two RCTs (A68, A69), no CCTs, and no non-randomised controlled trials of moxibustion for VaD were identified. Both RCTs were by the same group and used syndrome differentiation according to the following three syndromes:

- Liver and Kidney dual deficiency 肝肾亏虚.
- Turbid phlegm obstructing the Orifices 痰浊阻窍.
- *Qi* deficiency 气虚.

Table 7.21 Moxibustion vs. Piracetam: Mini-mental State Examination, Hasegawa Dementia Scale, and Activities of Daily Living

Outcome	No. of Studies (Participants), Duration	Effect Size (MD or SMD [95% CI], I^2)	Included Studies
MMSE	1 (86), 9 wks	MD: 5.31 [1.35, 9.27]*	A68
	1 (65), 16 wks	MD: 3.88 [0.29, 7.47]*	A69
MMSE total	2 (151), 9–16 wks	MD: 4.52 [1.87, 7.18]*, 0%	A68, A69
HDS	1 (86), 9 wks	MD: 3.29 [0.67, 5.91]*	A68
	1 (65), 16 wks	MD: 2.65 [–0.87, 6.17]	A69
HDS total	2 (151), 9–16 wks	MD: 3.06 [0.96, 5.17]*, 0%	A68, A69
'Lower is better' ADL	1 (86), 9 wks	SMD: –0.18 [–0.61, 0.24]	A68
	1 (65), 16 wks	SMD: –0.60 [–1.09, –0.10]*	A69
ADL total	2 (151), 9–16 wks	SMD: –0.37 [–0.77, 0.04]*, 35%	A68, A69

*Statistically significant. Abbreviations: ADL, activities of daily living; CI, confidence interval; HDS, Hasegawa dementia scale; MD, mean difference; MMSE, Mini-Mental State Examination; SMD, standardised mean difference; wks, weeks.

Both RCTs compared moxibustion to piracetam. In both studies, the main points for moxibustion were GV20 *Baihui* 百会, GV24 *Shenting* 神庭, and GV14 *Dazhui* 大椎. Additional points were added according to syndrome as follows: BL18 *Ganshu* 肝俞 and BL23 *Shenshu* 肾俞 were added for Liver and Kidney dual deficiency 肝肾亏虚, CV12 *Zhongwan* 中脘 and ST40 *Fenglong* 丰隆 were added for turbid phlegm obstructing the Orifices 痰浊阻窍, and CV6 *Qihai* 气海 was added for *qi* deficiency 气虚. Treatment involved the use of a moxa-stick with a slice of the herb *fu zi* 附子片 applied on each point. One session lasted 20 minutes and treatment was applied every day.

The studies differed by duration, so the results are presented separately and then pooled. In the pooled results (Table 7.21), there were significant improvements in the moxibustion groups based on the MMSE (MD: 4.52 [1.87, 7.18], $I^2 = 0\%$), HDS (MD: 3.06 [0.96, 5.17], $I^2 = 0\%$), and 'lower is better' ADL (SMD: –0.37 [–0.77, 0.04], $I^2 = 35\%$). Both studies were judged as 'low' risk for SG. Neither study reported on AEs.

Ear Acupuncture and Ear Acupressure

No studies of ear acupuncture for VaD were found, but one RCT of ear acupressure (A70) was identified. No non-randomised controlled studies or non-controlled studies of either intervention were found.

The single RCT of ear acupressure enrolled 180 people and compared ear acupressure to nimodipine for 12 weeks (A70). There was no mention of syndrome differentiation. Seeds from the herb *wang bu liu xing* 王不留行 (vaccaria seeds) were taped on four ear points, namely TF4 *Shenmen* 神门, AT3.4i *Naogan* 脑干, CO10 *Shen* 肾, and AT3 *Zhen* 枕. Seeds were changed every day and applied to alternate ears. Family members or caregivers were instructed to stimulate the points five times a day for five minutes each time. At the end of treatment, there were no significant differences between groups based on the MMSE (MD: 0.13 [–0.99, 1.25] n = 163 participants) or 'lower is better' ADL scores (SMD: 0.04 [–0.27, 0.35], n = 163 participants). Two people withdrew from the ear acupressure group due to allergic reactions to the tape used to hold the seeds in place. There was one case of mild dizziness and one case of diarrhoea in the nimodipine group.

Clinical Evidence for Commonly Used Acupuncture Interventions

Acupuncture therapies recommended in contemporary clinical guidelines include acupuncture (at traditional points), scalp acupuncture (using scalp zones), ear acupuncture, and moxibustion (see Chapter 2). The therapies assessed in the RCTs were acupuncture, scalp acupuncture, moxibustion, and acupressure on ear points.

Of the traditional points recommended in the guidelines, GV20 *Baihui* 百会, EX-HN1 *Sishencong* 四神聪, GV24 *Shenting* 神庭, GB20 *Fengchi* 风池, ST36 *Zusanli* 足三里, SP6 *Sanyinjiao* 三阴交, KI3 *Taixi* 太溪, GB13 *Benshen* 本神, HT7 *Shenmen* 神门, LR3 *Taichong* 太冲, ST40 *Fenglong* 丰隆, BL23 *Shenshu* 肾俞, and GV17 *Naohu* 脑户 were all used in multiple RCTs. The acupoint BL17 *Geshu* 膈俞 was used in one RCT. None of the RCTs included

LU7 *Lieque* 列缺, KI4 *Dazhong* 大钟, or HT5 *Tongli* 通里 as main points.

In the non-controlled studies, the recommended points, specifically GV20 *Baihui* 百会, EX-HN1 *Sishencong* 四神聪, GV24 *Shenting* 神庭, GB20 *Fengchi* 风池, ST36 *Zusanli* 足三里, SP6 *Sanyinjiao* 三阴交, KI3 *Taixi* 太溪, GB13 *Benshen* 本神, HT7 *Shenmen* 神门, LR3 *Taichong* 太冲, ST40 *Fenglong* 丰隆, and BL23 *Shenshu* 肾俞, were all used in multiple studies. The acupoint GV17 *Naohu* 脑户, KI4 *Dazhong* 大钟, and HT5 *Tongli* 通里 were used in single studies. No studies used LU7 *Lieque* 列缺 or BL17 *Geshu* 膈俞.

In the four RCTs of scalp acupuncture, the scalp zones MS1 *Ezhongxian* 额中线 and MS5 *Dingzhongxian* 顶中线 were used in two studies, while MS3 *Epangxian* 2额旁2线, MS4 *Epangxian* 3额旁3线, MS10 *Nieqianxian* 颞前线, and MS11 *Niehouxian* 颞后线 were each used in single studies. One of the RCTs (A66) and the single non-controlled study of scalp acupuncture (A67) used a different system of scalp acupuncture from that which was included in Chapter 2.

In the two RCTs of moxibustion, one of the main points, GV20 *Baihui* 百会, was included in the guidelines for moxibustion and for acupuncture, while GV24 *Shenting* 神庭 was included for acupuncture, as was the secondary point BL23 *Shenshu* 肾俞. The single RCT of ear acupressure used three of the points from the guidelines, namely TF4 *Shenmen* 神门, CO10 *Shen* 肾 (Kidney), and AT3 *Zhen* 枕 (occiput).

Overall, the main points used in acupuncture and scalp acupuncture interventions in the clinical trials were mostly the same as those recommended in the clinical guidelines. The points used in the ear acupressure study included a number of points indicated in the guidelines for ear acupuncture. Also, the frequently used acupuncture points in the RCTs included in this chapter are very similar to those found in a survey of all types of clinical studies of VaD,[7] indicating that the studies included in these meta-analyses used acupuncture interventions that were representative of acupuncture studies in China.

Summary of Clinical Evidence for Acupuncture and Related Therapies

The results of one small study (A1) suggested that real acupuncture utilising points typically used for dementia was better than needling at non-point locations, but the study was too small for any firm conclusions to be drawn. A larger study that compared similar points with no treatment reported that the acupuncture group showed improved results (A2), but when the data was analysed using the random effect model, this difference was not statistically significant. Such differences occurred several times in these meta-analyses and reflect the conservative random effects approach taken rather than any error on the part of the authors.

The majority of RCTs of acupuncture or electro-acupuncture involved comparisons with a variety of pharmacotherapies. Of these, only donepezil is recommended in international guidelines as an intervention for VaD, but only one small study tested donepezil (A3). For this study, the random effect model found no significant differences between groups after 12 weeks of treatment, suggesting that the acupuncture, which utilised points commonly used for dementia, had a similar effect to 5 mg donepezil based on MMSE, ADAS-cog, and 'lower is better' ADL outcomes.

For acupuncture vs. nimodipine, meta-analysis of three studies indicated a relative benefit for acupuncture based on MMSE scores, but heterogeneity was substantial. For electro-acupuncture vs. nimodipine, a pool of two studies also found a significant result in terms of MMSE scores without heterogeneity (Table 7.3). With HDS as an outcome, a pool of three studies of acupuncture vs. nimodipine found no significant difference between groups, but with substantial heterogeneity. A single study of electro-acupuncture found a similar result (Table 7.4). These similar measures of cognitive outcomes suggest that acupuncture and electro-acupuncture treatment may have similar levels of effectiveness relative to nimodipine for durations of up to six weeks. However, none of the studies were blinded.

Co-dergocrine mesylate was compared with acupuncture in multiple studies. For the MMSE, a meta-analysis of three studies indicated a significantly greater improvement in the acupuncture groups, but there was substantial heterogeneity (Table 7.3). Similar results were found for electro-acupuncture, but these were based on single studies of comparisons with co-dergocrine mesylate and nimodipine plus co-dergocrine mesylate (Table 7.3). With HDS as an outcome, the single study of electro-acupuncture vs. co-dergocrine mesylate revealed a similar result (Table 7.4).

Multiple studies provided comparisons with piracetam. For the MMSE, a pool of two studies found a significant benefit for the acupuncture groups with moderate heterogeneity, while a pool of two studies of electro-acupuncture found no significant difference between groups, without substantial heterogeneity (Table 7.3). With HDS as the outcome, the pools for acupuncture and electro-acupuncture vs. piracetam were both significant without heterogeneity (Table 7.4). When compared to co-dergocrine mesylate or piracetam, the meta-analysis results suggest that improvements in the cognitive outcome measures for the MMSE and HDS may be greater in the acupuncture and electro-acupuncture groups at up to 12 weeks of treatment. This result was similar to the total pool of comparisons with pharmacotherapies for these cognitive outcome measures (Tables 7.3 and 7.4).

For the measures of ADL, the meta-analysis was complicated by differences in scales which required the use of the SMD random effects model and the division of ADL pools into 'lower is better' and 'higher is better' types. Consequently, most subgroups only contained single studies. In the single comparison with donepezil, there was no difference between groups (Table 7.5). For two studies of electro-acupuncture compared to nimodipine, there was no difference between groups at six weeks without heterogeneity for 'lower is better' ADL, but a single study of acupuncture using 'higher is better' ADL revealed a significant benefit (Table 7.6). Overall, the total pools for acupuncture and electro-acupuncture vs. pharmacotherapies showed small but significant improvements with moderate heterogeneity.

In the integrative medicine studies, most subgroups contained single studies. For the MMSE, two studies that combined electro-acupuncture with nimodipine showed a significant benefit at six weeks without heterogeneity (Table 7.8). The total pools (acupuncture/electro-acupuncture) for the cognitive outcome measures MMSE and HDS showed significant benefits without substantial heterogeneity, but most studies lasted 12 weeks or shorter (Tables 7.8 and 7.9). For ADL outcomes, there were significant improvements in the total pools of integrative acupuncture/electro-acupuncture vs. pharmacotherapies for both types of scales, with no heterogeneity (Tables 7.10 and 7.11).

Overall, the meta-analyses of the outcomes of multiple RCTs suggest that the effectiveness of acupuncture and electro-acupuncture may be similar to or better than pharmacotherapies in terms of MMSE, HDS, and ADL outcomes. Furthermore, the addition of acupuncture or electro-acupuncture to a pharmacotherapy may provide additional benefit. However, the diversity in the pharmacotherapies used as comparators, variations between the acupuncture interventions, and differences in treatment durations limited our ability to pool the specific interventions and controls in order to determine which acupuncture interventions produced better outcomes.

The syndromes reported in the studies of acupuncture and electro-acupuncture were similar to those specified in the guidelines and textbooks in Chapter 2 — allowing for some differences in wording. The frequencies of points in the pools for RCTs of acupuncture/electro-acupuncture (Table 7.12) and integrative acupuncture/electro-acupuncture (Table 7.13) that reported improvements in cognitive and ADL outcomes were calculated to determine which points were used in studies showing evidence of effectiveness. The results indicated that the points frequently used in the studies that contributed to the overall results were typical of the points used for VaD and included many of the points recommended in guidelines and textbooks (Chapter 2). Therefore, the results of these analyses were based on studies of acupuncture interventions that were similar to those recommended for use in clinical practice.

It is notable that the points used frequently in non-controlled studies (Table 7.15) were similar to those generally used in RCTs

(Table 7.1) and those used in the studies that contributed to the meta-analysis pools that showed benefits for acupuncture (Tables 7.12 and 7.13). Nevertheless, it is important to note that the frequency of point usage is not a measure of efficacy and it remains unclear whether certain combinations of points are more effective than others. Further research is needed to determine optimum acupuncture interventions for VaD.

For scalp acupuncture, there were only four RCTs suitable for analysis and no studies reported ADAS-cog outcomes. In one study, scalp electro-acupuncture and scalp electro-acupuncture plus nimodipine showed benefits based on MMSE and ADL scores compared to no treatment. There were no comparisons with donepezil. The studies of comparisons with pharmacotherapies suggested that, based on MMSE and HDS outcomes, scalp acupuncture was not significantly different from nimodipine, but when compared to the pool of pharmacotherapies, scalp acupuncture showed a small but significant benefit with no heterogeneity (Table 7.17). For ADL outcomes, there was no difference in comparison with nimodipine, but this was based on a single study (Table 7.18). Conversely, there were significant differences in the pooled results for single studies of piracetam and citicoline (Table 7.19). In the single integrative medicine study, addition of scalp acupuncture to nimodipine produced no additional benefit at eight weeks for either the MMSE or the ADL (Table 7.20).

Due to the small number of studies on moxibustion and ear acupressure, it was not possible to make conclusions based on the meta-analysis results for these interventions.

When AEs were reported, these tended to be minor in the acupuncture groups, but AE reporting was inadequate in most studies, so it was not possible to draw any conclusions regarding the safety of acupuncture and related interventions based on the included studies.

There are a number of limitations that should be considered when interpreting the findings on acupuncture and related therapies. The durations of studies were relatively short (mainly 12 weeks or shorter) and only one study reported follow-up data. Therefore, the reported effects may not persist beyond these durations. In addition, all studies had inadequacies in methodological reporting and some meta-analysis pools showed considerable heterogeneity. Some studies did not employ proper randomisation or did not describe the method of randomisation used. Consequently, subgroup sensitivity analyses were conducted for studies judged as 'low' risk for SG when these were available. These analyses tended to reduce heterogeneity in the pools of acupuncture and electro-acupuncture vs. pharmacotherapy for cognitive and ADL outcomes without substantially changing effect sizes or overall outcomes, suggesting that this methodological weakness did not affect the overall results.

Only one study attempted to blind participants. It is possible that lack of blinding of participants, personnel, and outcome assessors in the majority of studies led to overestimations of effect sizes for the outcome measures. It should be noted that blinding of personnel delivering the acupuncture is difficult to undertake in any study. Nevertheless, blinding is not impossible and should be implemented in future studies.

In addition, differences between participant groups in relation to the duration and severity of VaD as well as the duration and frequency of treatment are likely to have affected results and led to heterogeneity. However, these aspects were not explored due to the relatively small number of studies in each meta-analysis pool. These factors limit our confidence in the results and contributed to the downgrading of the evidence according to GRADE. Further well-designed clinical trials are needed.

References

1. Peng WN, Zhao H, Liu ZS, Wang S. (2007) Acupuncture for vascular dementia. *Cochrane Database Syst Rev.* (2):CD004987.
2. 朱蔓佳, 张虹. (2009) 不同针刺方法治疗血管性痴呆meta分析. 辽宁中医杂志. **36**(9):1475–1477.
3. 辛明. 针灸治疗血管性痴呆的系统评价. 成都: 成都中医药大学 (2015).
4. 彭唯娜, 赵宏, 刘志顺, 刘保延. (2004) 电针治疗血管性痴呆的系统评价. 中国针灸. **24**(5):297–301.

5. 郭震浪, 苏振宁. (2016) 头针治疗血管性痴呆 meta 分析. 辽宁中医药大学学报. **18**(5):121–124.
6. Liu F, Li ZM, Jiang YJ, Chen LD. (2014) A meta-analysis of acupuncture use in the treatment of cognitive impairment after stroke. *J Altern Complement Med.* **20**(7):535–544.
7. Feng S, Ren Y, Fan S, *et al.* (2015) Discovery of acupoints and combinations with potential to treat vascular dementia: A data mining analysis. *Evid Based Complement Alternat Med.* **2015**:310591.

List of Clinical Studies Included in Chapter 7

Study Number	References
A1	陈艳霞，戴东，于涛，徐文贵，*et al.* (2011) "益气调血, 扶本培元" 针刺法对血管性痴呆患者脑葡萄糖代谢的影响. 中医杂志. **52**(13):1124–1127.
A2	孟迎春，韩景献. (2011) 益气调血扶本培元针法治疗血管性痴呆临床观察. 针灸临床杂志. **27**(9):35–37.
A3	文宰晟. (2012) 针药结合对气血亏虚型血管性痴呆治疗方案的优化研究. 学位论文. 南京中医药大学.
A4	包烨华，冯伟民，朱国祥，*et al.* (2004) 邹超. 头穴久留针治疗血管性痴呆的随机对照研究. 中国针灸. **24**(2):81–84.
A5	江红. (2006) 眼针治疗血管性痴呆的临床观察. 辽宁中医杂志. **33**(10):1333–1334.
A6	靳冬, 张玉莲, 王立存, 张连城. (2006) 头项针治疗血管性痴呆 26 例疗效观察. 中国临床医药研究杂志. (155):17.
A7	孟学峰，范晔，薛连峰. (2009) 调督醒神法针刺治疗血管性痴呆 30 例. 中医外治杂志. **4**:46–47.
A8	薛莉，康涛，张萍，杨元庆，张智龙 (指导). (2013) 调神益智针法治疗血管性痴呆患者 120 例临床观察. 四川中医. **31**(5):135–136.
A9	李佩芳，刘霞，王颖，王涛, *et al.* (2012) 刺督调神法对血管性痴呆患者智能水平及日常生活活动能力的影响. 中医药临床杂志. **24**(3):212–215.
A10	孔莉. (2013) 针刺治疗脑梗死后血管性痴呆的临床疗效观察. 天津中医药. **30**(12):726–728.
A11	李淑芝，鲁仲平，王东升，侯敬丽. (2006) 透穴治疗血管性痴呆 30 例临床观察. 中国中医药科技. **13**(4):233.
A12	孙善斌，杨骏，张闻东，陈幸生, *et al.* (2009) 辨经刺井法及颞三针治疗血管性痴呆临床观察. 上海针灸杂志. **28**(4):207–209.

(*Continued*)

(*Continued*)

Study Number	References
A13	李申林，李飞，程红亮，张闻东，(指导), *et al.* (2010) 辨经刺井配合颞三针治疗血管性痴呆临床研究. 中医药临床杂志. **22**(11):977–979.
A14	王立存，张玉莲，靳冬，郭家奎，*et al.* (2007) 头项针治疗血管性痴呆临床研究. 河北中医. **29**(10):923–925.
A15	于涛，石江伟，韩景献, (2007) 针刺治疗轻中度血管性痴呆临床观察. 辽宁中医杂志. **34**(7):978–980.
A16	赵建新，田元祥，程英武，马文香, *et al.* (2000) 益肾醒脑针法治疗血管性痴呆临床观察. 河北中医. **22**(11):844–846.
A17	彭晓虹，赵煜，刘耀，刘军, *et al.* (2009) 头电针对血管性痴呆认知功能影响的随机对照研究. 四川中医. **27**(2):113–115.
A18	张虹，赵凌，何成奇，胡卡明, *et al.* (2008) 头电针治疗血管性痴呆的临床多中心随机对照研究. 中国针灸. **28**(11):783–787.
A19	王惠明. (2007) 电针法治疗血管性痴呆临床疗效观察. 天津中医药. **24**(3):218–220.
A20	栗先增，周湘明，顾柏林. (2013) 电项针疗法对血管性痴呆患者认知功能影响临床研究. 辽宁中医药大学学报. **15**(6):190–192.
A21	徐丽红，庄礼兴 (指导). (2006) 电针四神聪等穴治疗老年血管性痴呆临床研究. 广州中医药大学，硕士学位论文.
A22	陈香妹，王德平，陈云龙. (2009) 针刺治疗血管性痴呆疗效观察. 甘肃中医学院学报. **26**(5):36–38.
A23	江钢辉，赖新生，莫飞智. (1998) 电针治疗血管性痴呆临床疗效对照观察. 广州中医药大学学报. **15**(2):110–113.
A24	莫飞智，李建强，储莉，雷立屏. (2000) 电针对血管性痴呆患者智力及其 P300 的影响. 中国针灸. **20**(11):687–690.
A25	江钢辉，陈振虎，赖新生. (2003) 针刺智三针和四神聪穴治疗血管性痴呆的临床研究. 广州中医药大学学报. **20**(4):271–273.
A26	陈振虎，赖新生，江钢辉. (2006) 电针对血管性痴呆患者认知功能的影响. 辽宁中医杂志. **33**(2):207–208.
A27	周颖，向诗余 (指导). (2012) 针刺结合西药治疗血管性痴呆的临床疗效观察. 湖北中医药大学，硕士学位论文.
A28	吴芙蓉. (2010) 针药结合治疗血管性痴呆. 针灸临床杂志. **26**(7):50–52.
A29	吴远华，朱广旗，邵勇，左彬. (2010) 督脉刺法治疗脑血管性痴呆的临床研究. 现代中西医结合杂志. **19**(7):794–795.

(*Continued*)

Study Number	References
A30	史洪润，何峰，窦伟，黄炳亮. (2009) 针刺井穴对血管性痴呆患者临床干预的疗效分析. 第四军医大学学报. **30**(7):667–669.
A31	戴晓红，郭玉红，张宏伟，邹伟. (2013) 头针快速提插捻转法为主治疗轻度血管性痴呆 35 例临床观察. 针灸临床杂志. **29**(8):10–11.
A32	戴晓红，郭玉红，张宏伟，邹伟. (2013) 头针快速提插捻转法为主治疗血管性痴呆疗效观察. 上海针灸杂志. **32**(9):709–710.
A33	王如杰. (2007) 针刺治疗血管性痴呆的临床分析. 辽宁中医药大学学报. **9**(1):128.
A34	王敏，王敏华，华启海，李震宇. (2005) 针刺“头三神”穴为主治疗血管性痴呆疗效观察. 上海针灸杂志. **24**(6):12–14.
A35	王雅君，朱茜，贾晓燕，李秉艳. (2005) 醒脑开窍针刺法配合神经活素对血管性痴呆康复效果对比观察. 现代康复. **5**(11):124.
A36	陆卫卫，周健. (2009) 针刺治疗血管性痴呆的临床观察. 辽宁中医杂志. **36**(10):1784–1785.
A37	王非，梁淼 (2003). 针刺配合胞二磷胆碱治疗血管性痴呆 32 例. 首都医药. **10**(24):33.
A38	王重新. (2007) 醒脑调神针法治疗血管性痴呆 30 例疗效观察. 中国中医急症. **16**(7):789–790.
A39	于颂华，王春梅，刘占芬，张智龙 (指导). (2005) “调神益智”针法治疗血管性痴呆 21 例临床观察. 针灸临床杂志. **21**(6):25–26.
A40	殷建权，李立红，冯爱春. (2011) 电针头穴对改善血管性痴呆患者症状的临床观察. 中华中医药学刊. **29**(2):415–416.
A41	赵宏，曹乃钊，刘志顺，王石. (2006) 电针治疗中重度血管性痴呆疗效观察. 针灸临床杂志. **22**(1):27–29.
A42	吴越，过婷，叶智存. (2009) 电针对血管性痴呆患者认知功能的影响. 临床精神医学杂志. **19**(1):36.
A43	朱蔓佳，张虹，赵凌. (2008) 头电针治疗血管性痴呆对脑功能成像的影响. 海南医学院学报. **14**(6):644–646.
A44	李艳慧，庄礼兴，郑琼，杨文辉. (1998) 针灸治疗血管性痴呆的临床观察. 中国针灸 **18**(11):645–647.
A45	唐强，张立雅，朱肖菊. (2005) 针灸治疗血管性痴呆 22 例. 陕西中医. **26**(4):360.

(*Continued*)

(*Continued*)

Study Number	References
A46	徐阜溧. (2012) 石杉碱甲配合针刺治疗脑梗死后血管性痴呆观察及护理. 实用中医药杂志. 28(1):32–33.
A47	张爱君. (2008) 五神针高压氧并用治疗血管性痴呆 42 例. 实用中医内科杂志. **22**(5):101.
A48	武连仲，侯庆，周新. (1998) 针刺治疗血管性痴呆的临床研究. 中国针灸. **18**(12):733–734.
A49	陈建宗，李刚，陈晓丽，梁红娟, *et al.* (2001) 针刺治疗脑血管性痴呆 30 例近期疗效. 安徽中医学院学报. **20**(2):36–37.
A50	陈邦国. (1999) 针刺治疗脑血管性痴呆 32 例疗效观察. 湖北中医杂志. **21**(1):39–40.
A51	陈俊琦，洪若熙，陈曦，苏尚贤, *et al.* (2008) "通督调神"法治疗血管性痴呆的临床观察. 时珍国医国药. **19**(2):300–301.
A52	陈玉宝. (2012) 针刺对血管性痴呆患者定量脑电图的影响. 现代中西医结合杂志. **21**(30):3368–3369.
A53	陈月琴. (2014) 针刺治疗血管性痴呆41例. 内蒙古中医药. **33**(2):28–29.
A54	樊小农，刘健，李平. (2005) 针刺影响不同程度血管性痴呆患者智能水平的实验观察. 中国临床康复. **9**(13):107–109.
A55	何希俊. (2001) 针药并用治疗血管性痴呆 20 例观察. 中医药学刊. **19**(3):267.
A56	华金双，孙忠人. (2003) 原络通经针法治疗 20 例血管性痴呆临床观察. 中医药学报. **31**(1):35.
A57	计毅，刘艳彬，郭振军. (2007) 电针治疗血管性痴呆的临床观察. 中华中医药学刊. **25**(5):1070–1071.
A58	刘智斌，牛文民，杨晓航，王渊, *et al.* (2011) 嗅三针治疗血管性痴呆嗅觉功能障碍的临床研究. 新中医. **43**(3):99–100.
A59	罗耀武，唐安戊，李东江. (2008) Position emission tomography (PET) 显像在血管性痴呆针刺治疗中的应用研究. 广东医学. **29**(12):2015–2016.
A60	马涛. (2007) "头项十八穴"治疗血管性痴呆 66 例. 江苏中医药. **39**(10):59.
A61	牟宪慧，王爱华. (2000) 针灸治疗血管性痴呆 26 例疗效观察. 针灸临床杂志. **16**(1):7.
A62	彭唯娜，马晓晶，刘志顺. (2005) 电针调理髓海方法治疗重度血管性痴呆 12 例. 针灸临床杂志. **21**(9):34–35.

(*Continued*)

Study Number	References
A63	刘军，彭晓虹，林大东，李常度, *et al.* (1998) 电针头穴治疗血管性痴呆临床研究. 中国针灸. **18**(4):197–200.
A64	李思康，丁定明，刘茜，李涛, *et al.* (2012) 头针治疗血管性痴呆随机对照研究. 上海针灸杂志. **31**(11):806–808.
A65	刘翼程，张红星，陈国华，吴文莉, *et al.* (2008). 头针治疗对脑梗死所致血管性痴呆的随机对照临床试验. 中西医结合学报. 2008; **6**(8): 806–809.
A66	于向华，张海峰. (2012) 头穴丛刺长留针法治疗血管性痴呆的临床观察. 上海中医药杂志. **46**(12):41–42.
A67	张立，关莹，邢艳丽. (2010) 头穴丛刺治疗血管性痴呆 32 例. 针灸临床杂志. **26**(6):18–19.
A68	王频，杨骏，杨帆，陈浩. (2009) 化瘀通络灸法治疗血管性痴呆临床观察. 中国中医急症. **18**(2):172–174.
A69	王频，杨骏，柳刚，陈浩，杨帆. (2010) 艾灸头部穴位为主对血管性痴呆患者脑脊液中生长抑素和精氨酸血管加压素水平影响的随机对照试验. 中西医结合学报. **8**(7):636–640.
A70	陈琪，黄宏敏，许玉皎，卢瑞丽 (2009) 耳穴贴压治疗血管性痴呆疗效对照观察. 中国针灸. **29**(2):95–97.

8

Clinical Evidence for Other Chinese Medicine Therapies

OVERVIEW

Along with Chinese herbal medicine and acupuncture therapies, other Chinese medicine therapies, such as *qi gong* 气功 and Chinese remedial massage, are alternatives or add-ons to the pharmacological treatment of symptoms in people with vascular dementia. Three clinical trials were identified for inclusion in this chapter. These were evaluated for the efficacy and safety of the interventions. The single randomised controlled trial of *Sun si miao*'s body strengthening exercises (*Sun si miao jian shen cao* 孙思邈健身操) found that it was beneficial for cognitive function and activities of daily living. Two non-controlled studies each reported that *hui chun gong* 回春功 and *tui na* 推拿 could improve clinical symptoms in patients with vascular dementia. Overall, there was very little evidence available for other Chinese medicine therapies for vascular dementia.

Introduction

In addition to Chinese herbal medicine and acupuncture therapies, Chinese medicine (CM) includes a range of other CM therapies to treat disease and maintain health. These include:

- Chinese exercise therapies include various styles of *tai chi* (*tai ji quan* 太极拳), various forms of *dao yin yang sheng gong* 导引养生功, and various types of *qi gong* 气功. These therapies tend to be holistic systems that coordinate body posture, movement, breathing, and meditation. They are generally used to maintain or restore health, develop spirituality, or as a component of martial arts training.

- Chinese remedial massage (*tui na* 推拿, *an mo* 按摩) involves using different parts of the palms and fingers and varying degrees of force to press, rub, or apply other manual techniques on meridians, acupuncture points, muscles, and skin areas.

Previous Systematic Reviews

A Cochrane review of exercise programs for people with dementia, including vascular dementia (VaD), found evidence that exercise is beneficial in terms of daily living activities but not cognitive functioning.[1] However, a subsequent systematic review reported that physical activity interventions, in particular aerobic exercises, had positive effects on cognitive functioning in people with multiple dementia types (including VaD).[2] A review of longitudinal studies found a significant association between physical exercise and a reduced risk of VaD development, suggesting a preventative effect.[3] However, these studies did not include subgroup analyses for *tai chi* 太极 or other Chinese exercises for dementia.

The effects of *qi gong* 气功 exercises, notably the 'eight brocades' *ba duan jin* 八段锦, has received considerable research attention.[4,5] In elderly people, *qi gong* 气功 has been documented to improve sleep quality,[6] promote health and well-being,[7] and reduce blood pressure.[8] However, no reviews of its application in VaD could be located. For various massage therapies, a Cochrane review found that studies of massage and other forms of touch did not provide definitive evidence of benefit for dementia.[9] However, a subsequent review of clinical studies found that massage was effective in managing agitation in people with dementia.[10] No reviews for the specific Chinese massages *tui na* 推拿 or *an mo* 按摩 for VaD were found.

Summary of the Clinical Evidence

Three clinical studies were included in this section. One was a randomised controlled trial (RCT) which explored the efficacy of

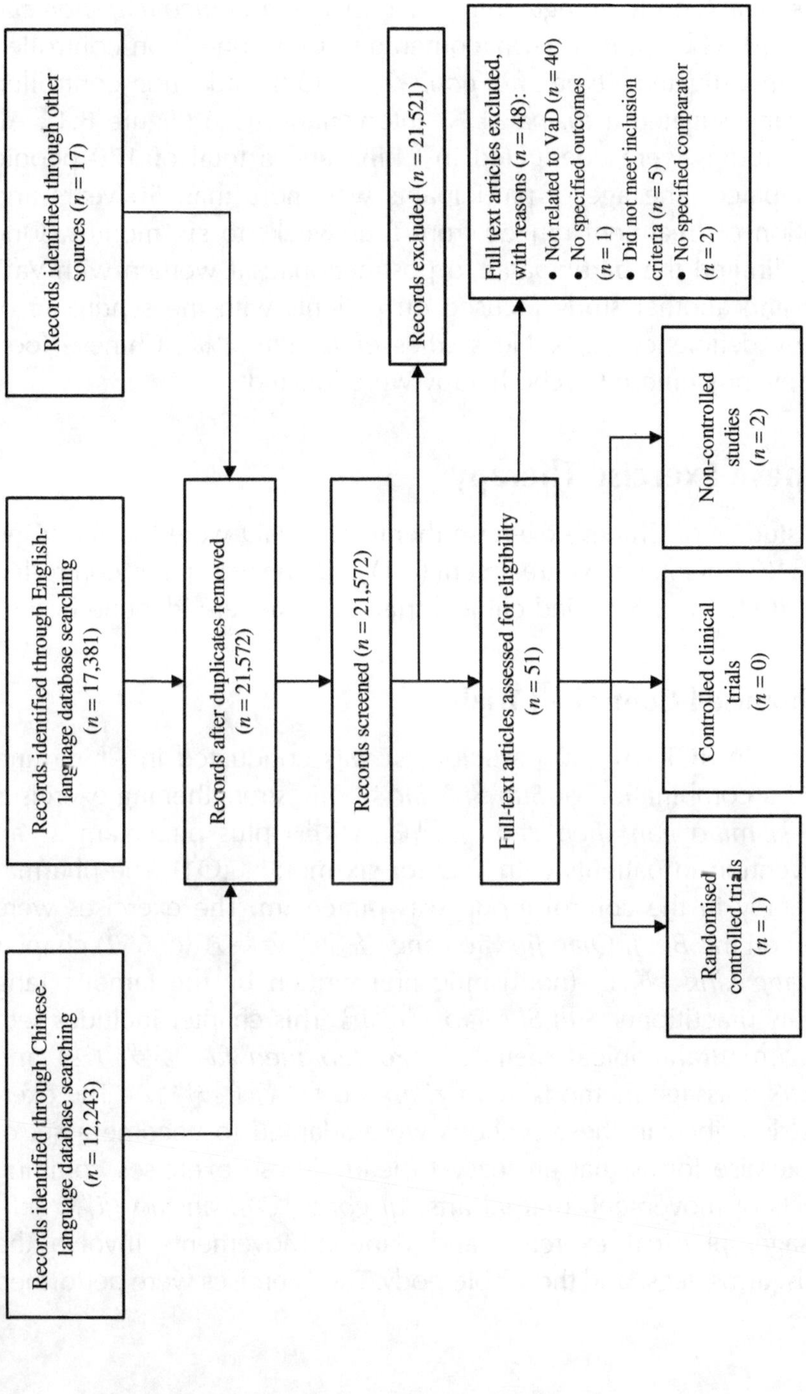

Figure 8.1 Flow Chart of Study Selection Process: Other Chinese Medicine Therapies

Sun si miao's body strengthening exercises (*Sun si miao jian shen cao* 孙思邈健身操) plus pharmacotherapy (O1), one non-controlled study investigated a type of *qi gong* 气功 (O2), and a non-controlled study investigated a *tui na* 推拿 intervention (O3) (Figure 8.1). All three studies were conducted in China and a total of 170 people participated. The age of participants was more than 50 years and duration of treatment ranged from four weeks to six months. One study limited the participants to postmenopausal women with VaD (O2) and another study focused on patients with the syndrome of Kidney deficiency (O3). No studies of *tai chi* 太极, Chinese food therapy, or Chinese psychotherapy were located.

Chinese Exercise Therapy

Two studies of Chinese exercise therapy for VaD were located. One was a RCT of integrative treatment (O1) and one was a non-controlled study (O2). No controlled clinical trials (CCTs) were identified.

Randomised Controlled Trials

The single RCT (n = 80 participants) was conducted in China and tested a combination of *Sun Si Miao*'s body strengthening exercises (*Sun si miao jian shen cao* 孙思邈健身操) plus piracetam as an intervention in patients with VaD for six months (O1). The pharmacotherapy in the control group was piracetam. The exercises were based on the *Bei Ji Qian Jin Yao Fang* 备急千金要方 (c. 652) chapter on *yang xing* 养性 (nourishing life) written by the famous Tang dynasty practitioner *Sun Si Miao* 孙思邈. This chapter includes sections on 'Brahmanical methods' (*Po luo men fa* 婆罗门法) and '*Laozi*'s massage methods' (*Lao zi an mo fa* 老子按摩法). The exercises described in these sections were adapted to become a set of 26 exercise forms that are easy to learn. These exercises combine aspects of movement, martial arts, *qi gong* 气功, *an mo* 按摩, self-massage, physical exercise, and dance. Movements involve the hands, arms, legs, and the whole body. The exercises were performed once a day for an hour each time. The efficacy of this trial was evaluated based on the Mini-Mental State Examination (MMSE) and activities of daily living (ADL).

Risk of Bias

Although the study was described as 'randomised', the method for sequence generation (SG) was not described nor was there any information on allocation concealment, so it was judged 'unclear' risk. It was assessed as having 'high' risk of bias in terms of blinding of participants and personnel and 'unclear' risk in terms of blinding of outcome assessors. As all data on the outcomes were available, the study was assessed as 'low' risk for incomplete outcome data. For selective outcome reporting, the study was assessed as having 'unclear' risk as no protocol was identified.

Results

Data suitable for analysis were available for the MMSE and ADL 'lower is better' scale.

Mini-Mental State Examination

At the end of six months of treatment, a significant benefit based on MMSE scores was found when *Sun Si Miao*'s body strengthening exercises were combined with piracetam (MD: 2.80, [1.43, 4.17]) versus piracetam alone (O1).

Activities of Daily Living

An ADL scale (14 items) whereby lower scores represented more improvement was used in this study. At the end of treatment, there was a significant difference between groups in ADL scores in favour of the combination of piracetam plus *Sun Si Miao*'s body strengthening exercises (MD: –4.10 [–6.46, –1.74]) (O1).

Non-controlled Studies

One non-controlled study assessed the efficacy of a form of *qi gong* 气功 called *Hui chun gong* 回春功 for VaD (O2). While there are a number of different types of *qi gong* 气功 that use the name *Hui chun gong* 回春功, the *Hui chun gong* 回春功 used in this study is a modern form of *qi gong* 气功 that was developed specially for postmenopausal women. It is a standing *qi gong* 气功 that involves six stages: (1) Adopting the basic horse stance posture with breathing and relaxation; (2) stretching various body parts; (3) visualising calmness; (4) progressive shaking of the abdomen, internal organs, muscles, and the whole body; (5) rotational movements of the shoulders; and (6) raising the arms above the head, then slowly lowering the arms with the palms together to conclude the set of exercises.

Results

The method described above was tested in 32 postmenopausal women with VaD who performed *Hui chun gong* 回春功 twice a day (O2). The outcome measure was an effective rate scale developed for dementia.[11] The study reported that the total effective rate was 87.6% after 4 weeks of treatment and most of the patients showed improved clinical symptoms. Statistical analysis was not conducted. In addition, measures of serum homocysteine and beta-amyloid showed reductions after treatment.

Safety of Chinese Exercise Therapy

Adverse events were not mentioned in the single RCT (O1) or in the non-controlled study (O2).

Chinese Remedial Massage Therapy

No RCTs or CCTs of Chinese remedial massage for VaD were found and only one non-controlled study was found. This study (O3) tested *tui na* 推拿, plus psychosocial support, and cognitive training in 58 patients with VaD for two months. Participants were required to have Kidney deficiency syndrome as the focus of the *tui na* 推拿 was on this syndrome as well as on VaD.

The *tui na* 推拿 method involved multiple stages and techniques as follows:

1. Press and roll (*an rou* 按揉) on the points: GV20 *Baihui* 百会, GB5 *Xuanlu* 悬颅, and the mastoid process, then apply separating-pushing (*fen tui* 分推) from EX-HN3 *Yintang* 印堂 to EX-HN5 *Taiyang* 太阳 to open the Orifices and arouse the Spirit (*kai qiao xing shen* 开窍醒神).
2. Knead (*ti na* 提拿) the GB21 *Jianjing* 肩井 area and the neck, then press hard on GB20 *Fengchi* 风池 and GV16 *Fengfu* 风府 to expel wind and transform phlegm (*qu feng hua tan* 祛风化痰).
3. Apply finger pressure (*dian an* 点按) to BL18 *Ganshu* 肝俞, BL19 *Danshu* 胆俞, BL23 *Shenshu* 肾俞, Ex-B7 *Yaoyan* 腰眼, BL54 *Zhibian* 秩边, and SP6 *Sanyinjiao* 三阴交 to nourish and tonify Liver and Kidney (*zi bu gan shen* 滋补肝肾), replenish essence, and nourish Marrow (*tian jing yi sui* 填精益髓).
4. Knead 提拿 the three *yin* and the three *yang* channels of the arm and leg. Press and roll (*an rou* 按揉) on ST31 *Biguan* 髀关, ST34 *Liangqiu* 梁丘, BL36 *Chengfu* 承扶, ST36 *Zusanli* 足三里, and ST40 *Fenglong* 丰隆 to course the channels, unblock the collaterals (*tong jing huo luo* 通经活络), and harmonise the circulation of *qi* and Blood (*tiao he qi xue* 调和气血).
5. Vigorously rub (*cuo yun* 搓运) along both sides of the spine (i.e., the *jia ji* point area 夹脊部) and the middle of the back to tonify the Kidney and nourish *qi* (*bu shen yi qi* 补肾益气) as well as transform phlegm and course the collaterals (*hua tan tong luo* 化痰通络).

The psychosocial support included explaining their condition and treatments to the patients, providing reassurance and care, and providing social support, including cultural activities and music.

The cognitive training involved memory training, arithmetic calculation, orientation training, and exercises that involved comprehension and reasoning.

Results

The effectiveness of the treatment was assessed using three self-made effective rate criteria for dementia, stroke, and Kidney deficiency. At the end of treatment, the total effective rate was over 90% on each of these criteria (O3).

Safety of Chinese Remedial Massage Therapy

The single included study did not mention adverse events.

Clinical Evidence for Other Chinese Medicine Therapies

Of the various other CM therapies used for VaD that were mentioned in Chapter 2 based on the guidelines and textbooks, clinical studies were located for one type of *dao yin yang sheng gong* 导引养生功 called *Sun Si Miao*'s body strengthening exercises (*Sun si miao jian shen cao* 孙思邈健身操), one type of *qi gong* 气功 (*Hui chun gong* 回春功), and a remedial massage intervention using *tui na* 推拿.

No studies of *tai chi* 太极, food therapy, or other CM therapies for VaD were located. However, one RCT of *tai chi* 太极 has been conducted on people with Alzheimer's disease[12] and another RCT investigated *tai chi* 太极 and the game mahjong (*ma jiang* 麻將) in people with dementia of various types.[13]

Summary of the Evidence for Other Chinese Medicine Therapies

Only three studies of other CM therapies for VaD met the inclusion and exclusion criteria. A single RCT found that *Sun Si Miao*'s body strengthening exercises combined with piracetam improved scores on the MMSE and ADL after 6 months of treatment compared to piracetam without an exercise program (O1). As only one non-blinded study was available, no conclusions can be made regarding the efficacy of this set of exercises in the treatment of

VaD. A non-randomised study of another Chinese exercise treatment, *Hui chun gong* 回春功, also reported improvements in dementia symptoms after four weeks of performing the exercises (O2). However, as there was no control group, the effectiveness of this intervention could not be evaluated.

For Chinese massage, a single non-controlled study was available (O3). This study reported that *tui na* 推拿 combined with psychosocial support and cognitive training improved the symptoms of dementia, stroke, and Kidney deficiency syndrome based on a self-made effective rate criteria. However, because other interventions were used in addition to *tui na* 推拿, there were no control groups, and the outcome measures were not validated, it was not possible to assess the efficacy of the *tui na* 推拿 massage method.

Overall, the findings based on studies of other Chinese therapies are encouraging, but the evidence is insufficient for firm conclusions to be made regarding their effectiveness and safety. Reviews of multiple studies of various exercise therapies have shown benefits in terms of ADL but not cognition in people with dementia[1] as well as cognitive benefits in people with mild cognitive impairment (MCI) but not in people with dementia.[14,15] In addition, a recent study found that long-term exercise using an exercise bike for at least 15 minutes a day for 15 months improved memory and neuropsychiatric symptoms in people with dementia.[16] *Tui na* 推拿 has been reported to improve symptoms in people with Alzheimer's disease[17] and other massage therapies have also reportedly benefited people with dementia in nursing homes.[18,19] Therefore, it is plausible that Chinese exercise and massage therapies could benefit people with VaD, provided that (1) patients' physical disability is not too severe so that they can safely perform the exercises and (2) patients are not severely cognitively impaired so they can learn the exercises.[20, 21] In such cases, Chinese remedial massage (*tui na* 推拿, *an mo* 按摩) could be used as a complementary measure for people with relatively mild VaD and varying degrees of disability, but the methods need to be adjusted to the needs of the individual. Nevertheless, more studies are needed to adequately assess the effects of these interventions in VaD.

References

1. Forbes D, Forbes SC, Blake CM, Thiessen EJ, *et al.* (2015) Exercise programs for people with dementia. *Cochrane Database Syst Rev* **4**:CD006489.
2. Groot C, Hooghiemstra AM, Raijmakers PG, *et al.* (2016) The effect of physical activity on cognitive function in patients with dementia: A meta-analysis of randomized control trials. *Ageing Res Rev* **25**:13–23.
3. Aarsland D, Sardahaee FS, Anderssen S, Ballard C, *et al.* (2010) Is physical activity a potential preventive factor for vascular dementia? A systematic review. *Aging Ment Health* **14**(4):386–395.
4. Cheng FK. (2015) Effects of baduanjin on mental health: A comprehensive review. *J Bodyw Mov Ther* **19**(1):138–149.
5. Zheng G, Huang M, Li S, *et al.* (2016) Effect of baduanjin exercise on cognitive function in older adults with mild cognitive impairment: Study protocol for a randomised controlled trial. *BMJ Open* **6**(4): e010602.
6. Chen MC, Liu HE, Huang HY, Chiou AF. (2012) The effect of a simple traditional exercise programme (baduanjin exercise) on sleep quality of older adults: A randomized controlled trial. *Int J Nurs Stud* **49**(3):265–273.
7. Zheng GH, Fang QY, Chen B, Yi HM, *et al.* (2015) Qualitative evaluation of baduanjin (traditional Chinese *qi gong*) on health promotion among an elderly community population at risk for ischemic stroke. *Evid Based Complement Alternat Med* **2015**:893215.
8. Xiao CM, Yang YQ, Zhuang YC. (2016) Effect of health *qi gong ba duan jin* on blood pressure of individuals with essential hypertension. *J Am Geriatr Soc* **64**(1):211–213.
9. Viggo Hansen N, Jorgensen T, Ortenblad L. (2006) Massage and touch for dementia. *Cochrane Database Syst Rev* (4):CD004989.
10. Moyle W, Murfield JE, O'Dwyer S, Van Wyk S. (2013) The effect of massage on agitated behaviours in older people with dementia: A literature review. *J Clin Nurs* **22**(5–6):601–610.
11. 郑筱萸. (2012) 中药新药临床研究指导原则. 北京: 中国医药科技出版社.
12. 谢多英. (2002) 体育疗法配合常规药物治疗痴呆精神行为症状的疗效观察. 中国民康医学. **24**(7):824–826.
13. Cheng ST, Chow PK, Song YQ, Yu ECS, *et al.* (2014) Can leisure activities slow dementia progression in nursing home residents? A cluster-randomized controlled trial. *Int Psychogeriatr* **26**(4):637–643.

14. Ohman H, Savikko N, Strandberg TE, Pitkala KH. (2014) Effect of physical exercise on cognitive performance in older adults with mild cognitive impairment or dementia: A systematic review. *Dement Geriatr Cogn Disord* **38**(5–6):347–365.
15. Zheng G, Xia R, Zhou W, Tao J, *et al.* (2016) Aerobic exercise ameliorates cognitive function in older adults with mild cognitive impairment: A systematic review and meta-analysis of randomised controlled trials. *Br J Sports Med* **50**(23):1443–1450.
16. Cancela JM, Ayan C, Varela S, Seijo M. (2016) Effects of a long-term aerobic exercise intervention on institutionalized patients with dementia. *J Sci Med Sport* **19**(4):293–298.
17. 黄霖. (1994) 点穴按摩治疗老年性痴呆临床观察. 按摩与导引. **4**:5–6.
18. Moyle W, Cooke ML, Beattie E, Shum DH, *et al.* (2014) Foot massage versus quiet presence on agitation and mood in people with dementia: A randomised controlled trial. *Int J Nurs Stud* **51**(6):856–864.
19. Harris M, Richards KC, Grando VT. (2012) The effects of slow-stroke back massage on minutes of nighttime sleep in persons with dementia and sleep disturbances in the nursing home: A pilot study. *J Holist Nurs* **30**(4):255–263.
20. Tadros G, Ormerod S, Dobson-Smyth P, *et al.* (2013) The management of behavioural and psychological symptoms of dementia in residential homes: Does *tai chi* have any role for people with dementia? *Dementia (London).* **12**(2):268–279.
21. Yao L, Giordani B, Alexander NB. (2008) Developing a positive emotion-motivated *tai chi* (pem-tc) exercise program for older adults with dementia. *Res Theory Nurs Pract* **22**(4):241–255.

List of Clinical Studies Included in Chapter 8

Study Number	References
O1	马学文, 刘万斌, 石新燕, 胡利勋. (2010) 孙思邈健身法对血管性痴呆康复的临床研究. 中国民康医学. 现代中医药. **30**(6):63–64.
O2	姬爱冬，柯冬云，邹缄. (2010) 气功对绝经后血管性痴呆患者HCY, Aβ干预作用的临床观察. 长春中医药大学学报. **26**(2):189–190.
O3	林超. (1999) 推拿治疗肾虚型中风痴呆58例临床观察. 河北中医. **21**(5):301.

9

Clinical Evidence for Combination Therapies

OVERVIEW

Two or more types of therapy are often used in combination in the clinical practice of Chinese medicine. Twenty randomised controlled trials, which used combinations of Chinese medicine therapies, were included. The most common combination therapy was Chinese herbal medicine combined with acupuncture or scalp acupuncture and one study also included rehabilitation therapy. The results showed that some combination interventions may be beneficial.

Introduction

Combination therapies are defined as two or more Chinese medicine (CM) interventions administered together, such as Chinese herbal medicine (CHM) and acupuncture. A previous systematic review of CHM combined with acupuncture for vascular dementia (VaD) included 17 studies and analysed data based on effective rate. The review found that combination therapies were more effective than control treatments comprising a variety of single therapy interventions.[1]

Randomised Controlled Trials of Combination Therapies

Our searches located 20 randomised controlled trials (RCTs) of CM combination therapy for VaD (Figure 9.1). Orally administered CHM

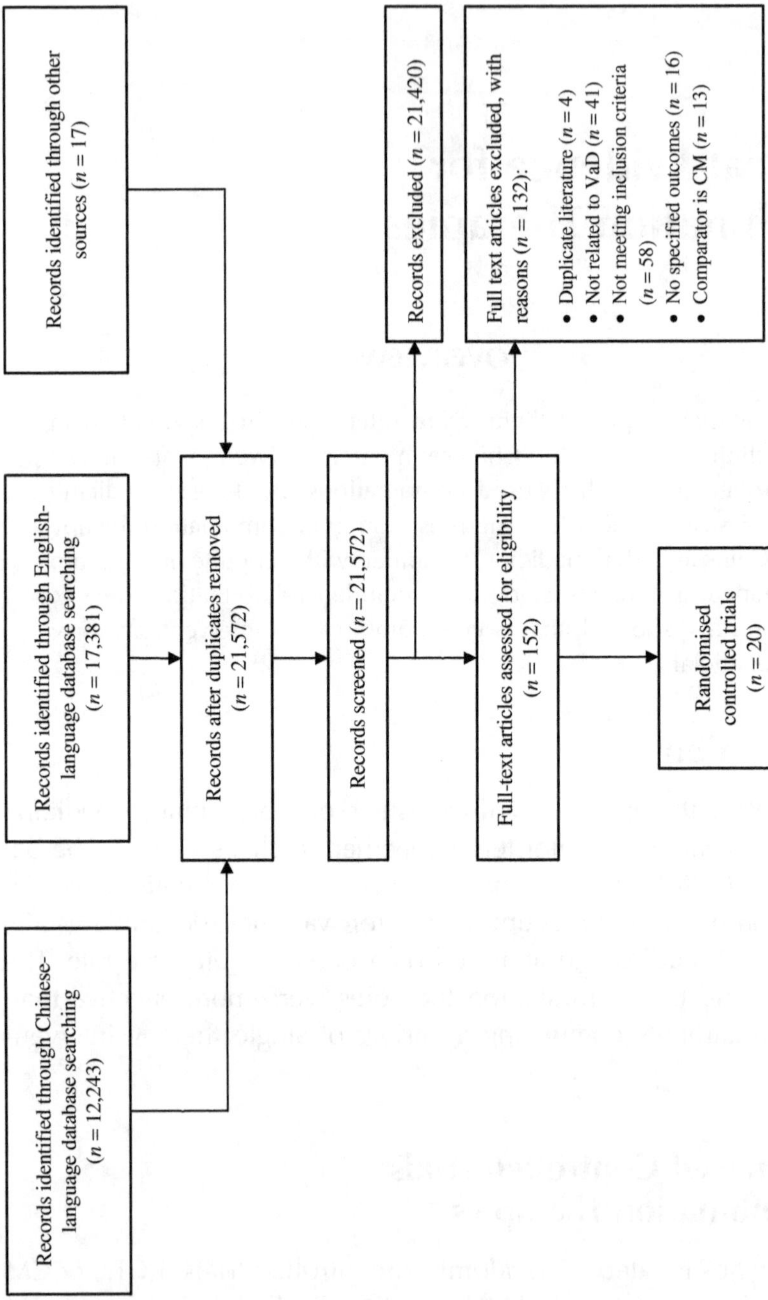

Figure 9.1 Flow Chart of Study Selection Process: Combination Therapies

Table 9.1 Summary of Combination Therapy Interventions

Combination Therapy Interventions	No. of Studies	Included Studies
CHM plus acupuncture*	14	C1–C14
CHM plus acupuncture* plus pharmacotherapy	4	C15–C18
CHM plus scalp acupuncture	1	C19
CHM plus scalp electro-acupuncture plus pharmacotherapy	1	C20
CHM plus acupuncture plus rehabilitation therapy	1	C8

*Including electro-acupuncture and acupuncture plus moxibustion. Abbreviations: CHM, Chinese herbal medicine.

plus acupuncture was investigated in 14 RCTs (C1–C14), one of which also used moxibustion (C14). Four RCTs used an integrative approach that combined CHM plus acupuncture with a pharmacotherapy (C15–C18), one of which combined the acupuncture with moxibustion (C18). Two RCTs tested oral CHM plus scalp acupuncture using modern scalp zones (C19, C20), one of which combined scalp electro-acupuncture with a pharmacotherapy (C20). One study tested various combinations of CHM, acupuncture, and rehabilitation therapy (C8) (Table 9.1).

One three-armed study used CHM plus acupuncture, huperzine A, and no pharmacological intervention for VaD (C3). Another four-armed study used CHM plus acupuncture, CHM plus rehabilitation therapy, CHM plus acupuncture plus rehabilitation therapy, and piracetam (C8). All the studies were conducted in China.

Risk of Bias

All of the 20 studies located were described as 'randomised', but only five described an appropriate method for sequence generation (SG). Two used the order in which patients visited, which is an inappropriate method. Thus, these were judged as 'high' risk for this item (Table 9.2). No study mentioned allocation concealment. Nineteen studies made no mention of blinding and one study used blinding of participants but only for the two test groups and not for the control (C1). Therefore, all

Table 9.2 Risk of Bias of Randomised Controlled Trials: Combination Therapies

Risk of Bias Domain	Low Risk *n* (%)	Unclear Risk *n* (%)	High Risk *n* (%)
Sequence generation	5 (25)	13 (65)	2 (10)
Allocation concealment	0 (0)	20 (100)	0 (0)
Blinding of participants	0 (0)	0 (0)	20 (100)
Blinding of personnel*	0 (0)	0 (0)	20 (100)
Blinding of outcome assessor	0 (0)	0 (0)	20 (100)
Incomplete outcome data	20 (100)	0 (0)	0 (0)
Selective reporting	0 (0)	20 (100)	0 (0)

*Blinding of personnel (acupuncturists) is challenging in manual therapies.

studies were assessed as having 'high' risk of bias in terms of blinding of participants, personnel, and outcome assessors. All studies were assessed as 'low' risk of bias for incomplete outcome data since drop-outs were few and balanced between groups. No protocols were identified for any included studies (either in electronic databases or clinical trial registers), but all reported data for the outcomes specified in the methods section, so all studies were assessed as having 'unclear' risk of bias for selective reporting. Overall, the methodological reporting was inadequate, so results should be interpreted with caution as none of the studies were free from potential bias.

Oral Chinese Herbal Medicine plus Acupuncture Therapy

Eighteen RCTs that investigated combinations of orally administered CHM plus acupuncture at traditional points were located. A total of 1,379 people enrolled in the intervention and control groups. Four of these studies used integrative medicine. In most studies, the mean ages of participants were between 55 and 75 years, but in one study the participants had mean ages of 42–45 years (C3). Treatment durations ranged from four to 12 weeks.

All studies used pharmacotherapy as a control and one study also included a comparison group which did not receive a pharmacotherapy for VaD (C3). The pharmacotherapies used in the control groups included donepezil, huperzine A, nimodipine, piracetam, oxiracetam, citicoline, co-dergocrine mesylate, and cerebroprotein hydrolysate. Studies that used almitrine-raubasine, which has been discontinued for dementia, were excluded.

Outcome measures included the Mini-Mental State Examination (MMSE), Alzheimer's Disease Assessment Scale — cognitive subscale (ADAS-cog), Hasegawa Dementia Scale (HDS), activities of daily living (ADL), Blessed Dementia Scale (BDS), and Blessed Behaviour Scale (BBS). Meta-analysis results are reported separately for the comparison with no pharmacotherapy, specific pharmacotherapies, and the integrative medicine studies.

Syndromes

Nine of the studies reported on CM syndromes. The four most frequently mentioned syndromes were:

- Turbid phlegm obstructing the Orifices 痰浊阻窍/痰浊蒙窍: 2 studies.
- Spleen and Kidney dual deficiency 脾肾两虚: 2 studies.
- *Qi* and Blood dual deficiency 气血亏虚: 2 studies.
- Kidney deficiency with Blood stasis 肾虚血瘀: 2 studies.

Frequently Used Herbs and Acupuncture Points

Two studies used the CHM formula *Huang di san ke li* 黄地散颗粒 combined with similar groups of acupuncture points (C1, C2). The other studies each used different CHMs. The most frequently used herbs in the formulae were *dan shen* 丹参, *shi chang pu* 石菖蒲, *di huang* 地黄 (mainly *shu di* 熟地), *chuan xiong* 川芎, *huang qi* 黄芪, and *gou qi zi* 枸杞子 (Table 9.3).

The most frequently used acupuncture points were GV20 *Baihui* 百会, EX-HN1 *Sishencong* 四神聪, ST36 *Zusanli* 足三里, SP6 *Sanyinjiao* 三阴交, KI3 *Taixi* 太溪, and GV26 *Shuigou* 水沟 (also known as *Renzhong* 人中).

Table 9.3. Acupuncture Points and Herbs Frequently Used in the Combined Interventions

Point Name	Frequency	Herb Name	Scientific Name of Herb	Frequency
GV20 *Baihui* 百会	16	*Dan shen* 丹参	*Salvia miltiorrhiza* Bge.	14
Ex-HN1 *Sishencong* 四神聪	12	*Shi chang pu* 石菖蒲	*Acorus tatarinowii* Schott.	10
ST36 *Zusanli* 足三里	9	*Di huang* 地黄	*Rehmannia glutinosa* Libosch.	10[2]
SP6 *Sanyinjiao* 三阴交	9	*Chuan xiong* 川芎	*Ligusticum chuanxiong* Hort.	8
KI3 *Taixi* 太溪	7	*Huang qi* 黄芪	*Astragalus membranaceus* (Fisch.) Bge.	7
GV26 *Shuigou* 水沟	7	*Gou qi zi* 枸杞子	*Lycium barbarum* L.	7
ST40 *Fenglong* 丰隆	6	*Shan zhu yu* 山茱萸	*Cornus officinalis* Sieb. et Zucc.	6
GB20 *Fengchi* 风池	6	*He shou wu* 何首乌	*Polygonum multiflorum* Thunb.	6
GV24 *Shenting* 神庭	6	—	—	—

Notes: (1) The use of some herbs may be restricted in some countries. Readers are advised to comply with relevant regulations and (2) *Shu di huang* 熟地黄 = 7, *sheng di huang* 生地黄 = 1, *di huang* 地黄 = 2.

Chinese Herbal Medicine plus Acupuncture vs. No Treatment

The single three-armed RCT included a comparison between a group (n = 20 participants) who received CHM plus acupuncture for four weeks and a group (n = 20 participants) who received no CHM or acupuncture treatment. Both groups received usual supportive care (C3).

The people in the CHM plus acupuncture group were all identified as having Kidney deficiency with phlegm turbidity and Blood stasis (*shen xu tan yu* 肾虚痰瘀). They received an unnamed herbal decoction for 'tonifying Kidney, mobilizing Blood, and dispelling phlegm' (*bu shen hua xue qu tan* 补肾活血祛痰) composed of *ba ji tian* 巴戟天, *tu si zi* 菟丝子, *ge gen* 葛根, *dan shen* 丹参, *shi chang pu* 石菖蒲, *tian zhu huang* 天竺黄, *shan zha* 山楂, *di long*

地龙, *gan cao* 甘草, and other herbs. They also received acupuncture at EX-HN1 *Sishencong* 四神聪, GV20 *Baihui* 百会, BL23 *Shenshu* 肾俞, SP10 *Xuehai* 血海, KI3 *Taixi* 太溪, SP6 *Sanyinjiao* 三阴交, ST36 *Zusanli* 足三里, and ST40 *Fenglong* 丰隆 every day for four weeks. At the end of treatment, there were significant improvements in the CM combination therapy group based on the MMSE (mean difference (MD): 10.20 [8.16, 12.24]), HDS (MD: 3.50 [2.24, 4.76]) and 'higher is better' ADL scores (standardised mean difference (SMD): 0.88 [0.23, 1.53]). The authors reported that there were no obvious adverse reactions.

Chinese Herbal Medicine plus Acupuncture vs. Pharmacotherapy

Fourteen RCTs compared the combination of oral CHM plus acupuncture with specific pharmacotherapies. Two of these studies used electro-acupuncture (C5, C7) and one study added moxibustion (C14). Five of the oral CHM interventions were not named and each of the named oral CHM interventions was different. The results of the meta-analyses are subgrouped according to the pharmacotherapies.

Mini-Mental State Examination

Thirteen studies reported data for the MMSE at the end of treatment (Table 9.4). The two studies that compared the CHM *Huang di san ke li* 黄地散颗粒 (main ingredients: *huang jing* 黄精, *shu di huang* 熟地黄, and other herbs) plus acupuncture with donepezil reported that there was a significant improvement in the combination groups relative to the controls (MD: 3.87 [1.99, 5.75], $I^2 = 0\%$) after 12 weeks of treatment. One of these studies also reported a significant difference at the six-month follow-up (MD: 3.68 [1.32, 6.04]) (C1). Significant benefits also were found for multiple studies comparing CHM plus acupuncture to huperzine A, piracetam, and co-dergocrine mesylate (Table 9.4). The total pool of 13 studies, that ranged in duration from four to 12 weeks, found a significant increase in MMSE outcomes in the CHM plus acupuncture groups compared

Table 9.4 Chinese Herbal Medicine plus Acupuncture vs. Pharmacotherapy: Mini-Mental State Examination at the End of Treatment

Pharmacotherapy	No. of Studies (Participants), Duration	Effect Size (MD [95% CI], I^2)	Included Studies
Donepezil	2 (68), 12 wks	3.87 [1.99, 5.75]*, 0%	C1, C2
Huperzine A	2 (100), 4 wks	4.00 [–3.15, 11.16], 97%	C3, C4
Nimodipine plus citicoline	1 (136), 4 wks	2.43 [0.82, 4.04]*	C5
Nimodipine plus piracetam	1 (56), 12 wks	1.20 [–0.19, 2.59]	C6
Piracetam	4 (311), 4–12 wks	1.12 [0.18, 2.05]*, 24%	C7–C10
Piracetam plus cerebroprotein hydrolysate	1 (76), 12 wks	3.58 [1.84, 5.32]*	C11
Co-dergocrine mesylate	2 (260), 4–8 wks	2.08 [0.64, 3.52]*, 89%	C12, C13
Total pool	13 (1,007), 4–12 wks	2.49 [1.59, 3.38]*, 80%	All above

*Statistically significant. Abbreviations: CI, confidence interval; MD, mean difference; wks, weeks.

to pharmacotherapy controls (MD: 2.49 [1.59, 3.38] I^2 = 80%); however, heterogeneity was substantial. In the sensitivity analysis of four studies (n = 204 participants) judged as 'low' risk of bias for SG, the significant difference remained with reduced heterogeneity (MD: 2.91 [1.26, 4.57], I^2 = 71%) (C1, C2, C11, C13).

Alzheimer's Disease Assessment Scale — Cognitive Subscale

One study provided data for the ADAS-cog in addition to the MMSE. This was a three-armed 12-week study (19 participants per group) with a six-month follow-up that compared acupuncture vs. donepezil (5 mg/day) vs. a combination of acupuncture and CHM (C1). All participants were required to have dual deficiency of *qi* and Blood (*qi xue kui xu* 气血亏虚) as a syndrome. The intervention in the combination therapy group (n = 19 participants) was *Huang di san ke li* 黄地散颗粒 plus acupuncture at the main points of CV17 *Danzhong* 膻中, CV12 *Zhongwan* 中脘, CV6 *Qihai* 气海, SP10

Xuehai 血海, ST36 *Zusanli* 足三里, TE5 *Waiguan* 外关, EX-HN1 *Sishencong* 四神聪, and GV20 *Baihui* 百会, with the addition of points based on syndrome differentiation (see details in Chapter 7).

Participants in the combination therapy group received acupuncture plus CHM plus a placebo for donepezil. Control group participants received donepezil plus a CHM placebo. At the end of 12-weeks treatment, there was a significant improvement in ADAS-cog scores (MD: –3.00 [–5.27, –0.73]) in the combination group compared to donepezil, and there was a similar result at a follow-up after six months (MD: –3.21 [–5.91, –0.51]). The result for the acupuncture-only group was not significant (see Chapter 7). This study was judged as 'low' risk of bias for SG. Four participants in the combination therapy group dropped out due to gastrointestinal disturbances arising from CHM, which the authors believed was due to the combination of *huang jing* 黄精 and *shu di huang* 熟地黄 being unsuitable for some people. Three people in the donepezil group died during the study, but there was no mention of the causes of death. It was also unclear whether intent-to-treat analysis was used.

Hasegawa Dementia Scale

Three studies using different pharmacotherapy controls each reported data for the HDS (Table 9.5).

In one study, the combination therapy (described above) was superior to huperzine A plus folic acid and vitamin B6 (C3). In another study (C14) that used a comparison with nimodipine, there was no significant difference between nimodipine and the combination therapy group. The combination therapy used two alternating groups of acupuncture points daily: (1) GV26 *Shuigou* 水沟, EX-HN1 *Sishencong* 四神聪, GV24 *Shenting* 神庭, GB13 *Benshen* 本神, ST36 *Zusanli* 足三里, KI3 *Taixi* 太溪, GB39 *Xuanzhong* 悬钟; and (2) GV20 *Baihui* 百会, GV14 *Dazhui* 大椎, GV4 *Mingmen* 命门, BL18 *Ganshu* 肝俞, and BL23 *Shenshu* 肾俞, with moxa added to limb points, plus a decoction of *lu rong* 鹿茸, *ren shen* 人参, *huang jing* 黄精, *gou qi zi* 枸杞子, *yi zhi ren* 益智仁, *dan shen* 丹参, and other herbs three times a day for eight weeks.

Table 9.5 Chinese Herbal Medicine plus Acupuncture vs. Pharmacotherapy: Hasegawa Dementia Scale at the End of Treatment

Pharmacotherapy	No. of Studies (Participants), Duration	Effect Size (MD [95% CI], I^2%)	Included Studies
Huperzine A (with folic acid and vitamin B6)	1 (40), 4 wks	2.10 [0.70, 3.50]*	C3
Nimodipine	1 (60), 8 wks	1.70 [–1.15, 4.55]	C14
Piracetam	1 (60), 12 wks	1.63 [–0.34, 3.60]	C9
Total pool	2 (160), 4–12 wks	1.91 [0.85, 2.97]*, 0%	All above

*Statistically significant. Abbreviations: CI, confidence interval; MD, mean difference; wks, weeks.

The result was similar for a study of combination therapy vs. piracetam (C9), which used a decoction of *shu di* 熟地, *shan zhu yu* 山茱萸, *gou qi zi* 枸杞子, *yuan zhi* 远志, *he shou wu* 何首乌, *dang gui* 当归, *bai shao* 白芍, *shi chang pu* 石菖蒲, *dan shen* 丹参, *chao zao ren* 炒枣仁, *sheng mu li* 生牡蛎, and other herbs according to syndrome plus acupuncture at EX-HN1 *Sishencong* 四神聪, GB20 *Fengchi* 风池, GV20 *Baihui* 百会, GV26 *Shuigou* 水沟, SP6 *Sanyinjiao* 三阴交, GB39 *Xuanzhong* 悬钟, LR3 *Taichong* 太冲, BL18 *Ganshu* 肝俞, KI3 *Taixi* 太溪, and BL23 *Shenshu* 肾俞, for 30 minutes a day and five times a week.

For the pool of three studies, there was a significant difference between groups in favour of combination therapy with no heterogeneity (MD: 1.91 [0.85, 2.97], $I^2 = 0$). None of the studies were judged as 'low' risk of bias for SG.

Activities of Daily Living

The ability to carry out daily living activities was assessed in seven studies using scales on which lower scores indicate higher levels of functioning ('lower is better') (Table 9.6). The pool of two studies that compared combination therapy with donepezil showed a significant improvement in the combination therapy groups. There was a similar

Table 9.6 Chinese Herbal Medicine plus Acupuncture vs. Pharmacotherapy: 'Lower is Better' Activities of Daily Living at the End of Treatment

Pharmacotherapy	No. of Studies (Participants), Duration	Effect Size (SMD [95% CI], I^2)	Included Studies
Donepezil	2 (68), 12 wks	–0.76 [–1.26, –0.27]*, 0%	C1, C2
Nimodipine plus piracetam	1 (56), 12 wks	–0.21 [–0.77, 0.34]	C6
Piracetam	2 (196), 4–2 wks	–0.58 [–0.86, –0.29]*, 0%	C7, C9
Piracetam plus cerebroprotein hydrolysate	1 (76), 12 wks	–0.21 [–0.67, 0.24]	C11
Co-dergocrine mesylate	1 (60), 8 wks	–0.00 [–0.51, 0.50]	C13
Total pool	7 (456), 4–12 wks	–0.42 [–0.64, –0.21]*, 19%	All above

*Statistically significant. Abbreviations: CI, confidence interval; SMD, standardised mean difference; wks, weeks.

significant benefit in the pool of two comparisons with piracetam, but none of the other comparisons showed significant differences. The total pool of seven studies with durations ranging from four to 12 weeks showed a significant difference between the combination therapy and pharmacotherapy groups (SMD: –0.42 [–0.64, –0.21], $I^2 = 19\%$). In the sensitivity analysis of four studies judged as 'low' risk of bias for SG ($n = 204$ participants), the significant difference remained with moderate heterogeneity (SMD: –0.36 [–0.72, 0.00], $I^2 = 38\%$) (C1, C2, C11, C13). No studies reported data using 'higher is better' ADL scales.

Blessed Dementia Scale

One study reported data for the BDS (C5). The combination of *Fu zhi tang* 复智汤 (main ingredients: *Ren shen* 人参, *lu jiao jiao* 鹿角胶, *gou qi zi* 枸杞子, *yi zhi ren* 益智仁, *dan shen* 丹参, *huang jing* 黄精, *shan zu yu* 山茱萸, *he shou wu* 何首乌, *shi chang pu* 石菖蒲, *chuan xiong* 川芎, and *niu xi* 牛膝) modified based on syndrome differentiation with electro-acupuncture once a day at GV20 *Baihui* 百会, BL23 *Shenshu* 肾俞, and BL17 *Geshu* 膈俞 was compared with a combination of nimodipine injection plus citicoline

Table 9.7 Chinese Herbal Medicine plus Acupuncture vs. Pharmacotherapy: Blessed Behaviour Scale at the End of Treatment

Pharmacotherapy	No. of Studies (Participants), Duration	Effect Size (MD [95% CI], I^2%)	Included Studies
Piracetam	1 (65), 12 wks	−0.11 [−1.86, 1.64]	C8
Co-dergocrine mesylate	1 (200), 4 wks	−2.67 [−3.01, −2.33]*	C12
Total pool	2 (265), 4–12 wks	−1.54 [−4.03, 0.95], 87%	All above

*Statistically significant. Abbreviations: CI, confidence interval; MD, mean difference; wks, weeks.

injection for four weeks (n = 136 participants). At the end of treatment, there was a significant improvement in the CM combination therapy group (MD: –3.08 [–5.12, –1.04]).

Blessed Behaviour Scale

Two studies reported results based on the BBS (Table 9.7). One study (C8) found that there was no difference between CHM plus acupuncture and piracetam (see integrative medicine below for further details). In the other study (C12), the combination of *Nao kang pian* 脑康片 (main ingredients: *Ren shen* 人参, *ling zhi* 灵芝, *shi chang pu* 石菖蒲, *chuan xiong* 川芎, and *yin yang huo* 淫羊藿, etc.) plus acupuncture at GV20 *Baihui* 百会, KI6 *Zhaohai* 照海, SP6 *Sanyinjiao* 三阴交, PC6 *Neiguan* 内关, GV24 *Shenting* 神庭, KI4 *Dazhong* 大钟, ST36 *Zusanli* 足三里, and HT7 *Shenmen* 神门 for four weeks was superior to co-dergocrine mesylate. The pool of two studies found no significant differences between groups, albeit with substantial heterogeneity (MD: –1.54 [–4.03, 0.95], I^2 = 87%).

Integrative Medicine: Chinese Herbal Medicine plus Acupuncture plus Pharmacotherapy

Four RCTs tested integrative medicine combination therapy in which the control groups received pharmacotherapy and the test groups received the same pharmacotherapy plus CHM and acupuncture

Table 9.8 Integrative Chinese Herbal Medicine plus Acupuncture vs. Pharmacotherapy: Mini-mental State Examination at the End of Treatment

Pharmacotherapy	No. of Studies (Participants), Duration	Effect Size (MD [95% CI], I^2%)	Included Studies
Huperzine A	2 (130), 4–8 wks	3.85 [2.08, 5.62]*, 26%	C15, C16
Oxiracetam plus citicoline	1 (70), 8 wks	3.14 [0.82, 5.46]*	C17
Total pool	3 (200), 4–8 wks	3.69 [2.43, 4.95]*, 0%	All above

*Statistically significant. Abbreviations: CI, confidence interval; MD, mean difference, wks, weeks.

(C15-C18). In one of these studies (C18), acupuncture was combined with stick moxibustion at GV20 *Baihui* 百会. Outcome data were available for the MMSE, HDS, and ADL.

Mini-Mental State Examination

Three integrative studies reported data for the MMSE (Table 9.8). The pool of two studies that combined CHM and acupuncture plus huperzine A found a significant increase in MMSE scores (MD: 3.85 [2.08, 5.62], $I^2 = 26$), with moderate heterogeneity.

One study (C17) that enrolled 70 people with Kidney deficiency, Blood stasis, and phlegm obstruction (*shen xu xue yu tan zu* 肾虚血瘀痰阻) used a combination of *Tong qiao huo xue bu nao tang* 通窍活血补脑汤 (main ingredients: *shi chang pu* 石菖蒲, *yu jin* 郁金, *chuan xiong* 川芎, *ren shen* 人参, *shan zhu yu* 山茱萸, *shu di huang* 熟地黄, *yi zhi ren* 益智仁, *dan shen* 丹参, *dan nan xing* 胆南星, *tu si zi* 菟丝子, *bu gu zhi* 补骨脂, *xian mao* 仙茅, *yin yang huo* 淫羊藿, *shan zhu yu* 山萸肉, *fu ling* 茯苓, *ba ji tian* 巴戟天, *jiu huang qi* 炙黄芪, *he tao ren* 核桃肉, and *di long* 地龙), electro-acupuncture at EX-HN1 *Sishencong* 四神聪, GB20 *Fengchi* 风池, GV20 *Baihui* 百会, ST36 *Zusanli* 足三里, ST40 *Fenglong* 丰隆, and BL20 *Pishu* 脾俞 and oxiracetam capsules plus citicoline injection. They compared this with a combination of the two pharmacotherapies. At the end of 8-weeks treatment, this study reported a significant increase in MMSE scores (MD: 3.14 [0.82, 5.46]) in the integrative medicine group (C17). The total pool of three studies revealed a significant benefit for integrative CM combination therapy groups compared to the pharmacotherapy control groups (MD: 3.69 [2.43, 4.95], $I^2 = 0\%$).

Hasegawa Dementia Scale

Three integrative studies reported outcomes for the HDS (Table 9.9). As in the meta-analysis of the MMSE, the pool of two studies of comparisons with huperzine A found a significant increase in HDS scores in the integrative CHM plus acupuncture groups, however with substantial heterogeneity (MD: 3.89 [0.91, 6.87], $I^2 = 84\%$).

For the comparison with nimodipine plus cerebroprotein hydrolysate injection (C18), the test group included these two pharmacotherapies plus: (1) the CHM *Bu shen xing nao tang* 补肾醒脑汤 with modifications based on syndrome; (2) acupuncture at GV26 *Shuigou* 水沟, GV20 *Baihui* 百会, EX-HN1 *Sishencong* 四神聪, GV24 *Shenting* 神庭, EX-HN3 *Yintang* 印堂, GV16 *Fengfu* 风府, GV14 *Dazhui* 大椎, GV9 *Zhiyang* 至阳, GV8 *Jinsuo* 筋缩, GV4 *Mingmen* 命门, GV3 *Yaoyangguan* 腰阳关, ST40 *Fenglong* 丰隆, SP6 *Sanyinjiao* 三阴交, and KI3 *Taixi* 太溪; and (3) stick moxibustion at GV20 *Baihui* 百会 once a day. After one month, there was a significantly greater increase in HDS scores in the combination therapy

Table 9.9 Integrative Chinese Herbal Medicine plus Acupuncture *vs.* Pharmacotherapy: Hasegawa Dementia Scale at the End of Treatment

Pharmacotherapy	No. of Studies (Participants), Duration	Effect Size (MD [95% CI], I^2%)	Included Studies
Huperzine A	2 (130), 4–8 wks	3.89 [0.91, 6.87]*, 84	C15, C16
Nimodipine plus cerebroprotein hydrolysate	1 (52), 4 wks	3.42 [1.40, 5.44]*	C18
Total Pool	3 (182), 4–8 wks	3.78 [1.90, 5.65]*, 70	All above

*Statistically significant. Abbreviations: CI, confidence interval; MD, mean difference, wks, weeks.

group compared to pharmacotherapy alone (MD: 3.42 [1.40, 5.44], $n = 52$ participants). The total pool of three studies found a significant improvement in the integrative CHM plus acupuncture groups relative to the pharmacotherapy groups (MD: 3.78 [1.90, 5.65], $I^2 = 70\%$). None of the studies were judged as 'low' risk of bias for SG.

Activities of Daily Living

One integrative study reported data for an ADL scale whereby lower scores indicate improvement ('lower is better') (C16). The CHM was *Bu shen huo xue hua tan fang* 补肾活血化痰方, which contained *huang qi* 黄芪, *yi zhi ren* 益智仁, *shan yu rou* 山萸肉, *gou qi zi* 枸杞子, *fu ling* 茯苓, *dan shen* 丹参, *xian ling pi* 仙灵脾, *niu xi* 牛膝, *di long* 地龙, *shi chang pu* 石菖蒲, *sheng di* 生地, *shu di* 熟地, *tu si zi* 菟丝子, *nv zhen zi* 女贞子, *shan yao* 山药, *cao shen qu* 炒神曲, *cao mai ya* 炒麦芽, and *cao shan zha* 炒山楂, with modifications based on syndrome differentiation. This was combined with acupuncture five times a week at GV20 *Baihui* 百会, GV26 *Renzhong* 人中, and HT7 *Shenmen* 神门 plus huperzine A. The control group received huperzine A alone. After 4 weeks of treatment, there was a significant improvement in the integrative CHM group (SMD: –0.61 [–1.18, –0.04], $n = 50$ participants) compared to the group that received huperzine A alone.

Another integrative study used a 'higher is better' ADL scale (C17) and found, after 8 weeks of treatment, a significant improvement in the group that received *Tong qiao huo xue bu nao tang* 通窍活血补脑汤, electro-acupuncture, oxiracetam capsule, and citicoline injection (SMD: 0.59 [0.11, 1.07], $n = 70$ participants) compared to the group that only received the two pharmacotherapies.

Safety of the Combination of Chinese Herbal Medicine plus Acupuncture

Most studies did not report adverse events (AEs). One study specified that there were no obvious AEs (C3) and another study mentioned two dropouts in the test group — one due to gastrointestinal symptoms and one due to pain from acupuncture and feeling cold — and one dropout in the donepezil control group for an unspecified reason (C2). In another study, there were four dropouts in the combination therapy group due to gastrointestinal symptoms associated with the CHM and three participants in the donepezil control group died during the study due to unspecified causes (C1).

Of the four integrative medicine studies, one reported that there were no AEs (C17) and two did not mention AEs (C15, C18). One study (C16) reported that two patients in the integrative medicine group had mild nausea and bloating and one had diarrhea, while in the pharmacotherapy-alone control group, three patients had nausea, two had mild dizziness and tinnitus, and one had insomnia.

Chinese Herbal Medicine plus Scalp Acupuncture Therapy

Two RCTs tested combinations of oral CHM plus scalp acupuncture. One was a comparison with pharmacotherapy (C19) and the other was an integrative medicine study (C20). The two studies used different systems of scalp acupuncture. Neither study used syndrome differentiation.

Chinese Herbal Medicine plus Scalp Acupuncture vs. Pharmacotherapy

One study involving 127 participants (C19) investigated the combination of the CHM *Bu shen huo nao wan* 补肾活脑丸 (main ingredients: *Yuan zhi* 远志, *shan zhu yu* 山茱萸, *he shou wu* 何首乌, *dan shen* 丹参, *huang jing* 黄精, *chuan xiong* 川芎, *chi shao* 赤芍, *shi chang pu* 石菖蒲, *bai jiang can* 白僵蚕, *and zhi gan cao* 炙甘草) plus scalp acupuncture at MS6 *Dingnieqianxiexian* 顶颞前斜线, MS7 *Dingniehouxiexian* 顶颞后斜线, MS1 *Ezhongxian* 额中线, and MS11 *Niehouxian* 颞后线 vs. nimodipine plus cerebrolysin injection. After 8 weeks of treatment, there were significant improvements in scores on the MMSE (MD: 2.68 [1.64, 3.72]), HDS (MD: 4.90 [3.90, 5.90]) and on a 'higher is better' ADL scale (SMD: 0.47 [0.12,

0.82]) for the combination therapy group compared to the group that received only the two pharmacotherapies.

Integrative Chinese Herbal Medicine plus Scalp Acupuncture vs. Pharmacotherapy

One study (n = 60 participants) tested a combination of the CHM *Yi zhi fang* 益智方 (main ingredients: *Ren shen* 人参*, huang qi* 黄芪*, shu di* 熟地*, shan zhu yu* 山茱萸*, cong rong* 苁蓉*, gou qi zi* 枸杞子*, yu jin* 郁金*, shi chang pu* 石菖蒲*, yi zhi ren* 益智仁*, dan shen* 丹参*, ge gen* 葛根*, shou wu* 首乌*, and gan cao* 甘草) plus scalp electro-acupuncture at the movement area *Dong qu* 动区, sensory area *Gan jue qu* 感觉区, and language area *Yu yan qu* 语言区 plus aniracetam for four weeks (C20). At the end of treatment, there were significant improvements in scores on the MMSE (MD: 4.47 [2.78, 6.16]), HDS (MD: 2.31 [0.61, 4.01]) and 'lower is better' ADL (SMD: –0.63 [–1.15, –0.11]) for the integrative combination therapy group compared to the group that received aniracetam alone.

Safety of the Combination of Chinese Herbal Medicine plus Scalp Acupuncture

Neither of the two studies that tested the combination of CHM plus scalp acupuncture reported any dropouts and neither reported on AEs. Therefore, the safety of this combination cannot be assessed.

Chinese Herbal Medicine plus Acupuncture plus Rehabilitation Therapy

One four-armed study included comparisons between various combinations of the CHM *Shen long jian nao tang* 参龙健脑汤 (main ingredients: *ren shen* 人参*, he shou wu* 何首乌*, yin yang huo* 淫羊藿*, di long* 地龙*, chuan xiong* 川芎*, yuan zhi* 远志*, and shi chang pu* 石菖蒲) plus acupuncture at GV20 *Baihui* 百会, GV16 *Fengfu* 风府, GB20 *Fengchi* 风池, EX-HN5 *Taiyang* 太阳, LI4 *Hegu* 合谷, LR3 *Taichong* 太冲, EX-HN1 *Sishencong* 四神聪, and EX-HN3

Yintang 印堂 plus a program of rehabilitation therapy that included attention training, improving thinking ability, piecing together patterns, drawing pictures, and counting balls for one hour a day, three times a week vs. piracetam tablets for 12 weeks (C8). Syndrome differentiation was not mentioned.

The authors reported some improvements after treatment in the CHM plus acupuncture, CHM plus rehabilitation therapy, and CHM plus acupuncture plus rehabilitation therapy groups compared to before treatment, but no improvements in the piracetam control group.

Meta-analysis of the end of treatment results for MMSE scores found no differences between CHM plus rehabilitation therapy (MD: 0.22 [−1.83, 2.27], $n = 64$ participants) or CHM plus acupuncture plus rehabilitation therapy (MD: 1.26 [−0.79, 3.31], $n = 69$ participants) and piracetam alone. Similarly, based on BBS scores, there were no significant improvements for CHM plus rehabilitation therapy (MD: −0.37 [−2.09, 1.35], $n = 64$ participants) or CHM plus acupuncture plus rehabilitation therapy (MD: −0.59 [−2.25, 1.07], $n = 69$ participants) when compared with the piracetam control group. There was no mention of AEs.

Clinical Evidence for Commonly Used Interventions

None of the herbal formulae included in the RCTs of the combination therapies were identical to those in the guidelines (see Chapter 2). However, the herbs *dan shen* 丹参, *shi chang pu* 石菖蒲, *shu di huang* 熟地黄, *chuan xiong* 川芎, *huang qi* 黄芪, *he shou wu* 何首乌, and *gou qi zi* 枸杞子 were all frequent ingredients in the formulae listed in Chapter 2.

A number of the acupuncture points listed in the guidelines were used frequently in the combination therapies assessed, including GV20 *Baihui* 百会, EX-HN1 *Sishencong* 四神聪, ST36 *Zusanli* 足三里, SP6 *Sanyinjiao* 三阴交, KI3 *Taixi* 太溪, GV26 *Shuigou* 水沟, GB20 *Fengchi* 风池, and ST40 *Fenglong* 丰隆. Overall, the combination therapy studies used formulae that contained herbs similar to those found in the RCTs in Chapter 5 and similar acupuncture points to those used in the RCTs in Chapter 7.

Summary of the Evidence for Combination Therapies

The majority of the combination therapies (14 RCTs) used CHM plus acupuncture or electro-acupuncture, with two studies also using moxibustion. Poolable data were available for outcomes based on the MMSE, HDS, ADL, and BBS. In the comparisons between combination CHM plus acupuncture and various pharmacotherapies, there were significant benefits in the combination therapy groups based on MMSE, HDS, and 'lower is better' ADL scores, but no differences were found between groups based on BBS scores. The included studies lasted four to 12 weeks, most had fewer than 100 participants, and none used blinding of participants. This limits our confidence in the results.

Four studies compared CHM plus acupuncture plus pharmacotherapy with the same pharmacotherapy alone. The pool of three studies of four to eight weeks duration found a significant benefit for this integrative approach based on MMSE scores. A similar result was found for the HDS. Although the ADL outcomes were not poolable, two studies reported that the integrative combination therapies led to significant improvements. Again, the studies were relatively small and not blinded.

Two studies tested the combination of CHM plus scalp acupuncture. A single eight-week study found improved outcomes compared to nimodipine alone based on the MMSE, HDS, and ADL. Another study found that CHM plus scalp acupuncture combined with aniracetam for four weeks was better than aniracetam alone based on the same outcome measures. In the single study that combined CHM, acupuncture, and rehabilitation therapy, there was no difference between this combination and piracetam after 12 weeks based on MMSE and BBS outcomes.

Overall, the results suggest that combination therapy may confer benefits in the treatment of VaD, at least in the short-term. However, the meta-analyses were based on small numbers of studies that were not adequately blinded and employed a diversity of interventions in the treatment groups. Consequently, it was not possible to determine which particular CHMs or acupuncture treatments contributed to the results. There was also considerable diversity in the pharmacotherapies used in the controls. Only two studies used donepezil as recommended in international guidelines.[2,3] Furthermore, lack of blinding, unclear reporting of methodological aspects, and inadequate reporting of safety data also increase the risk that the results were subject to bias. These issues all limit the strength of these conclusions.

References

1. 谢莹晔, 蔡琳, 谢美凤, 彭荣光, *et al.* (2014) 针灸结合中药治疗血管性痴呆 meta 分析. 新中医. **46**(2):200–202.
2. National Collaborating Centre for Mental Health. (2007) Dementia a NICE–SCIE guideline on supporting people with dementia and their carers in health and social care — Commissioned by the Social Care Institute for Excellence National Institute for Health and Clinical Excellence. The British Psychological Society and Gaskell, London.
3. National Institute for Health and Clinical Excellence (NICE) (2011). NICE technology appraisal guidance 217 — donepezil, galantamine, rivastigmine and memantine for the treatment of Alzheimer's disease (update). National Institute for Health and Clinical Excellence, London.

List of Clinical Studies Included in Chapter 9

Study Number	References
C1	文宰晟，李忠仁 (指导). (2012) 针药结合对气血亏虚型血管性痴呆治疗方案的优化研究. 南京中医药大学，博士学位论文.
C2	黄煜，刘跃光 (指导). (2011) 针刺结合中药治疗血管性痴呆的疗效比较性研究. 南京中医药大学，硕士学位论文.
C3	刘阳，王东浪. (2011) 针药结合治疗肾虚痰瘀互结型血管性痴呆的临床研究. 中国医药指南. **9**(20):141–142.
C4	卢昌均，周哲屹，刘国成，鹿俊磊，韦冰心，*et al.* (2013) 针药并用治疗血管性痴呆疗效观察. 上海针灸杂志. **32**(7):545–547.
C5	卢中莲，林豫路. (2006) 复智汤结合针刺治疗血管性痴呆的临床观察. 广西中医药. **29**(5):20–22.
C6	欧阳武，欧阳龙妹. (2012) 针药联合治疗血管性痴呆临床观察. 中医临床研究. **4**(22):35–36.

(*Continued*)

Study Number	References
C7	马云枝，沈晓明，杨泽锋. (2013) 通脉舒络胶囊结合针刺治疗血管性痴呆临床研究. 中国中医急症. **22**(3):381–383.
C8	Chen LP, Wang FW, Zuo F, Jia JJ, *et al.* (2011) Clinical research on comprehensive treatment of senile vascular dementia. *J Trad Chin Med.* **31**(3):178–181.
C9	王家祥，杜念念. (2013) 中药配合针刺治疗血管性痴呆（肝肾亏虚型）临床观察. 湖北中医杂志. **35**(7):3–4.
C10	邢越，王淑贤，周振坤. (2007) 针药结合治疗痰浊阻窍型轻度血管性痴呆 50 例临床观察. 黑龙江中医药. **36**(1):40–41.
C11	王庆向. (2012) 针药结合治疗血管性痴呆临床观察. 天津中医药. **29**(3):249–250.
C12	李万水，徐菊梅. (2002) 脑康片联合针刺疗法治疗血管性痴呆临床观察. 山东医药. **42**(30):42–43.
C13	王谨敏，王梅平，杜建，蔡晶，*et al.* (2007) 针灸结合康欣胶囊治疗肾虚血瘀型血管性痴呆的临床研究. 中西医结合心脑血管病杂志. **5**(5):398–400.
C14	郑谅，庄礼兴，李艳慧. (2000) 针药结合治疗血管性痴呆的临床研究. 上海针灸杂志. **19**(3):8–10.
C15	郝卫平，康美清，郭富城. (2012) 针药联合治疗血管性痴呆临床疗效观察. 中医药临床杂志. **24**(11):1048–1049.
C16	王文玉，钟凤芳，张京松. (2010) 中西医结合治疗老年血管性痴呆 25 例. 浙江中西医结合杂志. **20**(6):354–356.
C17	王子平. (2014) 通窍活血补脑汤配合电针治疗脑血管性痴呆疗效观察. 陕西中医. **35**(4):455–458.
C18	王强，胡蓉，仲秀艳，朱广旗. (2008) 补肾通督醒脑法治疗血管性痴呆 25 例 河南中医. **28**(4):38–39.
C19	吴军君，周启棣，王海燕. (2006) 中医补肾醒脑法治疗血管性痴呆 64 例的临床观察. 光明中医. **21**(8):64–65.
C20	苏保江. (2012) 中西医结合治疗血管性痴呆 30 例. 中国医学创新. **9**(4):44–45.

10

Summary and Conclusions

OVERVIEW

This chapter summarises the main findings of the previous chapters and provides cross-references between chapters for syndrome differentiation, herbal formulae, individual herbs, acupuncture and related therapies, acupuncture points, and other Chinese medicine therapies. The main results of the meta-analyses of the clinical trials are discussed, as well as the quality of the evidence and its limitations. The implications of the previous chapters' findings are discussed with regard to the clinical management of vascular dementia using Chinese medicine. Future directions are proposed for further clinical and experimental research.

Introduction

Chinese medicine (CM) therapies, usually in combination with pharmacotherapies and rehabilitation therapy, play an important role in the management of vascular dementia (VaD) in China. Current conventional management of VaD aims to reduce cardiovascular risk factors, prevent further strokes, and facilitate the recovery of cognitive and physical abilities. Dementia-specific pharmacotherapies, including acetylcholinesterase inhibitors and memantine, are considered first-line pharmaceutical interventions. However, their efficacy is limited. Therefore, adjunctive and supportive therapies, including Chinese herbal medicine (CHM) and acupuncture, have been used routinely in clinical practice.

In this monograph, a 'whole-evidence' approach has been taken to assess the state of the evidence for CM interventions in the management of VaD. Reviews of clinical guidelines and textbooks identified the main syndromes for dementia and VaD as well as a range of recommended or suggested CM interventions. These include oral CHM, acupuncture (including electro-acupuncture, scalp acupuncture, and ear acupuncture/acupressure), moxibustion, exercise therapies, and diet and lifestyle modifications (Chapter 2).

Analysis of records found in the classical literature identified CHMs and acupuncture therapies that have been used in the management of dementia and memory impairments associated with stroke. This provides historical evidence that such disorders have been treated using CM for close to two millennia (Chapter 3). With regard to evidence from clinical trials, numerous studies of CHMs have been conducted in China and other countries, and some of these studies have shown promising results (Chapter 5). The herbs used most frequently in the formulae tested in the randomised controlled trials (RCTs) have shown activity in experimental studies indicating their possible mechanisms of action (Chapter 6). The effectiveness of acupuncture and related therapies for VaD have received considerable clinical research and the available evidence suggests that acupuncture, electro-acupuncture, and scalp acupuncture are potentially beneficial (Chapter 7). Only a few studies have tested exercise and massage therapies and the results suggest that further study is warranted (Chapter 8). Combinations of CM therapies, mainly CHM plus acupuncture, have been investigated in a number of clinical trials. In general, the herbs and acupuncture points used in these combination therapies are consistent with those used in the studies listed in Chapters 5 and 7, and the results indicate some promising evidence of benefit (Chapter 9).

Chinese Medicine Syndrome Differentiation

Current clinical guidelines for all types of dementia highlight seven main syndromes based on combinations of signs and symptoms.[1] For each syndrome, one or two CHM formulae are suggested to guide clinical practice (Chapter 2) and these are typically modified according to the individual patient's clinical presentation.

Classical Literature

In the classical literature (Chapter 3), there were a few mentions of aetiology and syndrome differentiation. Wind was the main pathogenic factor that led to stroke (*zhong feng* 中风), although deficiency inside the body enabled wind to enter. In a few cases there were specific mentions of deficiency of *qi* and Blood and deficiency of the Liver and Kidney as aspects of aetiology. Although the citations tended to be brief, syndromes could often be inferred from the listed symptoms and the ingredients of the formulae used.

Clinical Studies

In Table 10.1, the main syndromes in Chapter 2 are cross-referenced to the syndromes mentioned in the clinical studies in Chapters 5, 7, and 9. High frequency syndromes from the RCT section of Chapter 5 have been added to the matrix, but it does not include every syndrome mentioned in every clinical study. In some cases, similar syndrome names have been grouped together. Of the seven syndromes listed in the guidelines for dementia (Chapter 2), turbid phlegm obstructing the Orifices 痰浊蒙窍 was mentioned in 11 CHM studies, including seven RCTs in Chapter 5, 11 RCTs in Chapter 7 (of which nine were for acupuncture/electroacupuncture and two were on moxibustion), as well as two RCTs of combination therapy in Chapter 9. Deficiency of 'Sea of Marrow' 髓海不足 was the next most frequently mentioned syndrome overall, appearing in 12 studies in Chapter 5 (including 6 RCTs), five RCTs in Chapter 7, and one RCT in Chapter 9. Spleen and Kidney dual deficiency 脾肾两虚 was mentioned in seven CHM studies, five acupuncture RCTs, and two RCTs of combination therapy. Heart and Liver fire 心肝火旺 was less frequent, with only two mentions in the CHM non-controlled studies (NCS), although it was more frequent in the acupuncture RCTs ($n = 5$). Blood stasis obstructing the Brain Collaterals 瘀阻脑络 was mentioned in three CHM RCTs, and two acupuncture RCTs mentioned the related syndrome Blood stasis obstructing the Collaterals 瘀血阻络. Endogenous toxins damaging the Brain Collaterals 毒损脑

Table 10.1 Summary of Syndromes Included in Chapters 2, 5, 7, and 9

Syndrome Name	Chapter 2	Chapter 5			Chapter 7			Chapter 9
		RCTs	CCTs	NCS	RCTs	CCTs	NCS	(RCTs)
Deficiency of 'Sea of Marrow' 髓海不足/脑髓不充	Yes	6	3	3	5	0	0	1
Spleen and Kidney dual deficiency 脾肾两虚	Yes	5	1	1	5	0	0	2
Turbid phlegm obstructing the Orifices 痰浊蒙窍/痰浊闭窍	Yes	7	3	1	11*	0	0	2
Blood stasis obstructing the (Brain) Collaterals 瘀阻脑络/瘀血阻络	Yes	3	0	0	2	0	0	0
Deficiency of *qi* and Blood 气血亏虚	Yes	0	0	0	2	0	0	2
Heart and Liver fire 心肝火旺	Yes	0	0	2	5	0	0	0
Endogenous toxins damaging the Brain Collaterals 毒损脑络	Yes	0	0	0	0	0	0	0
Liver and Kidney deficiency 肝肾亏虚	No	4	2	2	7*	0	1	1
Deficiency of the Kidney and Essence 肾精亏虚	No	5	0	0	3	0	0	1
Qi deficiency with Blood stasis 气虚血瘀	No	9	1	0	1	0	0	0
Qi stagnation with Blood stasis 气滞血瘀	No	3	0	1	6	0	1	0
Deficiency of the Kidney with Blood stasis 肾虚血瘀	No	8	0	0	0	0	0	1
Deficiency of the Kidney with phlegm turbidity and Blood stasis obstructing the Orifices 肾虚痰瘀阻窍	No	3	0	2	0	0	0	1

Table 10.1 (*Continued*)

Syndrome Name	Chapter 2	Chapter 5 RCTs	Chapter 5 CCTs	Chapter 5 NCS	Chapter 7 RCTs	Chapter 7 CCTs	Chapter 7 NCS	Chapter 9 (RCTs)
Spleen and Kidney deficiency with phlegm turbidity and Blood stasis obstructing the Collaterals 脾肾两虚, 痰瘀阻络	No	4	0	0	0	0	0	0
Phlegm turbidity and Blood stasis obstructing the collaterals 痰瘀阻络	No	3	1	0	0	0	0	0
Liver *yang* ascendant hyperactivity 肝阳上亢/肝阳暴亢	No	0	0	0	3	0	1	1

*Included in the two randomised controlled trials of moxibustion in Chapter 7. Abbreviations: CCTs, controlled clinical trials; NCS, non-controlled studies; RCTs, randomised controlled trials.

络 did not appear in any of the studies, but the related syndrome pathogenic toxins wrap and bind 邪毒缠结 appeared in two of the CHM controlled clinical trials (CCTs).

Other common syndromes included Liver and Kidney deficiency 肝肾亏虚 (8 CHM studies, 8 studies in Chapter 7) and insufficiency of Kidney and Essence 肾精亏虚 (5 CHM RCTs, 3 acupuncture RCTs). *Qi* deficiency with Blood stasis 气虚血瘀 was one of the most commonly mentioned syndromes in the CHM RCTs ($n = 9$), but it was only mentioned in one acupuncture RCT. Conversely, *qi* stagnation with Blood stasis 气滞血瘀 appeared in four CHM studies, but it featured in seven acupuncture studies. Another common syndrome in the CHM RCTs was deficiency of Kidney with Blood stasis 肾虚血瘀 ($n = 8$). While it was mentioned in one combination therapy RCT, it did not appear in the acupuncture studies. Another six studies mentioned the complex syndrome deficiency of Kidney with phlegm turbidity and Blood stasis obstructing the Orifices 肾虚痰瘀阻窍, while four studies mentioned Spleen and Kidney deficiency with phlegm turbidity and Blood stasis obstructing the collaterals 脾肾

两虚, 痰瘀阻络. These complex syndromes combine aspects of the syndromes listed in the guidelines, but we scored them separately for the purpose of illustration. Complex syndrome descriptions were not found in the acupuncture studies. The syndrome Liver *yang* ascendant hyperactivity 肝阳上亢/肝阳暴亢 did not appear in any of the CHM studies, but it was included in four studies in Chapter 7 and in one study of combination therapy.

Of the seven syndromes in the guidelines, four were used relatively frequently while three were less common. Of these, deficiency of *qi* and Blood 气血亏虚 was an underlying feature of more specifically named syndromes and this is a likely reason for its low frequency. In the case of endogenous toxins damaging the Brain Collaterals 毒损脑络, this is a relatively new syndrome specific to dementia.

Overall, because syndrome differentiation was mentioned in a minority of studies, Table 10.1 should not be interpreted as an indication of how frequent certain syndromes appeared in participants. One survey of 83 people with post-stroke dementia found that most had more than one syndrome, with insufficiency of the Kidney and Essence 肾精亏虚 being the most common, followed by ascendant hyperactivity of Liver *yang* 肝阳上亢 and deficiency of *qi* and Blood 气血亏虚.[2] A study of 63 people with VaD found that 27% had insufficiency of the Kidney and Essence 肾精亏虚, 25% had turbid phlegm obstructing the Orifices 痰浊蒙窍, 19% had ascendant hyperactivity of Liver *yang* 肝阳上亢, 13% had deficiency of *qi* and Blood 气血亏虚, while the reminder had other syndromes.[3] The authors reported that acupuncture treatment was better at improving the full-type syndromes of ascendant hyperactivity of Liver *yang* 肝阳上亢 and turbid phlegm obstructing the Orifices 痰浊蒙窍, than the empty-type syndromes such as insufficiency of the Kidney and Essence 肾精亏虚.

In the present analysis, turbid phlegm obstructing the Orifices 痰浊蒙窍 was the predominant syndrome in both CHM and acupuncture studies while ascendant hyperactivity of Liver *yang* 肝阳上亢 was relatively uncommon and appeared mainly in the acupuncture studies. In the studies that used syndrome differentiation and/or adjustment of the intervention according to syndrome, outcome data were reported as aggregates. Therefore, it was not possible to determine whether there were any differences in outcomes based on the syndrome.

Chinese Herbal Medicine

This section summarises the evidence from Chapters 2, 3, 5, and 9 in relation to CHM. Current clinical guidelines recommend the use of multi-ingredient formulae prescribed according to syndrome differentiation and modified according to the signs, symptoms, and needs of the individual person (Chapter 2) as a component of VaD management.

Classical Literature

In the classical and pre-modern era, CHM was frequently used in the management of memory impairments, dementia, stroke (*zhong feng* 中风), and its sequelae (Chapter 3). There were no specific terms for VaD during that time, so it was not possible to directly identify citations in classical books that correspond to VaD. Nevertheless, it is probable that VaD was included within the scope of these disorders. Therefore, descriptions of memory impairments that appeared to be associated with stroke and/or paralysis were selected as possible instances of VaD. The requirement for multiple symptoms to be present limited the available data, so the results should be considered as relevant to post-stroke dementia with symptoms of paralysis and not to other types of VaD.

The formulae used in the classical literature were not typical of those used in modern CHM (Chapters 2 and 5), although there were similarities in some formulae. The most distinct difference was the frequent use of herbs to expel wind, such as *fang feng* 防风 and *du huo* 独活, in the formulae identified in Chapter 3, which reflects pre-modern theories of stroke as being due to external pathogenic wind. Such herbs, in combination with herbs for warming and coursing the channels, are also used for impairments of movement, such as those that occur in stroke sequelae. In contrast, contemporary CHM formulae tend to focus on strengthening the body and dispelling internal blockages of *qi*, Blood, and phlegm. Nevertheless, commonalities with contemporary CHM were also evident. Herbs for tonifying *qi* and Blood, such as *ren shen* 人参, *fu ling* 茯苓, and *dang gui* 当归, were common in both classical and modern formulae (Chapter 5), as were herbs to remove Blood stasis such as *chuan xiong* 川芎, nourish Liver and Kidney such as *shu di huang* 熟地黄, and herbs to improve cognition such as *yuan zhi* 远志.

Clinical Studies

With regard to the clinical trial evidence for the efficacy of CHM for VaD, 180 RCTs were included (Chapter 5). There were only a few RCTs of CHMs versus placebo or no treatment. These showed benefits at 8–12 weeks for cognitive outcomes measured using the Mini-Mental State Examination (MMSE), Hasegawa's Dementia Scale (HDS), and for Activities of Daily Living (ADL). In general, ethical considerations weigh against giving placebo interventions to people with dementia, so most data were for comparisons with pharmacotherapies and integrative therapies that combined a CHM and a pharmacotherapy.

In the comparisons with a variety of pharmacotherapies, CHM showed overall effectiveness at the end of treatment based on MMSE, HDS, and/or ADL outcomes. The meta-analyses of subgroups of RCTs ranging in duration from eight to 24 weeks found that CHM did not produce any significant improvement compared to donepezil in terms of MMSE, ADAS-cog, or 'lower is better' ADL outcomes. There was no heterogeneity for the MMSE or ADAS-cog results and moderate heterogeneity for ADL scores. In the comparisons with nimodipine, there were significant differences in favour of CHM based on the MMSE, HDS, and 'lower is better' ADL. However, there was considerable heterogeneity in the meta-analysis results for outcomes on the MMSE and ADL. Similar meta-analysis results were evident for CHM compared to huperzine A and co-dergocrine mesylate on the MMSE with moderate heterogeneity and HDS with substantial heterogeneity, but there were no significant differences between groups on outcomes for 'lower is better' ADL.

When CHMs were combined with conventional pharmacotherapies using an integrative treatment approach, the pooled meta-analysis results suggested that the addition of CHM produced significant additional benefits in terms of outcomes for the MMSE, HDS, and ADL. The combination of CHM with donepezil showed a significant benefit based on MMSE outcomes without heterogeneity and ADL outcomes with substantial heterogeneity. The result for ADAS-cog was not significant, but this was based on only two studies. Benefits were evident when CHMs were combined with nimodipine, huperzine A, and co-dergocrine mesylate based on the MMSE with moderate to substantial heterogeneity. For 'lower is better' ADL, there was a benefit for nimodipine but not huperzine A or co-dergocrine mesylate. However, few studies were available and heterogeneity was considerable.

These results suggest that the effects of the CHMs were similar to those of a variety of pharmacotherapies at durations of up to 24 weeks. In a number of comparisons, there were statistically significant differences in favour of CHM, but the magnitudes of the differences were small. In addition, there was considerable heterogeneity in the meta-analysis results in some subgroups. In none of the comparisons was there a significant difference in favour of a specific pharmacotherapy. In the studies of integrative medicine, the combination of CHM plus pharmacotherapy was generally better than the pharmacotherapy alone. However, the considerable heterogeneity in some of the meta-analysis results indicates that there was substantial variability between the studies included in the pooled results. Heterogeneity was reduced in some of the subgroups based on specific pharmacotherapies, but this was not always the case. This suggests that at least part of the variability in outcomes was due to differences in the CHMs used. However, it was not possible to determine which CHMs were more effective since most studies tested different formulae, even though many were based on similar ingredients.

Inadequate reporting of adverse events (AEs) was evident in many studies. The reported AEs in the CHM groups tended to be gastrointestinal and not serious, but inadequacies in the data prevented us from conducting further analyses to verify this.

Our interpretation of the clinical study results was limited by the relatively poor methodological reporting, lack of blinding in most studies, small size of some studies, and heterogeneity in meta-analysis results. These aspects reduced our confidence in the precision of the reported results and the consequent outcomes of the meta-analyses. Based on the Grading of Recommendations Assessment, Development, and Evaluation (GRADE) assessments, we downgraded the certainty of the evidence from 'moderate' to 'low' for the comparisons with placebo controls (Chapter 5, Table 5.20), 'low' to 'very low' for the comparisons with donepezil (Chapter 5, Table 5.21), and 'low' to 'very low' for the comparisons with CHM plus donepezil (Chapter 5, Table 5.21).

Chinese Herbal Medicine Formulae in Clinical Guidelines and Textbooks, Classical Literature, and Clinical Studies

To provide an overview of which CHM formulae appeared in multiple chapters, Table 10.2 lists all the CHM formulae described in clinical guidelines and textbooks (Chapter 2) plus the formulae used in multiple RCTs in Chapter 5. These are cross-referenced to formulae in the classical literature (Chapter 3), formulae in CCTs and NCS in Chapter 5, and formulae in RCTs in Chapter 9. Assessment was based on formula name rather than ingredients, so un-named formulae are excluded while modified forms of a formula are grouped together.

Eight formulae included in Chapter 2 were recommended for the management of dementia, including VaD, based on syndrome differentiation. None of these appeared in the classical literature citations for 'possible' VaD, but some similar formulae did (see Chapter 3).

In the RCTs in Chapter 5, four of the seven formulae from Chapter 2 were used at least once. Modified *Bu yang huan wu tang* 补阳还五汤加减 was used in four RCTs, one CCT, and one NCS. *Tong qiao huo xue tang* 通窍活血汤 was used in one RCT and one NCS while *Huan shao dan* 还少丹 and *Qi fu yin* 七福饮 were each used in one RCT. The other three formulae in Chapter 2 did not appear in any of the included clinical studies. Of these formulae, modified *Bu yang huan wu tang* 补阳还五汤加减, provided data suitable for meta-analysis. The results showed that, when combined with a pharmacotherapy, this formula was associated with a significant improvement in HDS scores based on three RCTs, with moderate heterogeneity (Chapter 5, Table 5.23).

Table 10.2 Summary of Oral Chinese Herbal Medicine Formulae Included in Chapters 2 to 9

Formula Name	Chapter 2	Chapter 3 (No. Citations)	Chapter 5 (No. of Studies) RCTs	CCTs	NCS	Chapter 9 (No. of Studies)
Modified *Bu yang huan wu tang* 补阳还五汤加减	Yes	0	4	1	1	0
Bu *chang nao xin tong* jiao nang 步长脑心通胶囊	No	0	4	0	1	0
Fu *fang hai she jiao nang* 复方海蛇胶囊	No	0	3	0	0	0
Cong sheng jiao nang 聪圣胶囊	No	0	3	1	0	0
Kang xin jiao nang 康欣胶囊	No	0	3	1	0	1
Tian zhi ke li 天智颗粒	No	0	3	1	0	0
Modified *di huang yin zi* 地黄饮子加减	No	0	2	0	2	0
Qi fu yin 七福饮	Yes	0	1	0	0	0
Tong qiao huo xue tang 通窍活血汤	Yes	0	1	0	1	0
Huan shao dan 还少丹	Yes	0	1	0	0	0
Huang lian jie du tang 黄连解毒汤	Yes	0	0	0	0	0
Xi xin tang 洗心汤	Yes	0	0	0	0	0
Gui pi tang 归脾汤	Yes	0	0	0	0	0
Tian ma gou teng yin 天麻钩藤饮	Yes	0	0	0	0	0

Abbreviations: RCTs, randomised controlled trials; CCTs, controlled clinical trials; NCS, non-controlled studies.

Of the other multi-ingredient formulae tested in several RCTs, five were modern commercial formulations. *Bu chang nao xin tong jiao nang* 步长脑心通胶囊, which is based on the traditional formula *Bu yang huan wu tang* 补阳还五汤, was used in four RCTs and one NCS. *Kang xin jiao nang* 康欣胶囊 was used in three RCTs and one NCS in Chapter 5 plus one RCT in Chapter 9. *Cong sheng jiao nang* 聪圣胶囊 and *Tian zhi ke li* 天智颗粒 were each used in three RCTs and one NCS, and *Fu fang hai she jiao nang* 复方海蛇胶囊 was tested in three RCTs. Modified *Di huang yin zi* 地黄饮子加减 was based on a traditional formula and was tested in two RCTs and two NCS in Chapter 5. Of these studies, three of the RCTs of *Bu chang nao xin tong jiao nang* 步长脑心通胶囊 provided data suitable for pooling. The meta-analysis results found that the groups that used this formula showed small but significant increases in MMSE scores compared to the groups that used pharmacotherapy, with very little heterogeneity (Chapter 5, Table 5.23).

GRADE Assessment

The GRADE assessments found the certainty of the evidence for modified *Bu yang huan wu tang* 补阳还五汤加减 compared to nimodipine to be 'low' based on the MMSE and 'lower is better' ADL in one RCT (Chapter 5, Table 5.24). In addition, the quality of the evidence was 'very low' for modified *Bu yang huan wu tang* 补阳还五汤加减 combined with pharmacotherapies for the HDS based on three RCTs (Chapter 5, Table 5.26). For *Bu chang nao xin tong jiao nang* 步长脑心通胶囊 versus pharmacotherapies, the GRADE assessment was 'low' for the MMSE, HDS, 'lower is better' ADL, and FAQ based on one to three RCTs. The certainty of evidence was also 'low' for the integrative use of this formula with donepezil based on MMSE and 'lower is better' ADL outcomes.

The clinical trials tested both traditional formulae and modern formulations, but only a few formulae were tested in multiple studies that provided data suitable for pooling in a meta-analysis. However, it should be noted that the variety in formula names tends to mask the similarity in the ingredients of many formulae and these analyses do not include un-named formulae that may be similar to named formulae.

Formula Ingredients

When the herbs used in the formulae are considered, those found to be high frequency ingredients in the RCTs in Chapter 5 were also frequent in the formulae used in the NCS (Chapter 5, Table 5.35) as well as in the formulae used in the combination therapies (Chapter 9). A number of these herbs were also frequent in the formulae used in the classical literature, such as *chuan xiong* 川芎, *dang gui* 当归, *ren shen* 人参, *huang qi* 黄芪, and *di huang* 地黄. However, there were also notable differences, such as the relatively high frequencies of *fang feng* 防风 and *du huo* 独活 in the classical formulae.

Acupuncture and Related Therapies

This section summarises the evidence from Chapters 2, 3, 7, and 9 (Table 10.3). Acupuncture using traditional points was recommended

Table 10.3 Summary of Acupuncture and Related Therapies Included in Chapters 2 to 9

Intervention	Chapter 2	Chapter 3 (No. of Citations)*	Chapter 7 (No. of Studies)			Chapter 9 (No. of Studies)*
			RCTs*	CCTs*	NCS*	
Acupuncture/Electro-acupuncture	Yes	34	39	2	20	18
Electro-acupuncture	Yes	0	13	2	1	4
Scalp acupuncture	Yes	0	4	0	1	2
Moxibustion	Yes	21	2	0	2	2
Ear acupuncture/acupressure	Yes	0	1	0	0	0

*Some studies used more than one intervention (e.g., acupuncture plus moxibustion). These are counted separately in this table. Abbreviations: RCTs, randomised controlled trials; CCTs, controlled clinical trials; NCS, non-controlled studies.

in the guidelines for the management of dementia, including VaD (Chapter 2), and acupuncture was used in the classical literature (Chapter 3). Acupuncture was tested in multiple controlled and uncontrolled clinical trials (Chapter 7) and was the most common among the interventions combined with CHM in the 14 studies of combination therapy (Chapter 9). Electro-acupuncture was recommended in Chapter 2 and was tested in multiple clinical studies.

Scalp acupuncture using modern scalp zones (not including acupuncture on the head using traditional points) was included in Chapter 2. It was used in four RCTs and one NCS (Chapter 7) and was combined with CHM in four RCTs in Chapter 9. Modern ear points for acupuncture or acupressure were listed in Chapter 2, but only one clinical study used ear points. In this case, ear acupressure was used (Chapter 7).

Moxibustion is frequently combined with acupuncture or used alone in clinical practice. In the classical literature, a number of points were mentioned as suitable for moxibustion (Chapter 3) and Chapter 2 included moxibustion as one of the listed therapies. In the clinical studies, two RCTs tested moxibustion alone and two NCS used moxibustion in combination with acupuncture (Chapter 7). Two RCTs combined CHM with moxibustion plus acupuncture (Chapter 9).

Therefore, clinical evidence based on multiple studies was available for acupuncture using traditional points, electro-acupuncture, and scalp acupuncture.

Clinical Evidence for Acupuncture and Electroacupuncture

In one small RCT, a comparison between acupuncture and sham-acupuncture reported higher MMSE scores in the real acupuncture group after eight weeks of treatment (Chapter 7). Another study showed no difference between acupuncture and conventional therapy based on MMSE outcomes after six weeks, but the nature of the conventional therapy was not defined, so the results were difficult to interpret.

The majority of the studies (24 RCTs) compared acupuncture, with or without electro-stimulation, with a pharmacotherapy that is used in the treatment of VaD. Most studies also specified that other supportive therapies, such as anti-hypertensive and/or lipid lowering drugs, were used as needed in both groups. Based on MMSE results, 18 studies showed that the acupuncture groups tended to have significantly better outcomes (Chapter 7, Table 7.3). The results were similar for the HDS based on 12 studies (Chapter 7, Table 7.4) and ADL scores based on eight studies (Chapter 7, Table 7.5) at treatment durations of up to 12 weeks. However, the pooled results showed considerable heterogeneity and there were no significant differences between groups for the comparisons with donepezil.

An integrative approach that combined acupuncture or electro-acupuncture with a pharmacotherapy was used in 17 RCTs. In 13 of these studies, which ranged from two to 24 weeks, there was a significant increase in MMSE scores without substantial heterogeneity (Chapter 7, Table 7.8). Similar results were found for the HDS based on seven studies (Chapter 7, Table 7.9) and ADL based on six studies (Chapter 7, Table 7.10).

GRADE Assessments

Only one study, which provided a comparison with donepezil using outcomes for the MMSE, ADAS-cog, and ADL, was assessed with GRADE. No significant differences were found between groups, but the small sample size and inadequacies in reporting led to the certainty of the evidence being downgraded to 'low'.

AE reporting was not adequate in most acupuncture and electro-acupuncture studies, so an assessment of the safety of the acupuncture intervention was not possible.

Scalp Acupuncture

In the four RCTs of scalp acupuncture, one included a comparison with conventional treatment and reported significant benefits in the scalp acupuncture group in terms of MMSE and ADL outcomes after eight weeks of treatment. All four studies tested comparisons with specific pharmacotherapies and the pool of four studies showed a small, but significant, increase in MMSE scores in the scalp acupuncture groups (Chapter 7, Table 7.17) without heterogeneity, but no difference in ADL scores based on a single study. Only one four-armed study included groups for integrative scalp acupuncture. This study found scalp electro-acupuncture plus nimodipine to be superior to conventional therapy in terms of the MMSE and ADL but there was no significant difference between groups when compared to nimodipine. As only one study reported on AEs, it was not possible to assess the safety of scalp acupuncture.

Moxibustion

For moxibustion, both studies were conducted by the same research group and both employed a similar design. When compared with piracetam, significant improvements were found in the moxibustion groups in terms of MMSE, HDS, and ADL outcomes (Chapter 7, Table 7.21).

Ear Acupressure

The single study comparing ear acupressure with nimodipine enrolled 180 participants and employed an intervention very similar to that as recommended in the guidelines. After 12 weeks, there were no significant differences between groups based on the MMSE or ADL. The only AEs reported in the ear acupressure group were two allergic reactions to the tape used to hold the Vaccaria seeds on the points.

For the acupuncture therapies, most of the evidence was based on acupuncture at traditional points with or without electrostimulation. The evidence suggested that acupuncture was as effective as, or more effective than, a diverse pool of pharmacotherapies for cognitive and ADL outcomes. However, none of these studies were blinded and many provided inadequate detail regarding methodological aspects, so the quality of this evidence was generally 'low'. For the other acupuncture-related therapies, there were too few studies for any conclusions to be made.

Acupuncture Points Used in Key Clinical Guidelines, Textbooks, Classical Literature, and Clinical Studies

To provide a summary and comparison of which traditional acupuncture points were commonly used, all the points that were recommended in Chapter 2 plus the points most frequently used in Chapter 3 ('possible' VaD) and the RCTs in Chapter 7 were included in Table 10.4. The use of these points was cross-referenced to other clinical trial types in Chapters 7 and 9. Separate sections are presented for points that are recommended for acupuncture/electro-acupuncture and moxibustion treatment.

GV20 *Baihui* 百会 was the most commonly used point for acupuncture in the classical literature (Chapter 3), in clinical trials of acupuncture/electro-acupuncture (Chapter 7), and in acupuncture interventions of combination therapies (Chapter 9). Of the other points included in the clinical guidelines, EX-HN1 *Sishencong* 四神聪 was not included in the results for Chapter 3, but the point was frequently used in the RCTs and NCS in Chapters 7 and 9. The acupoints GV24 *Shenting* 神庭, GB20 *Fengchi* 风池, ST36 *Zusanli* 足三里, and SP6 *Sanyinjiao* 三阴交 were all used frequently in the acupuncture RCTs and other clinical studies.

Frequency analyses were limited by the small number of classical literature citations for 'possible' VaD. Among the most common points, both GV20 *Baihui* 百会 and PC6 *Neiguan* 内关 were also common in the RCTs while GB39 *Xuanzhong* 悬钟 was an occasional inclusion in the clinical studies.

Of the points commonly used in clinical studies that were not listed in Chapter 2, the most notable were GV26 *Shiugou* 水沟, PC6 *Neiguan* 内关, and SP10 *Xuehai* 血海. Conversely, some of the points listed in the clinical guidelines were not commonly used in the clini-

Table 10.4 Summary of Acupuncture Points Included in Chapters 2 to 9

Acupuncture Point	Chapter 2	Chapter 3 (No. of Citations)	Chapter 7 (No. of Studies)			Chapter 9 (No. of Studies)
			RCTs	CCTs	NCS*	
Acupuncture						
GV20 *Baihui* 百会	Yes	17	27	1	14	16
EX-HN1 *Sishencong* 四神聪	Yes	0	26	0	8	12
KI3 *Taixi* 太溪	Yes	0	4	0	9	7
KI4 *Dazhong* 大钟	Yes	0	0	0	1	1
ST36 *Zusanli* 足三里	Yes	0	11	1	9	9
BL23 *Shenshu* 肾俞	Yes	0	3	0	6	5
HT7 *Shenmen* 神门	Yes	0	4	1	5	4
GB20 *Fengchi* 风池	Yes	0	14	1	8	6
GV24 *Shenting* 神庭	Yes	0	16	0	6	6
GV17 *Naohu* 脑户	Yes	0	2	0	1	0
LU7 *Lieque* 列缺	Yes	9	0	0	0	0
ST40 *Fenglong* 丰隆	Yes	0	3	0	4	6
SP6 *Sanyinjiao* 三阴交	Yes	0	7	0	7	9
HT5 *Tongli* 通里	Yes	0	0	0	1	0
LR3 *Taichong* 太冲	Yes	0	4	1	7	3
BL17 *Geshu* 膈俞	Yes	0	1	0	0	1
GV26 *Shiugou* 水沟	No	0	12	0	8	7
PC6 *Neiguan* 内关	No	1	10	1	5	5
GB13 *Benshen* 本神	No	0	8	0	6	1
SP10 *Xuehai* 血海	No	0	7	0	2	3
GB39 *Xuanzhong* 悬钟	No	1	1	1	2	3
Moxibustion						
HT3 *Shaohai* 少海	Yes	0	0	0	0	0
GV20 *Baihui* 百会	Yes	8	2	0	1	1
ST36 *Zusanli* 足三里	Yes	0	0	0	2	1
LU7 *Lieque* 列缺	No	8	0	0	0	0

*Some studies used more than one intervention (e.g., acupuncture plus moxibustion). These are counted separately in this table. Abbreviations: RCTs, randomised controlled trials; CCTs, controlled clinical trials; NCS, non-controlled studies.

cal studies. The acupoint LU7 *Lieque* 列缺 was listed in Chapter 2 and used in the classical literature but not in the RCTs. The acupoints HT5 *Tongli* 通里 and KI4 *Dazhong* 大钟 were included in Chapter 2 but did not appear in the RCTs in Chapter 7, although they were used in one or two other clinical studies.

Moxibustion was relatively infrequent in the clinical studies. Of the three points listed for moxibustion in the clinical guidelines (Chapter 2), GV20 *Baihui* 百会 was frequent in the classical literature and clinical studies, whereas ST36 *Zusanli* 足三里 was used in only a few clinical studies. Moxibustion on *Lieque* 列缺 appeared in the classical literature but not in any of the clinical studies.

Of the seven scalp acupuncture zones listed in the guidelines (Chapter 2), all were used in at least one RCT in Chapter 7, whilst MS1 *Ezhongxian* 额中线 and MS11 *Niehouxian* 颞后线 were also used in studies that were included in Chapter 9 (Table 10.5). The scalp zones MS6 *Dingnieqianxiexian* 顶颞前斜线 and MS7 *Dingniehouxiexian*

Table 10.5 Summary of Scalp Acupuncture Zones Included in Chapters 2 to 9

Scalp Zone	Chapter 2	Chapter 7 (No. of Studies)			Chapter 9 (No. of Studies)
		RCTs	CCTs	NCS*	
MS1 *Ezhongxian* 额中线	Yes	2	0	0	1
MS2 *Epangxian* 1 额旁 1 线	Yes	1	0	0	0
MS3 *Epangxian* 2 额旁 2 线	Yes	1	0	0	0
MS4 *Epangxian* 3 额旁 3 线	Yes	1	0	0	0
MS5 *Dingzhongxian* 顶中线	Yes	2	0	0	0
MS6 *Dingnieqianxiexian* 顶颞前斜线	No	2	0	0	1
MS7 *Dingniehouxiexian* 顶颞后斜线	No	1	0	0	1
MS10 *Nieqianxian* 颞前线	Yes	1	0	0	0
MS11 *Niehouxian* 颞后线	Yes	1	0	0	1

Note: A few studies used a different system of scalp zones. These are not included in this table (see Chapter 7). Abbreviations: RCTs, randomised controlled trials; CCTs, controlled clinical trials; NCS, non-controlled studies.

顶颞后斜线 were used in multiple RCTs but were not mentioned in the guidelines.

Ear points were used in the single RCT of ear acupressure. This study used three of the ear points from Chapter 2, namely TF4 *Shenmen* 神门, CO10 *Shen* 肾 (Kidney), and AT3 *Zhen* 枕 (occiput).

In general, the traditional points recommended for acupuncture and electro-acupuncture in Chapter 2 were also used frequently in clinical trials, with a few exceptions. Conversely, a few points frequently used in clinical studies were not included in the guidelines. However, considering the number of points that could be used to treat the cognitive and physical symptoms associated with VaD, some differences were to be expected. For scalp acupuncture, there was considerable overlap between the zones listed in the guidelines and those used in clinical studies, but this was based on a small number of studies. There was very little clinical research on ear points for VaD.

Other Chinese Medicine Therapies

This section summarises the evidence from Chapters 2, 3, 8, and 9 for other CM therapies in the treatment of VaD (Table 10.6). The clinical guidelines suggested that exercise therapies, including *tai chi*太极, *qi gong* 气功, and Chinese remedial massage, including *tui na* 推拿 and *an mo* 按摩, could be used as adjunctive therapies for dementia.

Table 10.6 Summary of Other Chinese Medicine Therapies in Chapters 2 to 9

Intervention	Chapter 2	Chapter 3 (No. of Citations)	Chapter 8 (No. of Studies)			Chapter 9 (No. of Studies)
			RCTs	CCTs	NCS	
Chinese exercise therapy (*qi gong* 气功)	yes	0	1	0	1	0
Remedial massage (*tui na* 推拿, *an mo* 按摩)	yes	0	0	0	1	0

Abbreviations: RCTs, randomised controlled trials; CCTs, controlled clinical trials; NCS, non-controlled studies.

In the classical literature (Chapter 3), no citations were located for the use of these therapies for VaD, but it should be noted that there were relatively few citations identified as 'possible' VaD. In the modern clinical trial literature, there was only one controlled study available for meta-analysis. In the single RCT of exercise therapy, which tested *Sun Si Miao*'s body strengthening exercises 孙思邈健身操, there were significant improvements in terms of cognitive function and ADL (Chapter 8). In the NCS, the authors reported benefits from one form of *qi gong* 气功 (*hui chun gong* 回春功) and a *tui na* 推拿 intervention, but meta-analysis was not feasible. No studies of *tai chi* 太极 that were specific to VaD were identified.

Other Chinese Medicine Therapies in Key Clinical Guidelines and Textbooks, Classical Literature, and Clinical Studies

Although none of the exercise, remedial massage, or food therapy methods included in Chapter 2 appeared in the classical literature for VaD, *Sun Si Miao*'s body strengthening exercises 孙思邈健身操 were based on classical methods for promoting health and longevity and the study of *Hui chun gong* 回春功 included a number of commonly used *qi gong* 气功 methods. In addition, the study of *tui na* 推拿 employed established techniques (Table 10.6).

Of the foods suggested in Chapter 2 as potentially beneficial for people with dementia, some were ingredients in the classical formulae (Chapter 3) and in the formulae tested in clinical studies, but no clinical trials of food therapy for VaD were found. Overall, there were few clinical studies of other CM therapies for VaD.

Limitations of the Evidence

In each chapter, we aimed to provide a comprehensive survey of the topic area based on data from multiple sources, but there may have been omissions and oversights. Due to the range and amount of data available, analyses and discussions may not have been sufficiently detailed for all readers.

In Chapter 2, we examined a range of clinical guidelines and textbooks but limited the scope of the chapter to those that were current and authoritative at the time of writing. Hence, the number of syndromes and guiding formulae listed are fewer than if we had included every guideline and recommendation. Consequently, this chapter should be regarded as an overview of current practice and not a complete survey.

Evidence from Classical Literature

The searches of the classical literature in Chapter 3 were limited to the books included in the *Zhong Hua Yi Dian* 中华医典 version 5. While this was the largest single digital resource available at the time of writing, it does not include every Chinese medicine book published in the pre-modern era, nor does it include all the fragmentary texts recovered in archaeological excavations. Therefore, the results inevitably include omissions. The search and data filtering processes aimed to capture all citations relevant to post-stroke VaD. However, these were based on a limited number of terms and criteria, so some may have been missed. Certain citations are also open to interpretation, so while they may have contained possible references to VaD, they may also have been relevant to other conditions.

The categorisation of results into 'possible' VaD and 'likely' VaD was based on the information available in the citations only. Since many citations were brief and may not have mentioned the terms used in the selection criteria, these would have been eliminated through our categorisation process. Moreover, it was not possible to make definitive diagnoses of VaD retrospectively, so these categories should be regarded as tentative. Issues such as these reflect the limitations inherent in screening large samples of predominantly unstructured pre-modern literature. Therefore, we suggest that readers who have specific interests in the classical CM literature should consult the original sources. With regard to the frequency lists of CHMs and acupuncture points, these provide points of comparison between the classical and modern literature and should not be interpreted as definitive summaries of how VaD was treated in the past. In addition, the botanical identity of herbs can change from region to region and over time, so there may have been regularisation errors in the allocation of scientific names.

Evidence from Clinical Studies

The evidence from the modern literature is based mainly on meta-analyses of the outcomes of controlled clinical trials. While these were identified by searching multiple databases written in Chinese and English, we did not conduct searches in other languages, so some studies may have been missed. The criteria for inclusion in the analyses were pre-specified and the eliminated studies either did not provide diagnostic criteria for VaD, used comparators other than pharmacotherapies in current use, or did not include pre-specified outcome measures. In addition, studies in which there appeared to be data errors and the authors could not be contacted for clarification were excluded from analyses. Consequently, the meta-analyses were based on a subset of published studies and not on all the clinical studies identified in the searches. Since we aimed to provide summaries of the current state of the evidence, we endeavoured to compare like with like, as far as possible, to provide the reader with meaningful data.

Meta-analysis results were based on aggregate data from multiple studies and there were limits to how many subgroup analyses were feasible in the exploration of variables within the datasets. It is important to note that each study had its individual features and variations existed in the conditions under which the trials were conducted, the age and severity of the participants, the dosage and form of the interventions, and the procedures used in data collection and analysis. Therefore, statistical heterogeneity in the results of our meta-analysis pools was not surprising. In recognition of the likelihood of heterogeneity, random effects models were used throughout the analyses in order to provide conservative effect size estimates. Sensitivity analyses based on risk-of-bias judgements were used to mitigate the effects of the generally 'low' quality of methodological reporting in the clinical trials. Although these tended to reduce heterogeneity, few studies employed blinding, so these results still require careful interpretation.

Meta-analysis results were presented for test groups versus control groups at the end of the longest treatment period. Too little data were available for meta-analyses to be conducted at follow-up. When the result was significant with a 95% confidence interval, this indicates that the difference between the groups was unlikely to be due to chance. However, it does not tell us whether this difference is clinically meaningful. When compared with a placebo, the result provides an estimate of how much improvement can be attributed to the test intervention over and above any placebo effect. This may or may not be clinically meaningful depending on the outcome measure and the duration of the treatment period. In the comparisons between a CM test intervention and a pharmacotherapy control, a very small difference or no difference may still be meaningful since it indicates that both interventions had similar effects. However, we do not provide measures of the before-versus-after changes within the two groups, so it may be difficult to determine whether the result was clinically meaningful in the control group.

In the case of integrative medicine, the studies aimed to assess whether combining a CM therapy with a pharmacotherapy provided an additional benefit. A significant difference between groups was evident in many studies, but most studies did not employ placebos for the CM therapy in the control group, so it would have been evident to participants that one group was receiving additional therapy. Therefore, the results of studies employing this design are biased in favour of the integrative group. Consequently, the effect size found in the meta-analysis may be inflated. These issues need to be considered when interpreting the meta-analysis results and in clinical decision making.

It was not feasible to include the details of every intervention used in every study due to the large number of included studies. The frequency tables for herbal formula names, herbal ingredients used in the formulae, acupuncture points, and scalp zones aim to summarise the main features of the CM interventions and facilitate comparisons between different categories of clinical trials and different chapters. Higher frequency herbs or acupuncture points should not be considered as more effective for VaD than lower frequency items. Some herbs are typical inclusions in formulas for a wide range of disorders. Additional details for some individual studies are also provided in the current text for the purpose of illustration, but this does not mean that these studies are better or more important than other studies.

Implications for Practice

The clinical guidelines and expert recommendations in Chapter 2 provide the basis for syndrome differentiation and formula selection in clinical practice. However, it should be noted that these guidelines can apply to a variety of dementia types, which include, but are not limited to, the various categories of VaD. The results from the classical literature provide an overview of how post-stroke VaD was viewed and managed in the past and illustrate how concepts and clinical therapy have changed over time. These changes have been considerable and the information contained in this chapter should not be used as a basis for contemporary treatment.

From the viewpoint of evidence-based CM, the clinical trials and RCTs in particular provide the best available evidence of the effectiveness of CM interventions for VaD. However, the diversity of the RCTs makes the translation of this evidence into clinical practice difficult. In general, RCTs that employed rigorous methodology, had longer durations, and tested larger and more representative samples of participants should be afforded more weight. In addition, interventions that have been tested in multiple high quality studies with consistent outcomes should be preferred over interventions whose evidence is derived from single studies.

Herbal Formulae

In the case of oral CHMs, the available evidence for specific formulae is limited in amount and quality. *Bu yang huan wu tang* 补阳还五汤 is a traditional formula from the Qing dynasty book

Yi Lin Gai Cuo 医林改错 (c. 1830) that is currently being used to promote Blood circulation, remove Blood stasis, supplement *qi*, and unblock the collaterals. In modern CM, it has been modified and used for post-stroke disorders, including VaD and multi-infarct dementia,[4] and was tested in six clinical studies, including four RCTs. The meta-analysis results of three RCTs indicate that there were improvements in cognition when combined with pharmacotherapy (Chapter 5). The manufactured product *Bu chang nao xin tong jiao nang* 步长脑心通胶囊, which is based on *Bu yang huan wu tang* 补阳还五汤, was tested in five clinical studies. The pooled result for three RCTs showed benefits for cognition. Although other formulae have been tested in multiple studies (Table 10.2), the results could not be pooled.

Herbs in Formulae

While the formulae have a diversity of names, many share the same ingredients. Analysis of the herbs in the formulae that were included in meta-analysis pools and showed a significant benefit for cognitive outcomes found the most commonly tested herbs to be *shi chang pu* 石菖蒲, *he shou wu* 何首乌, *chuan xiong* 川芎, *huang qi* 黄芪, *dang gui* 当归, *dan shen* 丹参, and *yuan zhi* 远志 (Chapter 5, Table 5.28). Of these, *huang qi* 黄芪, *dang gui* 当归, and *chuan xiong* 川芎 are core ingredients of *Bu yang huan wu tang* 补阳还五汤 and *Bu chang nao xin tong jiao nang* 步长脑心通胶囊, while *shi chang pu* 石菖蒲 and *yuan zhi* 远志 are typical additions to formulae when there are symptoms of memory impairment. In addition, the experimental studies summarised in Chapter 6 indicate that a number of these herbs have shown effects on vascular and neurological systems that may explain their clinical effects. Nevertheless, it is important to note that the clinical practice of CHM is based on syndrome differentiation (Chapter 2) and prescription according to the needs of the individual, so the above formulae and herbs will not be appropriate for all VaD sufferers.

Acupuncture Therapies

The clinical trial evidence for acupuncture and electro-acupuncture suggests that both approaches can result in improvements on cognitive and ADL outcome measures, at least in the short term. Although there was considerable diversity in the specific acupuncture interventions tested in the clinical trials, certain points were used in multiple studies. Of the points used in the RCTs for which cognitive benefits were evident, EX-HN1 *Sishencong* 四神聪, GV20 *Baihui* 百会, GV24 *Shenting* 神庭, and GB20 *Fengchi* 风池 were the most frequently applied (Chapter 7, Table 7.12). Each of these points was included in the clinical guidelines (Chapter 2) and GV20 *Baihui* 百会 was the most frequent point in the classical literature (Chapter 3). A few RCTs of scalp acupuncture indicated that this approach may be beneficial, but there were only two studies in the meta-analyses. Similarly, the evidence for ear acupuncture and moxibustion was based on too few studies for any conclusions to be made.

Combination Therapies

For the combination of CHM plus acupuncture, the meta-analyses indicated improvements in cognitive and ADL outcomes (Chapter 9). Although the Chapter 2 formulae were not tested in any of these RCTs, the frequent herbal ingredients were similar to those in the RCTs in Chapter 5. Of the frequently used acupoints, GV20 *Baihui* 百会, EX-HN1 *Sishencong* 四神聪, ST36 *Zusanli* 足三里, and SP6 *Sanyinjiao* 三阴交 were all included in Chapter 2 and were frequently used in the acupuncture RCTs (Chapter 7). This suggests that the combinations of CHM plus acupuncture were based on interventions that were similar to those tested in the CHM and acupuncture RCTs. However, it was not possible to directly compare results from Chapters 5 and 7 with the meta-analysis results in Chapter 9 to determine if any additional benefit was gained when CHM was combined with acupuncture.

Safety

With regard to the safety of the CHM interventions, the herbs used frequently in the clinical studies are commonly used today and the risk of AEs should be low, provided that the herbs are of good quality, used within the recommended dosage ranges, appropriate for the person for whom they are prescribed, and not used for prolonged periods without assessment. The frequently used acupoints are also commonly used points that should present little risk as long as the acupuncture is administered by properly trained practitioners, the needles are sterile, and adequate care is taken when performing the acupuncture, electro-acupuncture, or moxibustion.[5,6] When herbs are combined with pharmacotherapies, additional care is required as there is potential for adverse interactions.[7] Herb-drug interactions were not reported in the clinical studies, but given that people with VaD may consume a variety of medications, clinicians should consider any possible interactions when prescribing CHMs, monitor responses to the combination, and take appropriate action if interactions are suspected.[8,9]

Implications for Research

Although numerous studies have evaluated the effects of CM interventions for VaD, more rigorously designed studies are needed. Trials should be registered and detailed protocols should be available. It is important that the enrollment of participants, the generation of randomisation sequence, and the process of allocation concealment be conducted independently in order to reduce the risk of bias. Similarly, outcome assessors and those conducting statistical analyses should be blind to group allocation. Safety should be monitored by an independent committee to ensure that data on AEs and dropouts are adequately collected and reported.[10]

It is difficult to blind participants and investigators in studies of CHM, particularly when decoctions are used. However, blinding becomes feasible when the CHM has been manufactured into a pill or capsule.[11] Acupuncture and other manual therapies present unique challenges with regards to blinding, but considerable progress has been made in the development of sham-acupuncture devices for use in clinical trials.[12,13] Besides these aspects of the design and management of clinical trials, improvements are needed with regard to the provision of data on the quality of CHM interventions and their constituent ingredients, details of how the CHMs were prepared or manufactured, as well as details of any placebo control interventions used.[14,15]

Although syndrome differentiation is an important feature of CM, many studies did not mention whether syndrome differentiation was used as a selection criterion or as a basis for selecting or modifying formulae. In the studies that did use syndrome differentiation, details of the criteria used to define the syndromes were inadequate. Furthermore, when syndrome differentiation is used as the basis for selecting the most appropriate intervention, it is important to provide separate data for the syndrome subgroups and not just aggregate data.[16] In addition, pragmatic comparative effectiveness studies could be used to assess the effects of CM interventions that are adjusted to individual needs, as in clinical practice.[17,18]

There is considerable scope for improvement in the reports on clinical trials. These tended to be brief and did not provide all the information required by the Consolidated Standards of Reporting Trials[19] and the extensions for herbal medicine,[20] traditional CM,[21] and acupuncture.[22,23] Poor reporting of the methods and conduct of trials as well as inadequate safety data both reduce the credibility of the outcomes. In such cases, the study has low impact and contributes little to scientific knowledge, so researchers and journal editors need to cooperate in order to raise the standard of CM clinical research.[10,24,25]

The reviews of the experimental studies of the frequently used herbs and their constituents (Chapter 6) indicate that these herbs show activities in models relevant to VaD. These studies have identified a number of pathways through which the herbs may exert clinical effects and there is considerable scope for further research in this field, especially with regard to the combined effects of multiple compounds on the numerous degenerative processes involved in VaD.

References

1. 田金洲，韩明向，涂晋文，杨承芝，*et al.* (2000) 血管性痴呆的诊断、辨证及疗效评定标准. 北京中医药大学学报. **23**(5):16–24.
2. Tang NY, Liu CH, Liu HJ, Li TC, *et al.* (2012) Chinese medicine patterns in patients with post-stroke dementia. *J Tradit Complement Med* **2**(2): 123–128.
3. Shi GX, Liu CZ, Guan W, Wang ZK, *et al.* (2014) Effects of acupuncture on Chinese medicine syndromes of vascular dementia. *Chin J Integr Med* **20**(9):661–666.
4. 周庚生, 胡紀明. (1985) 中西医临床精神病学. 北京 中国中医药出版社.
5. Witt CM, Pach D, Brinkhaus B, Wruck K, *et al.* (2009) Safety of acupuncture: Results of a prospective observational study with 229,230 patients and introduction of a medical information and consent form. *Forsch Komplementmed* **16**(2):91–97.
6. McCulloch M, Nachat A, Schwartz J, Casella-Gordon V, *et al.* (2015) Acupuncture safety in patients receiving anticoagulants: A systematic review. *Perm J* **19**(1):68–73.
7. Izzo AA, Hoon-Kim S, Radhakrishnan R, Williamson EM (2016). A critical approach to evaluating clinical efficacy, adverse events and drug interactions of herbal remedies. *Phytother Res* **30**(5):691–700.
8. Shaw D. (2010) Toxicological risks of Chinese herbs. *Planta med* **76**(17):2012–2018.
9. Zhang L, Yan J, Liu X, Ye Z, *et al.* (2012) Pharmacovigilance practice and risk control of Traditional Chinese Medicine drugs in China: Current status and future perspective. *J Ethnopharmacol* **140**(3):519–525.
10. Ellenberg SS. (2012) Protecting clinical trial participants and protecting data integrity: Are we meeting the challenges? *PLoS Med* **9**(6): e1001234.
11. Bian ZX, Moher D, Dagenais S, Li YP, *et al.* (2006) Improving the quality of randomized controlled trials in Chinese herbal medicine, Part II: Control group design. *Zhong Xi Yi Jie He Xue Bao* **4**(2):130–136.
12. Zhang CS, Yang AW, Zhang AL, May BH, *et al.* (2014) Sham control methods used in ear-acupuncture/ear-acupressure randomized controlled trials: A systematic review. *J Altern Complem Med* **20**(3):147–161.
13. Lin JG, Chen CH, Huang YC, Chen YH. (2012) How to design the control group in randomized controlled trials of acupuncture? *Evid Based Compl Alt* **2012**:875284.

14. Wolsko PM, Solondz DK, Phillips RS, Schachter SC, *et al.* (2005) Lack of herbal supplement characterization in published randomized controlled trials. *Am J Med* **118**(10):1087–1093
15. Leung KS, Bian ZX, Moher D, Dagenais S, *et al.* (2006) Improving the quality of randomized controlled trials in Chinese herbal medicine, Part III: Quality control of Chinese herbal medicine used in randomized controlled trials. *Zhong Xi Yi Jie He Xue Bao* **4**(3):225–232.
16. Jiang M, Lu C, Zhang C, Yang J, *et al.* (2012) Syndrome differentiation in modern research of traditional Chinese medicine. *J Ethnopharmacol* **140**(3):634–642.
17. Witt CM. (2011) Clinical research on acupuncture — Concepts and guidance on efficacy and effectiveness research. *Chin J Integr Med* **17**(3):166–172.
18. Witt CM, Aickin M, Cherkin D, Che CT, *et al.* (Collaborators) (2014) Effectiveness guidance document (EGD) for Chinese medicine trials: A consensus document. *Trials* **15**:169.
19. Schulz KF, Altman DG, Moher D, Grp C. (2010) CONSORT 2010 Statement: Updated guidelines for reporting parallel group randomised trials. *Trials* **24**;11.
20. Gagnier JJ, Boon H, Rochon P, Moher D, *et al.* (2006) Reporting randomized, controlled trials of herbal interventions: An elaborated CONSORT statement. *Ann Intern Med* **144**(5):364–367.
21. Bian Z, Liu B, Moher D, Wu T, *et al.* (2011) Consolidated standards of reporting trials (CONSORT) for traditional Chinese medicine: Current situation and future development. *Front Med* **5**(2):171–177.
22. MacPherson H, White A, Cummings M, Jobst K, *et al.* (STRICTA Group) (2002) Standards for reporting interventions in controlled trials of acupuncture: The STRICTA recommendations. Standards for Reporting Interventions in Controlled Trials of Acupuncture. *Acupunct Med* **20**(1):22–25.
23. MacPherson H, Altman DG, Hammerschlag R, Youping L, *et al.* (Group SR) (2010) Revised STandards for Reporting Interventions in Clinical Trials of Acupuncture (STRICTA): Extending the CONSORT statement. *J Evid Based Med* **3**(3):140–155.

24. Manheimer E, Wieland S, Kimbrough E, Cheng K, *et al.* (2009) Evidence from the Cochrane Collaboration for Traditional Chinese Medicine therapies. *J Altern Complement Med* **15**(9):1001–1014.
25. Bian ZX, Li YP, Moher D, Dagenais S, *et al.* (2006) Improving the quality of randomized controlled trials in Chinese herbal medicine, Part I: Clinical trial design and methodology. *Zhong Xi Yi Jie He Xue Bao* **4**(2):120–129.

Glossary

Terms	Acronym	Definition	Reference
95% Confidence Interval	95% CI	A measure of the uncertainty around the main finding of a statistical analysis. Statistics such as risk ratio (RR) are usually presented as a point estimate and a 95% confidence interval. This means that if someone were to keep repeating a study in other samples from the same population, 95% of the confidence intervals from those studies would contain the true value of the unknown quantity.	http://handbook.cochrane.org/ v.5.1; pt2, 12.4.1
Acetylcholinesterase inhibitor	AChE inhibitor	A class of drugs used for dementia, such as donepezil.	—
Acupressure	—	Application of pressure on acupuncture points.	—
Acupuncture	—	The insertion of needles into humans or animals for remedial purposes.	World Health Organisation. (2007). WHO International Standard Terminologies of Traditional Medicine in the Western Pacific Region.
Alzheimer's Disease Assessment Scale–cognitive subscale	ADAS-cog	Outcome measure of cognitive function.	Mohs RC, Rosen WG, Davis KL. (1983) The Alzheimer's disease assessment scale: An instrument for assessing treatment efficacy. *Psychopharmacol Bull* **19**(3):448–450.

(*Continued*)

(Continued)

Terms	Acronym	Definition	Reference
Alzheimer's disease	AD	A degenerative brain disease that involves progressive decline in memory, language, problem-solving, and other cognitive skills due to neuronal damage. Named after the anatomist Alois Alzheimer.	Goedert M, Spillantini MG. (2006) A century of Alzheimer's disease. *Science* **314**(5800):777–781.
Activities of daily living	ADL	Outcome measure of the ability to perform normal, everyday activities.	—
Allied and Complementary Medicine Database	AMED	Alternative medicine bibliographic database.	https://www.ebsco.com/products/research-databases/allied-and-complementary-medicine-database-amed
Australian New Zealand Clinical Trial Registry	ANZCTR	Clinical trial registry based in Australia.	http://www.anzctr.org.au/
Cerebral autosomal-dominant arteriopathy with subcortical infarcts and leukoencephalopathy	CADASIL	A rare genetic disorder leading to early onset vascular dementia.	Gorelick PB, Counts SE, Nyenhuis D. (2006) Vascular cognitive impairment and dementia. *Biochim Biophys Acta* **1862**(5):860–868.
Cerebral autosomal recessive arteriopathy with subcortical infarcts and leukoencephalopathy	CARASIL	A rare genetic disorder leading to early onset vascular dementia.	Gorelick PB, Counts SE, Nyenhuis D. (2016) Vascular cognitive impairment and dementia. *Biochim Biophys Acta* **1862**(5):860–868.
Cerebrovascular disease	CVD	Various medical conditions, including stroke, that affect the blood vessels of the brain and cerebral circulation.	Roman GC, Tatemichi TK, Erkinjuntti T, *et al.* (1993) Vascular dementia: Diagnostic criteria for research studies. Report of the NINDS-AIREN international workshop. *Neurology* **43**(2):250–260.

(Continued)

Terms	Acronym	Definition	Reference
China National Knowledge Infrastructure	CNKI	Chinese language bibliographic database.	www.cnki.net
Chinese Biomedical Literature Database	CBM	Chinese language bibliographic database.	www.imicams.ac.cn
Chinese Clinical Trial Registry	ChiCTR	Chinese clinical trial registry.	http://www.chictr.org
Chinese herbal medicine	CHM	Chinese herbal medicine.	—
Chinese medicine	CM	Traditional system of medicine native to China.	—
Chongqing VIP Information Company	CQVIP	Chinese language bibliographic database.	www.cqvip
ClinicalTrials.gov	—	Clinical trial registry based in the USA.	https://clinicaltrials.gov/
Cochrane Central Register of Controlled Trials	CENTRAL	Bibliographic database that provides a highly concentrated source of reports of controlled trials.	http://community.cochrane.org/editorial-and-publishing-policy-resource/overview-cochrane-library-and-related-content/databases-included-cochrane-library/cochrane-central-register-controlled-trials-central
Combination therapies	—	Two or more Chinese medicines from different therapy groups (e.g. Chinese herbal medicine, acupuncture therapies, or other Chinese medicine therapies) administered together.	—
Convention on International Trade in Endangered Species of Wild Fauna and Flora	CITES	International convention aimed at preventing or regulating trade in threatened and endangered species of plants and animals.	https://www.cites.org/eng/disc/text.php
Cumulative Index of Nursing and Allied Health Literature	CINAHL	Bibliographic database.	https://www.ebscohost.com/nursing/about

(Continued)

(*Continued*)

Terms	Acronym	Definition	Reference
Cupping therapy	—	Suction through the use of a vaccuumised cup or jar.	World Health Organisation. (2007). WHO International Standard Terminologies of Traditional Medicine in the Western Pacific Region.
Diagnostic and Statistical Manual of Mental Disorders	DSM	Manual issued by the American Psychiatric Association. It has multiple editions including DSM-IV and DSM-5.	American Psychiatric Association. (2010) Diagnostic and statistical manual of mental disorders, fifth edition (DSM-5). American Psychiatric Association, Washington, DC
Effect size	—	A generic term for the estimate of the effect of a study's treatment.	—
Effective rate	—	A measure of the proportion of participants who achieved an improvement, as outlined in Chapter 4.	—
Electro-acupuncture	—	Electric stimulation of the acupuncture needle following insertion.	WHO International Standard Terminologies of Traditional Medicine in the Western Pacific Region. World Health Organisation. (2007)
EU Clinical Trials Register	EU-CTR	European clinical trial registry.	https://www.clinicaltrialsregister.eu
Excerpta Medica database	Embase	Bibliographic database.	http://www.elsevier.com/solutions/embase
Grading of Recommendations Assessment, Development, and Evaluation	GRADE	Approach used to grade the quality of evidence and strength of recommendations.	http://www.gradeworkinggroup.org/

(*Continued*)

Terms	Acronym	Definition	Reference
Health-related quality of life	HR-QoL	A conceptual or operational measurement that is commonly used in a health care setting as a means to assess the impact of disease on the person.	Brooker C. (2010) Mosby's dictionary of medicine, nursing and health professions. Elsevier, United Kingdom.
Heterogeneity	—	Used in a general sense to describe the variation in or diversity of participants, interventions, and measurement of outcomes across a set of studies, or the variation in the internal validity of those studies. When used specifically as statistical heterogeneity, it describes the degree of variation in the effect estimates from a set of studies. Also used to indicate the presence of variability among studies beyond the amount expected due to chance.	http://handbook.cochrane.org/ v.5.1; pt2, 9.5.1
Hasegawa Dementia Scale	HDS	Outcome measure of cognitive function. The revised version, HDS-R, is typically used.	Imai Y, Hasegawa K. (1994) The Revised Hasegawa Dementia Scale (HDS-R) — Evaluation of its usefulness as a screening test for dementia. *J Hong Kong Coll Psychiatr* **4**(2):20–24.
I^2	—	A measure of study heterogeneity that indicates the percentage of variance in a meta-analysis.	http://handbook.cochrane.org/ v.5.1; pt2, 9.5.2
Integrative medicine	—	Chinese herbal medicine combined with pharmacotherapy or other conventional therapy.	
Mean difference	MD	In meta-analysis: A method used to combine measures on continuous scales where the mean, standard deviation, and sample size in each group are known.	http://handbook.cochrane.org/ v.5.1; pt2, 9.4.5.1

(*Continued*)

(***Continued***)

Terms	Acronym	Definition	Reference
Meta-analysis	—	The use of statistical techniques in a systematic review to integrate the results of included studies. Sometimes misused as a synonym for systematic reviews, where the review includes a meta-analysis.	—
Mini-Mental State Examination	MMSE	Outcome measure of cognitive function.	Folstein MF, Folstein SE, McHugh PR. (1995) Mini-mental state. A practical method for grading the cognitive state of patients for the clinician. *J Psychiatr Res* **12**(3):189–198.
Moxibustion	—	A therapeutic procedure involving ignited material (usually moxa) to apply heat to certain points or areas of the body's surface to manage disease.	World Health Organisation. (2007). WHO International Standard Terminologies of Traditional Medicine in the Western Pacific Region.
National Institute for Health and Clinical Excellence and Social Care Institute for Excellence Guideline	NICE-SCIE Guideline	Joint project by the National Institute for Health and Clinical Excellence (NICE) and the Social Care Institute for Excellence (SCIE), in conjunction with the National Collaborating Centre for Mental Health (NCCMH) in the UK.	National Collaborating Centre for Mental Health. (2007) Dementia a NICE–SCIE guideline on supporting people with dementia and their carers in health and social care. The British Psychological Society and Gaskell, London, UK.

(*Continued*)

Terms	Acronym	Definition	Reference
National Institute of Neurological Disorders and Stroke (NINDS) and the Association Internationale pour la Recherche et l'Enseignement en Neurosciences (AIREN)	NINDS-AIREN	The agencies that jointly developed the diagnostic criteria for vascular dementia.	Roman GC, Tatemichi TK, Erkinjuntti T, *et al.* (1993) Vascular dementia: Diagnostic criteria for research studies. Report of the NINDS-AIREN international workshop. *Neurology* **43**(2):250–260.
Non-controlled studies	NCS	Observations made on individuals, usually receiving the same intervention, before and after the intervention but with no control group.	—
Controlled clinical trial	CCT	A study in which people are allocated to different intervention groups using methods that are not random.	—
Other Chinese medicine therapies	—	Other Chinese medicine therapies include all traditional therapies except Chinese herbal medicine and acupuncture/moxibustion, such as *tai chi*, *qi gong*, *tui na*, and cupping.	—
PubMed	PubMed	Bibliographic database.	http://www.ncbi.nlm.nih.gov/pubmed
Qi gong 气功	—	Physical exercises and breathing techniques.	—
Randomised controlled trial	RCT	Clinical trial that uses a random method to allocate participants to treatment and control groups.	—
Risk of bias	—	Assessment of clinical trials to indicate if results overestimate or underestimate the true effect because of bias in study design or reporting.	http://handbook.cochrane.org/ v.5.1; pt2, ch.8
Risk ratio (Relative risk)	RR	The ratio of risks in two groups. In intervention studies, it is the ratio of the risk in the intervention group to the risk in the control group. A risk ratio of one indicates no difference between comparison groups. For undesirable outcomes, a risk ratio	http://handbook.cochrane.org/ v.5.1; pt2, 9.2.2.2

(*Continued*)

(Continued)

Terms	Acronym	Definition	Reference
		that is less than one indicates that the intervention was effective in reducing the risk of that outcome.	
Summary of findings	SoF	Presentation of results and ratings of the quality of evidence based on the GRADE approach.	http://www.gradeworkinggroup.org/
Standardised mean difference	SMD	Similar to mean difference (MD). Used when different instruments measure the same construct. The SMD expresses the intervention effect in standard units rather than the original units of measurement. As a rule of thumb, a SMD of 0.2 represents a small effect, 0.5 a moderate effect, and 0.8 a large effect.	http://handbook.cochrane.org/ v.5.1; pt2, 9.2.3.2; 12.6.2
Tai chi 太极 (*tai ji* 太极)	—	A Chinese martial art with health benefits.	—
Transcutaneous electrical nerve stimulation	TENS	Application of transdermal electrical current to acupuncture points via conducting pads.	—
Tui na 推拿	—	Chinese massage involving rubbing, kneading, or percussion of the soft tissues and joints of the body with the hands, usually performed by one person on another, especially to relieve tension or pain.	World Health Organisation. (2007). WHO International Standard Terminologies of Traditional Medicine in the Western Pacific Region.
Vascular dementia	VaD	Dementia associated with cerebrovascular disease.	Roman GC, Tatemichi TK, Erkinjuntti T, *et al.* (1993) Vascular dementia: Diagnostic criteria for research studies. Report of the NINDS-AIREN international workshop. *Neurology* **43**(2):250–260.
Wangfang database	Wanfang	Chinese language bibliographic database.	www.wanfangdata.com

(*Continued*)

Terms	Acronym	Definition	Reference
World Health Organisation	WHO	WHO is the directing and coordinating authority for health within the United Nations system. It is responsible for providing leadership on global health matters, shaping the health research agenda, setting norms and standards, articulating evidence-based policy options, providing technical support to countries, and monitoring and assessing health trends.	http://www.who.int/about/en/
Zhong Hua Yi Dian 中华医典	ZHYD	The ZHYD 'Encyclopaedia of Traditional Chinese Medicine' is a comprehensive series of electronic books stored on compact disk. The collection was put together by the Hunan electronic and audio-visual publishing house. It is the largest collection of Chinese electronic books and includes the major Chinese ancient works, many of which are from rare manuscripts and are the only existing copies. These books cover the period from ancient times up to the period of the Republic of China (1911–1948).	Hu R, ed. (2000) Zhong Hua Yi Dian [Encyclopaedia of Traditional Chinese Medicine]. 4th ed. Electronic and Audio-Visual Publishing House Changsha.
Zhong Yi Fang Ji Da Ci Dian 中医方剂大辞典	ZYFJDCD	Compendium of Chinese herbal formulae with over 96,592 entries derived from classical Chinese books. The Nanjing Chinese Medicine Institute compiled the ZYFJDCD and first published it in 1993.	Peng HR, ed. (1994) Great Compendium of Chinese Medical Formulae, 1st ed. [in Chinese]. People's Medical Publishing House, Beijing.

Index

Evidence-based Clinical Chinese Medicine

Print ISSN: 2529-7562
Online ISSN: 2529-7554

Series Co Editors-in-Chief

Charlie Changli Xue *(RMIT University, Australia)*
Chuanjian Lu *(Guangdong Provincial Hospital of Chinese Medicine, China)*

Published

Vol. 1 *Chronic Obstructive Pulmonary Disease*
by Charlie Changli Xue and Chuanjian Lu

Vol. 2 *Psoriasis Vulgaris*
Lead Authors: Claire Shuiqing Zhang and Jingjie Yu

Vol. 3 *Chronic Urticaria*
Lead Authors: Meaghan Coyle and Jingjie Yu

Vol. 4 *Adult Asthma*
Lead Authors: Johannah Shergis and Lei Wu

Vol. 5 *Allergic Rhinitis*
Lead Authors: Claire Shuiqing Zhang and Qiulan Luo

Vol. 6 *Herpes Zoster and Post-herpetic Neuralgia*
Lead Authors: Meaghan Coyle and Haiying Liang

Vol. 7 *Insomnia*
Lead Authors: Johannah Shergis and Xiaojia Ni

Vol. 8 *Alzheimer's Disease*
Lead Authors: Brian H May and Mei Feng

Vol. 9 *Vascular Dementia*
Lead Authors: Brian H May and Mei Feng

Vol. 10 *Diabetic Kidney Disease*
Lead Authors: Johannah Shergis and Lihong Yang

Vol. 11 *Acne Vulgaris*
Lead Authors: Meaghan Coyle and Haiying Liang

More information on this series can also be found at https://www.worldscientific.com/series/ebccm

Vol. 12 *Post-Stroke Shoulder Complications*
Lead Authors: Claire Shuiqing Zhang and Shaonan Liu

Vol. 16 *Atopic Dermatitis*
Lead Authors: Meaghan Coyle and Junfeng Liu

Forthcoming

Vol. 13 *Post-Stroke Spasticity*
Lead Authors: Claire Shuiqing Zhang and Shaonan Liu

Vol. 14 *Unipolar Depression*
Lead Authors: Yuan Ming Di and Lingling Yang

Vol. 15 *Chronic Heart Failure*
Lead Authors: Claire Shuiqing Zhang and Liuling Ma

Vol. 17 *Colorectal Cancer*
Lead Authors: Brian H May and Yihong Liu